Not Pregnant

Not Pregnant

Cathie Quillet
with Dr. Shannon Sutherland

.

Copyright © 2016 Cathie Quillet
All rights reserved.
ISBN-13: 9781534639904
ISBN-10: 153463990X
Library of Congress Control Number: 2016912107
CreateSpace Independent Publishing Platform
North Charleston, South Carolina

What People Are Saying About
Not Pregnant

If you are going through infertility, **Not Pregnant** will speak to your soul! It reads like a good conversation with a close girlfriend.

Infertility makes you feel alone; no one and nothing is safe. **Not Pregnant** helps you work through that, giving you tools to help start the conversation so those around you can understand this season of your life better. It's the best of both worlds: relatable stories from others going through the same thing yet [it includes] the medical aspect to help you understand what is going on with you physically.

—Katie, experienced secondary infertility

This book has the power to meet people in their pain, to show them they are not alone and that they are not without hope. There are real-life examples of others who have walked this road, as well as tools and wisdom to navigate this journey in a healthy way. And all of this is done in a very readable, chatting-with-a-dear-friend-over-coffee kind of way!

—Wendy Gapastione, pastor's wife

Cathie's vulnerable story of miscarriages and infertility spoke directly to my soul. Every woman should read **Not Pregnant**—not only to find permission and grace and compassion for your own journey but to connect to the greater human experience of loss and hope. Her insightful wisdom and courageous words inspire me to step out of my circumstances and understand infertility—not as a label but as a brave journey, one that I have much to learn from.

—Bekah Pogue, author of *Choosing Real*

As the founder of an organization that works with families who experience not only the loss of their children but also secondary infertility, as well as those who are unable to carry viable babies to term, I found **Not Pregnant** to be an amazing resource of real-life information for families longing to have a baby. Reading this book felt comfortable and comforting, like an old friend chatting on the patio. There are so few resources in existence for mothers and fathers walking this agonizing path. And those that do exist often fail to capture the honest struggles faced by couples. **Not Pregnant** helps couples feel less alone on the journey and offers some hope and joy along the way…even in the face of very real, raw pain and longing. I especially enjoyed hearing the male perspective, often overlooked but no less essential. I look forward to sharing this amazing resource with our clients. Well done to Cathie and all who contributed your sacred stories to this project.

—Kelly Gerken, founder of Sufficient Grace for Women, Inc., contributor for *Still Standing Magazine*, and author of *Sufficient Grace*

As someone who has walked this journey myself, I know that good resources are hard to find. This book is practical and helpful and provides a space to identify and feel the experiences that come with infertility. I'm excited about the many women who will be comforted and guided by Cathie's powerful story.

—Amanda Caldwell, marriage and family therapist

To my Tyler:
You are God's greatest gift to me.

To our boys:
You are the silver lining to our not-pregnant journey.

In Memory of my Beautiful Mother:
Who passed away during the completion of this project.
I will love you and miss you forever.
I love you MORE.

Contents

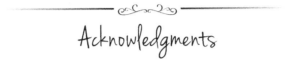

Acknowledgments

THANK YOU, LORD, for having plans for our lives, which—even though we may never understand this side of eternity—are good. This is my offering to you.

Thank you, Shannon, for partnering in this journey with me. While I never imagined that a book is what you would help me birth, I am forever grateful to you for faithfully supporting us through our *Not Pregnant* journey.

Thank you to each and every person who contributed to the writing of this book by sharing your story. Your voices are an integral part of the mission of *Not Pregnant*.

Thank you to our family who supported us during our *Not Pregnant* journey and throughout the writing of this book. To Mom and Dad L, Mom and Dad Q, Bob, Steph, Cody, Bill, Nese, Aydin, Ashley, Jacob, Noah, Dylan, Hudson, and Austin—thank you for praying for us and cheering us on in life.

To our four babes whom our arms and hearts ache for...know that we will never live a day without love for you. While you only lived a matter of weeks with us, we will hold the memory of those days forever in our hearts.

To our precious children who made us parents...you are an answer to prayer and so much longing. People always tell us how lucky you two are to have Daddy and me, but Daddy and I truly are the lucky ones! We love you to Africa and back!

Finally, thank you to my main man—Tyler, you are God's greatest gift to me, my best friend, my rock when the storm hits, and the supporter of my dreams. Thank you for helping make this dream come true. I love you, always and forever.

Foreword

NOT PREGNANT EXPLORES the profound sadness of infertility with kindness, wit, humor, and good science. It brings out feelings that most of us want to ignore, deny, or repress. The sorority/fraternity of those who have not been able to have children is a quiet, hidden group. People practically never talk about miscarriages, the struggle to have a baby, and the toll it takes on a marriage and on other relationships. *Not Pregnant* addresses this conspiracy of silence in the best possible way: by incorporating a blend of frank truth talking with genuine caring, concern, and understanding. No blaming allowed.

Cathie speaks both from her own experience and from the research and interviews she has conducted to make certain that she describes the experience of many infertile couples. Her grasp of the slippery feelings that hurt people and of the ways our society addresses (or doesn't address) infertility is deep and gentle. Her comments are so genuine and can be so funny that you are pleased to see someone dealing with deep wounds while still allowing life to happen around her.

This difficult subject needs the hand of a person with experience who also has the clinical background to speak objectively about what happens to us when we lose a pregnancy or never have one. Her ability to talk about and to normalize the bewildering array of feelings that come and go—anger, shame, jealousy, sadness, and hopelessness—is impressive. She has blended both personal experience and expertise expertly.

Cathie brings out issues that many never even think about, such as secondary infertility: being able to have one child but not another. This is another group whose experience is invisible to the rest of society. Her use of language is deft and precise, and she gives us aha moments in every section of the book.

The book exudes warmth and compassion and is a sounding board for every feeling a not-expectant parent might have. It gives people permission to feel what they feel. It also provides a wealth of information on how to live through this experience that we never expect to happen to us. This book will become a valuable resource to those who are struggling with infertility and for those who experienced the physical, emotional, and psychological tsunami long ago but whose feelings have never been validated.

Dr. Ellen Anderson, Psychologist

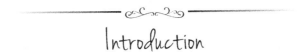

Introduction

I REMEMBER WHEN my husband and I came home from our honeymoon. We had just spent a week in paradise. Two blissful kids skipped off that plane in anticipation of their new lives together—and without a clue of what to expect. Off the plane and into the real world.

Call us old-fashioned, but we did not live together before we got married. This decision made our transition all the more profound.

It had been a beautiful whirlwind. He flew me to San Francisco to propose at the foot of the Golden Gate Bridge at sunset. Hello? Talk about a fairy tale! There were months of wedding planning and then the day itself...my dream come true. Not just the wedding day but the man, too! Then off we had gone to Jamaica for a week of sunshine and adventure.

We returned home to be hit upside the head with reality.

I remember wishing that there had been a book warning me of what came next. Perhaps I am a tad sentimental, but surrendering my maiden name felt like a big deal. In the past few years, we had welcomed two sisters-in-law into the family who had taken our name. Now I was losing mine. Joining bank accounts? Yeah, we were "becoming one," but where did my individuality go? All these transitions were welcome changes—changes that I had waited for since puberty—however, they were still profound, as I had not anticipated the emotional accompaniment.

I wanted there to be a book to tell me that I was normal for feeling all those obscure feelings that I felt. I wanted to know that I was typical. Validated. I wanted to feel a tad less crazy. A virtual high five or an "I totally understand" would have been sufficient.

Fast forward a few years.

All of a sudden, we were standing face-to-face with another change—this one as exciting as the last. We decided it was time to add to our family. There was a whole new set of things to learn. Many things to process. Many things that made me feel the need for some validation.

But months turned into years. Years turned into heartache. Yearning. Longing. That is when Shannon and I met, and she became an integral part of our journey.

My husband and I sat as patients in her office, with a notepad of questions, trying to make sense of the storm we had just found ourselves smack-dab in the middle of.

Am I normal? What next? Why is this so painful?

How can the absence of something you never had hurt so bad?

What is it about an expectation not coming to fruition that causes such traumatic, life-paralyzing grief? The expectation of this dream coming true—simply and romantically—is what cut the deepest when it did not happen.

When the expectation that a baby comes after meeting the man of your dreams intersects the reality that infertility also writes itself into your story, you get emotional stretch marks and unwelcome anguish.

I perused many a bookstore in an attempt to find a book to help me feel less marginalized, less ostracized, and a tad more validated during our struggle. I had never been much of a reader; however, during life-changing seasons of life, I run to the closest bookshelf in order to assure myself that I am not the only one who has treaded these waters. I need some validation every now and again. I looked, and I came up empty.

My motivation for writing *Not Pregnant* is to give people a book that I wish I had found when my husband and I were wading through the crashing waves of infertility. I wanted a book warning me about what to expect when you are not expecting.

In high-school health class, no one warns you that a baby may not come easily. No one teaches you how to deal with unexpected seasons of grief and the fact that sometimes life hurts in unexpected ways. No one talks about infertility until you are standing face-to-face with it.

Infertility is the inability to achieve a clinical pregnancy after twelve months of trying.

Infertility may mean something more personal to you.

You may call infertility the thing that cost you your marriage. You may call infertility the thing that robbed you of pleasure in the bedroom. To you and your spouse, infertility may be the source of your tears, greatest torment, and frustration. Infertility may have intruded enough to become a pickpocket raiding your bank account as you pay for medicinal interventions that you struggle to pronounce.

This journey is riddled with sadness, loneliness, anger, grief, depression, misunderstanding, resentment, and bitterness. We write this book having been there. Infertility. Miscarriage. Surgery. Diagnoses. More surgery. Pain. Grief. Struggle. Hysterectomy. I'll tell you more about that later.

The pain is real. The pain is lonely. Let's be honest: the pain drives you crazy.

I remember when I was pursuing my marriage and family therapy license and preparing for the national exam. There, tucked in the middle of other marital struggles, was a brief excerpt on infertility.

I'll admit it; I skimmed it. My answer at the time was, "That's not a struggle. All it means is that the couple gets to have more sex—yay for them." Go ahead and shake your head at me. My past ignorance makes me shake my head at myself.

I walked into our own struggle with that same amount of ignorance. The only thing that changed my perspective was the reality that abruptly met us.

Unfortunately for us—but fortunately for them—those who have never met the reality of the ugliness of infertility are also innocently ignorant. Those around us who haven't experienced the struggle can make it exponentially lonelier and more difficult for us. Can I get an amen?

(I would be remiss if I suggested that those fighting infertility were alone in this fight. Let's not forget those tirelessly fighting against mental illness and chronic disabilities; those currently surviving abuse, addiction, and lengthy singleness that extends past the social average; and those silently waging the war of living a marginalized life. My examples only scratch the surface. Can we pinky swear, knowing how we feel in the loneliness of infertility, that we will not be the perpetrators of pushing those farther to the periphery of society? Ignorance of our situation is hard to live with. Let us not make others feel alone because of our ignorance of their situation.)

Dr. Shannon Sutherland fights the medicinal struggle against infertility and for women's health daily. Like her colleagues, she battles on the front lines to help make couples' dreams come true. Medicinally, she fights. Emotionally, she supports. That is why I asked her to be a part of this project. She is an advocate for women's health and gives much of who she is to supporting couples' journeys.

I have women who are struggling to conceive walk into my office on a weekly basis, merely seeking some validation for the plethora of experiences that they encounter during any given moment. Tears are abundant as they search for understanding in an act of desperation. Brokenness, anger, sadness, fear, and hopelessness all intermingle in a sacred dance while they attempt to hold their hope of motherhood within arm's reach.

At the end of our journey together, Shannon and I want you to walk away with two things: permission and validation.

We want you to feel like there is an army of women around you, having walked a similar road, cheering you on as you experience every emotional nook and cranny of your heart. We hope that *Not Pregnant* will help you feel less ostracized from the rest of femininity and more confident in your story.

We want you to know that it is OK to grieve. You have permission to be angry. We want you to feel the freedom to ask your doctor the hard questions. You are validated if you want to quit, or you can try as long as you want. You have the right to do what is best for you and your spouse.

Throughout the course of this book, you will notice that I refer to the life growing inside one's womb as a *baby*. I do so unabashedly and without compromise. My desire was for a baby. I had four positive pregnancy tests, four heartbeats, and, therefore, I believe I had four babies temporarily growing in my womb.

Dr. Sutherland, however, writes from a scientific perspective, and her contributions will, therefore, use medical terminology to discuss the baby-making process (how's that for scientific?) and early life.

We write from these perspectives not for argument's sake or for political division.

This book is not intended to be a medical companion to your journey or an answer to those burning questions. It is intended to be an emotional companion to validate your emotional and relational burdens from the unexpected obstacles that too many women encounter.

While Shannon and I have experienced our own journeys, we recognize that not everyone has a journey that mirrors ours. In an effort not to pigeonhole everyone into our own stories, we have surveyed countless women who have shared similar experiences and added snippets of their hearts throughout the book. In the appendices in the back, we have also given a voice to the male experience in the hopes of bridging the gap in the male-female emotional divide. In all cases throughout this book, names and identifying information have been changed.

Before we embark on this journey together, lean in for one bit of truth.

To the woman wondering when it will be your turn...

To the woman who feels trepidation about being with family during the holidays due to the addition of new babes who aren't yours or whose family tiptoes around you leaving you feeling invisible because they just don't know what to say...

To the woman who can't avoid shopping areas where kids' clothes, toys, and other paraphernalia are sold and secretly wipes away a glistening tear before the dam breaks in the middle of Target...

To the woman who doesn't want to look in the mirror anymore because you are doubting your femininity...

To the woman who cries alone in what you hope will one day be a nursery...

To the woman who is still longing. *Still*...

To the woman going through the motions, praying desperately that tomorrow will bring something different, and hoping that this year this prayer will be answered because it hasn't been in yesterdays past...

To the woman who is nodding her head and silently screaming, "Amen"...

To the desperate woman, the lonely woman, the barren woman, the waiting woman, the cautiously hopeful woman…

You are seen. You are heard. We stand alongside you.

We write this for you. We write in an effort to validate your emotions, ease your pain, make you feel more comfortable in your own skin, and give you a giant, virtual, it's-going-to-be-OK hug. We write this for you because your story and your heart matter.

Blessings to you as you commence this pilgrimage toward healing, dear one.

PART 1

Infertility

CHAPTER 1

—— ✤ ——

Infertility

"HELLO?"

All I heard was crying on the other end of the phone.

"Are you there?"

All she could muster was a gentle, "I'm here."

More crying.

"They're pregnant," she said.

Both of us were silent.

The pain was too familiar.

Through the course of a few more sobs, I learned that my dear, cherished, infertile friend was sitting in the bathroom stall at her work. Hiding with tear-stained cheeks was an all-too-common occurrence at this point in her pursuit of a viable pregnancy.

She sat alone.

She wept.

Questioned.

Coveted.

"I'm happy for them," she tried to convince me. "They said it wasn't planned. They were kind of shocked, like they didn't know how it happened. We've been trying to make it happen for years, and they don't know how it happened!"

I've been there.

Have you?

With nothing but dreams set before you and hopes of exercising your God-given right to bear children, you are left with empty arms and a broken heart and clinging to shattered hope.

As she sat on the cold, tile flooring of her office building, there was nothing for me to say.

I wanted to fix it. I wanted to fly cross-country to squeeze her distressed shoulders and repair her broken spirit. I wanted to find the right thing to say. I was desperate for a miracle for my friend, who I am confident would be a wonderful mother if she were only given the opportunity.

Eventually we hung up the phone. No answers found. No change in circumstances. This wasn't the first time in the past months of her own negative pregnancy tests that she had learned a dear friend was expecting. With a heart growing increasingly calloused, she picked herself up off the cold floor, blotted the mascara that had traveled halfway down her cheek, pulled herself together, and got back to work.

That's how we do it, right? We learn somewhere along the path that you are allowed moments to grieve and then you have to pull yourself together so that people around you do not have to be pulled into your sad world of pregnancy tests, progesterone suppositories, and disappointment.

By some point in this journey of infertility, we learn how to securely fasten our masks in place so that we can go about the regularly scheduled programming in our lives without disturbing those around us. Why would they want to talk about your misshapen uterus, your dysfunctional egg production, or your husband's slow swimmers?

Infertility says that we have to cry alone in bathroom stalls while our colleagues go about their business in the cubicle right down the hall.

Infertility says that we plaster on a smile as we walk through our church's lobby while all the little children who we wished called us "Mommy" run around our ankles. The blissful mamas-to-be glowingly walk into the auditorium while we avoid the children's wing of the church altogether. Guilty as charged. For years you would not have seen me anywhere close to that side of the building. It just hurt too bad.

Infertility makes us stand alone in the middle of Times Square on New Year's Eve, eagerly waiting for the ball to drop. Millions of people are packed like cattle into those few blocks to experience this time-honored tradition. Merry people all around are ringing in the new year while reminiscing about the year now falling behind. They cheer and lovingly embrace those around you. You smile like the rest while crying silent tears in your soul because you only wish you were at home with your new little bundle of joy sleeping quietly beside you.

Infertility makes us different. It changes people. Men and women. Old and young. Optimists and pessimists. Religious and nonreligious. Throughout the course of this pilgrimage toward parenthood, wannabe parents transform. Hope turns into pain. Pain turns into brokenness. Brokenness turns into bitterness. Bitterness hopefully does not lead to permanent change.

It is not just a woman's body that changes. She begins to see the world in a different light. All of a sudden, everything is hard. Everything hurts. She dares not turn to the right or to the left for risk of being exposed to something that will prick the dam that she has built to protect herself.

Marriage changes. Sex changes. Dreams change. Relationships change. Self-image changes. Bank accounts change.

The little girl who, once upon a time, loved playing mommy with all of her little girlfriends after school is now a woman who dreads reading the result on the pregnancy test because fairy-tale land may be the only place where she will get to play mommy.

The empty room in your house that you dreamed about changing into a nursery morphed into an underutilized workout room and is now a junk room you avoid opening the door to. If you were to open the door, boxes wouldn't fall out, but the hopes and dreams of becoming a family of three, four, or five certainly would.

The bank account that was supposed to be spent on a ten-year-anniversary trip to the coast of Greece is now being spent on your second round of IVF treatment.

Your biological clock may be ticking, and people around you are wondering why you were so focused on your career instead of starting a family when your sisters did. After all, if you had, you might not be forced to scale this Everest in front of you.

Beloved, lean in closely for this one: You, my new friend, are not alone. I promise you that.

No matter how many times the stick has read *not pregnant*, we are here with you, grieving for you, only wishing we could carry you through this until you carry that healthy baby out of your neighborhood hospital.

Trust me; I imagined this scene for years: My husband and I are at the hospital. I'm all sweaty with that soon-to-be-maternal glow, proving that I have been in labor for hours. My treasured teammate husband is holding my hand next to me—holding in his need to pee so that he doesn't miss a thing. Our four parents are outside the waiting-room doors, waiting for my husband to carry the baby out to meet them like Steve Martin does in *Father of the Bride Part II*. Shannon is there, cheering us along, telling me it's time to push. She successfully helps us deliver a healthy baby and puts the baby on my chest. Tears. Tears. More elated tears.

But for me, the stick still reads *not pregnant*.

The feeling of loneliness as you go around your daily activities or touch your stomach haunts you, but hear me when I tell you this: There is a sisterhood of women with aching hearts around the world beckoning you into this most unfortunate of sororities. It is such a sad club to be a part of; however, there is comfort to be found in mere belonging.

I suppose that's why we're here. To be a cheerleader for you as you experience cramping and fatigue during your own journey. The road may be long, my friend, but our hope is that there are glimmers of hope, peace, and strength for you along that road.

From Shannon

Realize that no two people have the exact same issues or story. We are individuals and must be treated as such. You have options, no matter what your situation may be. Start with a conversation with your significant other: How far are you willing to go? There is so much testing available and even more complex treatment options… even experimental treatments in foreign countries. Where to start? Talk about your preferences, the amount of money you can spend, and whether or not your insurance will cover any reproductive medicines or therapies. What about your religious views? Be open and honest with each other. You don't need any more surprises going through this rigorous journey. When you have decided to seek medical advice, make sure your provider is comfortable evaluating and treating infertility. This field is part science and part art. Not everyone likes or wants to pursue this type of practice. Also remember that not all providers will practice the same way. Some will be aggressive and others more reserved. You should find one you and your significant other are at peace with and relate to, whether it is a primary-care physician, OBGYN, or reproductive endocrinologist.

Before you go to your appointment, make a menstrual journal. Include when you bleed, for how long, and if you have pain and when. Journal for at least three months. If you have been using ovulation-predictor kits, please include the days the kits say you are ovulating. Explain your daily diet and exercise. Write down all of your medications, vitamins, and herbal supplements, both for you and your spouse. Be prepared to answer a lot of questions about your history. Don't take any of the questions personally or feel embarrassed; some of the questions can be in depth. Expect a physical exam, a very thorough one. Tests may include vaginal cultures, blood work, and a pelvic ultrasound. You may be offered a hysterosalpingogram (a test to look for fallopian-tube potency) or surgery. Oh, and, gentlemen, we don't want you to feel left out, so you may be asked to get a semen analysis.

Personal Inventory

1. In what area is infertility hardest for you? Where is your loneliness?
2. In what part of your life are you hiding yourself from pain?
3. In what part of this journey do you need to find validation?

CHAPTER 2

Cathie's Story

MY HUSBAND AND I got married and had a plan for how we were going to build our family.

We were going to enjoy wedded bliss for at least two years. (Poor, little, naïve, unassuming younger me.) At least that was the script that we agreed to tell people when they asked when we were going to add children to our family.

At first that question is cute. When asked, you stare lovingly into your spouse's eyes and you answer together that you are just going to enjoy each other for a while before you start trying. Once you've been trying for a while, those glances turn into painful, I-need-a-hug-once-this-person-walks-away looks.

We made it to our year-one wedding anniversary, and then it started—the pain, that is. Terrible, stabbing, debilitating, don't-touch-me pain. Pelvic pain that caused me to avoid anything that had to do with intimacy or pants that needed to be buttoned.

This is when Shannon and I met. Thank heaven, too. She was a glimmer of light in the midst of darkness. I went into her office as a naïve quasi newlywed, still with the hope of children standing before me.

I learned a new word that day: *hysteroscopy.* Surgery. By this point in my life, I had already experienced a surgery, thanks to the softball that collided with and subsequently relocated my nose a tad to the right. I had a cast on my nose that, in sixth grade, felt boy repellant. The day I went back to school sporting my new facial decoration, unbeknown to my parents and me, we had year-book pictures for the basketball and volleyball teams I was on taken. There, in the middle of the black-and-white photographs, was a white, circular focal point, documenting my injury for years to come. You are welcome for the laugh, dear reader.

But back to the story…

Shannon's hypothesis was that I had endometriosis.

∽∾∾

From Shannon

A relatively common and complex disease, endometriosis is primarily a pelvic condition usually resulting in painful menses or painful intercourse. No one knows what endometriosis is exactly or why it is found where it is. There are many theories as to how tissue that resembles the inside lining of the uterus is found in odd places like the bladder, colon, brain, and lung. Those areas are, thankfully, less commonly affected than pelvic endometriosis. We do see endometriosis in multiple family members at times, so there could be a loose hereditary component. Some theories include retrograde menstruation and lymphatic spread. Other thoughts exist but are not proved.

Once thought to be a major cause of infertility, we now know that this relatively minor disease usually does not affect fecundity rates. However, more aggressive, extensive disease causes adhesion formation, fallopian-tube damage, and anatomic distortion, thus decreasing successful conception. Endometriosis is staged as levels one through four: one being a very mild disease and four being aggressive. Diagnosis is made primarily by evaluating symptoms of dysmenorrhea (painful periods) and dyspareunia (painful intercourse) and findings on a physical exam. A pelvic ultrasound can visualize a large collection of endometriosis called an *endometrioma*, but it cannot detect small, individual areas of endometriosis or adhesion formation. Definitive diagnosis is made by visualization through a diagnostic laparoscopy (surgery) and biopsy of tissue. Treatment options are difficult when dealing with fertility because a lot of the therapies inhibit the ability to conceive. Medical therapy, along with physical therapy, acupuncture, and musculoskeletal manipulation, can help control symptoms while a patient is trying to get pregnant. Surgical treatment may prove more beneficial in some circumstances.

Six years ago I went in for surgery and woke up to my husband's kind eyes telling me that Shannon was correct and that I did indeed have endometriosis. Everywhere. Uterus. Bowels. Bladder. Pelvis. I don't even know what else is down there, but if there is anything, it was covered. I continued gathering information as I drifted in and out of consciousness.

At our post-op appointment, Shannon gave us three options. Due to the rate of endometriosis growth, as well as the amount of real estate it already occupied in my girly region, we had to make a decision.

First, we could choose birth control. Due to my family history of breast cancer and my personal history of erratic hormonal changes—which made my emotional state that of a bipolar Chihuahua—we decided that was not a decent option. Please tell me I am not alone!

Second, we were told that I could start taking Lupron, a medicine that would temporarily throw my body into menopause. My husband was not particularly fond of this idea due to the whole bipolar Chihuahua problem. Truthfully, living inside those emotions did not seem particularly inviting to me either, so that option ruled itself out for us also.

Our third option was to start trying for a baby. Eek! We were a little ahead of our two-year schedule, but this option seemed like the least of the three evils.

That January, just a year and a half after we got married, we started trying to conceive. My brain struggles to remember if we told anyone that we were going to start trying, but the questions about our plans were already in full swing since we had been married for a while.

During my eighth-grade camping trip, I first started my period. Clearly junior high was a completely unfortunate time in my life. (You can laugh; it's funny to me now, too.) I had never had a regular period from that time since. During those first menstrually blessed years, I had experienced a ninety-day period as well as ninety days without a period. I was the full spectrum of crazy. That being said, my husband and I had no idea at how to embark on this process of conceiving.

Counting days, ovulation sticks, and temperature readings were all new to us. There is a learning curve that no one tells you about while you awkwardly sit in ninth-grade health class.

While each month did not bring its own visit from Aunt Flo, the days seemed to drag. Every cramp, every bit of nausea, every hormonal fluctuation, and every sexual encounter with my husband seemed to bring with it its own set of emotions. (We'll explore all those lovely emotions in another chapter, so hold tight!)

I'll fast forward through all the details to month eight when we found out that we were pregnant.

Once upon a time, my husband made me promise that I would never pee on a stick without him, so he was present when we found out. Let's just talk about that for a moment, shall we? Why is it that we have to find out something so beautifully wonderful by urinating on a piece of plastic over a place that collects all of our human waste? Who wants to photograph that moment for the baby book?

Our stick read *pregnant* that Saturday morning, and with tearstained cheeks, my husband got down on his knees in front of me and said, "I'm so excited, but what on earth did we just do?" He tenderly wiped the tears off my face, and we embraced.

That's when adrenaline kicked in. He started pacing. We agreed not to call our parents or tell anyone until we had reached thirteen weeks. That lasted about thirteen minutes.

After we called everyone to tell the news, my husband—glowing and oozing testosterone out every single pore—had to go do something manly. Like every expectant father does, he grabbed our chainsaw, carried it to the backyard like a lumberjack, and cut down a tree. Why not, right?

That first trimester was pretty textbook. I was exhausted, sleeping in Walmart parking lots and on the side of the road to and from work. I vomited up a bottle of juice, which I will not name— nor will I ever drink it again. It was glorious, even the upchuck experience. We shopped for nursery-room bedding, thought of names, dreamed about future family events, and whimsically went about our business.

I loved being pregnant.

Around week ten I noticed a change. My energy level was coming back, I was able to keep down food better than I had in the past month, and I no longer felt pregnant. I don't know how to describe it, but something was wrong.

Our concern took us to the hospital for an ultrasound. Still not really able to fathom the idea that something could be wrong, we waited in a cold and stale room. Weeks ago the stick had told us that we were pregnant, and a couple of weeks ago, we'd had our first prenatal appointment and ultrasound where junior had had a heartbeat—strong, resilient. Baby was growing. Inside me. I was a mommy. There was our baby, so full of life. We should have only been thirty weeks from meeting our dream come true.

Now we sat, fingers interlocked, and fearfully waited for the ultrasound tech to tell us the fate of this sweet life.

"I'm sorry. The heartbeat has stopped. I don't see your baby anymore."

Even now almost five years later, my lips quiver and my eyes well up with tears.

I don't know if you felt it, but the earth fell off its axis a little bit that day. I'm sorry if it disrupted your activities momentarily. It changed us and our world permanently.

The tech excused herself.

Draped in unattractive hospital garb, I fell into my husband's arms.

What kind of a mother can't keep her child alive? What kind of a woman was I? I felt like I needed to be exiled into a defective women's camp.

Again my husband grabbed my face tenderly, like he had when we had found out about this life. "Promise me," he said. "Promise me this isn't going to change us."

Through sobs, I promised.

We left that room different people. Hopes shattered. Life lost. Dreams changed. Innocence gone.

We spent a few months trying to collect ourselves as we waited for the green light to try again. During this time, my pain and crazy cycle lengths led me back to Shannon's office, and I was eventually diagnosed with polycystic ovary syndrome. I felt like I was collecting diagnoses every time I went in there; however, new diagnoses meant new treatment options, which meant that perhaps we were closer to becoming parents.

⊙⟶⟵⊙

From Shannon

Polycystic ovary syndrome (PCOS), or Stein-Leventhal syndrome, is a multifactorial condition with autosomal-dominant inheritance. Environmental factors revolving around diet and exercise can contribute to the severity of the disease and the extent to which it can affect ovulation and, therefore, fertility. Anovulation, or the lack of being able to release an egg from an ovary every month in a timed pattern, is one of the most common reasons for impaired fecundity. Some patients will go in and out of ovulation with a seven-to-twelve pound weight gain or loss. Other patients may never control their symptoms, no matter what their diet and exercise program consists of. Historically the general population thought of this condition as only affecting women who were significantly overweight; we now know that is just not correct. PCOS can afflict women of all body types.

The primary dysfunction of PCOS is altered hormonal regulation. This creates an imbalance in the follicle-stimulating hormone (FSH) and luteinizing hormone (LH), as well as in insulin and glucose metabolism. Sometimes you will hear of this as a prediabetic condition: insulin resistance. Some patients experience symptoms that consist of difficulty with weight management, hirsutism (hair growth in nontraditional places), acne, and abnormal vaginal bleeding. Women may also have pelvic pain due to a multitude of small cysts on the ovaries. Common treatments should include an explanation of the condition and options—such as a referral to a nutritionist for a PCOS diet and exercise program—and possibly medications to override the insulin resistance and anovulation.

Surgery, such as ovarian driving or wedging, was once done but is no longer the mainstay of treatment; however, it may be offered in certain circumstances. Rates of successful conception can be fairly high if a woman suffers from this condition alone and if the condition is managed aggressively.

◦◦C◦◦2◦◦

Thirteen months later—after two Clomid (oral medication prescribed for infertility) cycles, countless negative pregnancy tests and ultrasounds, and tears and more tears—we were able to conceive again. I remember Shannon looking my husband, Tyler, in the eyes and warning him that this pregnancy was going to be worse. She lovingly said, "If you think she was neurotic last time, she is going to be even worse this time." Ha! That's why I love her; she speaks it like it is. She was so right. I was paranoid, looking for any physical sign to indicate whether or not I was still pregnant.

Five weeks into this pregnancy, we found out that we miscarried again—on New Year's Eve, no less.

Just a few months later, at six weeks pregnant, we lost Baby Quillet number three.

Finally that summer we lost baby number four.

If you drew my emotions that year, they would look something like a roller coaster, defined by the highest peaks, drastic breathtaking drops, and endless nauseating loops. By our fourth wedding anniversary, we had been trying to make a family for more months than not. Progesterone suppositories, appointments with reproductive endocrinologists, visits with Shannon, Clomid, hormones, and HCG tests had become our life. We had other stuff going on in life; however, it all seemed to orbit around the missing piece of our family.

I'll tell you, our story hasn't been written the way we thought it would be when I walked down the aisle toward Tyler on that May day in 2008. I never suspected that we would have children who didn't share our DNA or that I would be classified medically as barren or infertile.

But I am. I am barren.

I remember a day when I was in high school and I asked my mom why my hips were so pronounced in comparison to my girl-friends. My pear shape had me contemplating my design.

"Those are birthin' hips, Cath," she said. I am glad that even then, we were close enough friends that she could joke with me like that. Infertility means that these "birthin' hips" did me no good.

I realize that you pick up a book like this hoping for an opti-mistic story that ends with a quiverful of children. Ours doesn't end like that.

In case you are wondering why we gave up on trying for bio-logical children, let me tell you. My endometriosis continued to grow. My polycystic ovaries continued to be problematic.

Also it appears that miscarriage one or two ruined my uterus. I had atypical symptomology during those miscarriages. I had a second hysteroscopy (remember the surgery I had that kicked off this whole endeavor?) that diagnosed me with a wicked case of adenomyosis. While we will never be completely sure what hap-pened exactly, it appears that an early miscarriage saturated into my uterus and caused it to be more like a wet sponge than a firm balloon, as Shannon once described it. This caused prolapse, *more* pain, and now a secondary bladder disease. Needless to say, I no longer have my uterus. We have a whole chapter on hys-terectomies, if you're interested.

From Shannon

Adenomyosis is an anatomical and medical condition of the uterus. The once tight and firm, muscular uterus with an evolving endometrial lining is transformed into a soggy, spongelike, irritated organ, due to the invasion of that endometrial lining into the muscular layer of the uterus. Although this condition causes a myriad of symptoms such as pelvic pain, heavy or irregular bleeding, and dyspareunia (painful intercourse), it is usually not a primary cause of infertility. Diagnosis can be aided by the patient's history of symptoms, a pelvic ultrasound, and the surgical visualization of the uterus. There is no known lab work to diagnose adenomyosis. Treatments are geared toward control of the symptoms. This can be difficult when fertility is desired, because many of the therapies inhibit pregnancy. Pain control can be found with physical therapy, musculoskeletal manipulation, massage, nonsteroidal pain medications, and acupuncture. Hormones can be given to help with symptoms but may prohibit pregnancy for a short time while on the therapy. There is not a definite surgical treatment that preserves the uterus. There may be a slight increase in early miscarriage rates with adenomyosis.

꩜

I love stories. A client who had taken a break from therapy came back after a two-year hiatus. When I asked why she returned, she said, "Because no one knows my story like you do." It is such an honor to be welcomed into someone's story. If you are like me and have any interest in hearing the end of ours, keep reading. You'll get there!

PART 2

I Wish I Would Have Known

CHAPTER 3

How Much It Was Going to Hurt

THE ROLLERCOASTER STOOD before me in all its radiant glory. I had examined it. Towering above me the sun shone behind my Everest with its scarlet paint job and sleek lines; it was my Goliath. I had waited for this time for what felt like forever.

Adorned with a neon LA Gear fanny pack and a liberal spray of Aqua Net, I stood there; my moment had arrived. That day the Viper roller coaster at Magic Mountain welcomed me in, as my head finally reached above the designated height to ride.

I stood below the ride and anticipated my chance to walk through the turnstiles. I had waited long enough for my cheeseburger to digest so that I would not to lose it, and I had chosen my riding partner. I was ready.

Finally my group was at the front of the line. I stepped into the cart, pulled the lap belt across my lap, and wondered how that small strap was going to keep me from flying into oblivion when we plummeted for stories. I wondered why this moment had caused me so much anticipation and questioned what on earth I was doing.

As the train inched forward, my palms started getting sweaty and the cheeseburger didn't feel so settled anymore. We reached the first crest, and I could see all the splendor of Valencia in Southern California. Anticipatory panic met jitters and a healthy smattering of consternation. I was ready for the thrill of a lifetime.

We passed over the top of the hill and plunged down several stories to what felt like our death below. Much to my surprise, we survived the fall and progressed along the track to the double loop and the corkscrew. In a matter of forty-five seconds, I experienced a plethora of emotions that left my legs weak and my adrenaline clamoring for more punishment.

Little did I know that years later I would be standing toe-to-toe with another behemoth. It carried with it a similar allure and beckoned me with a promise that my dream would come true—a dream that my quiver would be full. I had watched others enjoy the same ride. I felt like I had been patient waiting for my opportunity. The time was right.

Fifteen years after my moment at Magic Mountain, my husband and I embarked on another adventure, with hands clasped, unaware of what was ahead.

As we strapped in for the ride, we knew the possibility of bumps and hoped for nausea. What we did not fully foresee was the overabundance of emotions that would confront us along the way. This new roller coaster did not boast a forty-five second ride; instead, it was a twenty-eight-day cycle.

I rode the ride and subsequent emotions consecutively for months on end. Days one through fourteen, I was blissfully hopeful. I harnessed into the roller coaster with butterflies in my stomach, awaited the journey ahead, and anticipated that this would be the month. The dream was birthed anew at the start of every cycle, and I would be gaily optimistic. A glutton for emotional punishment.

Then came the sex. The we're-making-a-baby kind of sex that was a juxtaposition of "I have never felt so connected to you" and "This is just a means to an end to make us a family of three" and every complexity in between. I would approach the first crest of the roller coaster and would wait, about to drop into apathy, fear, and emotions masquerading as hope.

I would arrive at the corkscrew, and upside down, I would go. I didn't know which way was up anymore. I would covertly touch my breasts throughout the day, hoping that I would find some new tenderness. Nausea and exhaustion were welcome guests that I may have psychosomatically generated in my hopeful reality. I remember wishing that my husband would notice changed emotions and extra hormones, suggesting that we had triumphantly changed our lives. For the first time in my life, I hoped that my pants would be too snug. I remember wishing that there was a more obvious signal that would announce that one's womb was full of life. Why couldn't my belly button just turn purple, my eyes change color, or my perspiration smell like a lily field? No? Too much to ask? Awesome, I'll just wait to pee on a stick instead.

Inevitably, one of two outcomes happened. Either my monthly visitor obnoxiously arrived, much to my chagrin, or Aunt Flo was postponed and we dipped into our lifetime supply of pregnancy sticks to test the successful meeting of my egg and his sperm. Those moments squatting over the plastic stick confront you with their own set of optimism and fear. The minutes waiting for the stick to react to your HCG seem like an eternity and seem to dictate your forever.

If the test reads *pregnant,* off the roller coaster you go, skipping arm-in-arm into your future dream come true. If the test reads *not pregnant*, then you have to endure the pain of your menses while you wait in line to get back on the roller coaster.

Each month the cycle and the romanticism of the process lose its appeal more and more. It becomes less of an experience to anticipate and more of a practice of dread.

Each woman on this roller coaster shares the experience of the cycle. What differs, however, is how she experiences it and what emotions she encounters.

Tangled Ball of Emotions

As I started graduate school, I did not know what I wanted to specialize in, and I thought that I would pigeonhole myself later, years into my professional journey. I wanted to experience it all prior to figuring out where I belonged.

Enter H. Norman Wright, stage right. That's when my passion for the hard things in life began to emerge.

When I was in my first semester of graduate school, we had a seminar forced upon us that inadvertently birthed a new passion in me. Norm Wright came to our little seminary and spoke on grief. He is a marriage, family, and child therapist who specializes in trauma work. He spoke in detail about his experience with grief and trauma, and he caught this green therapist hook, line, and sinker. I bought several books and dived right into them the second I got home. I found my niche that day, and I found a mentor in Mr. Wright—even if he did not know it! (If you have any interest in understanding the process of grief, read his books.)

Professionally, I use H. Norman Wright's *tangled ball of emotions*[1] quite frequently. Look at the ball like a skein (or ball) of yarn. Exposed on the outside are the complexities of emotions that one experiences while grieving. The longer you have been on this roller coaster of infertility, the more of these emotions you have most likely experienced.

These are just the emotions that you can see, though. Lying beneath are the emotions that you do not want anyone to observe. After all, you might feel that people would be entitled to judge you for those inner emotions.

Denial? Check! Apathy? Check, check! Yearning. Inadequacy. Disappointment. This tangled ball of grief looked like my heart on a monthly basis. At any moment my life could be turned upside

---

1 Wright (2003).

down by my changing emotions. No wonder those closest to us have a difficult time trying to support us. How can they know where we are if where we are changes so rapidly?

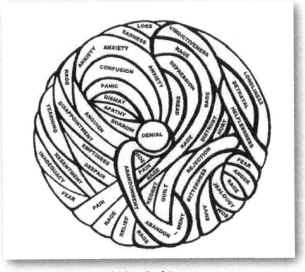

Tangled Ball of Emotions

Let's take a look at some of these emotions.

Pain

How can anyone go through this life-altering experience without encountering any pain? Pain becomes a traveling companion that finds its way into the story line too often.

Pain is around every corner in the form of pregnancy tests, baby showers for friends, disagreements with your spouse, and questions (or the absence thereof) from friends and family.

Infertility is a journey of self-awareness and personal discovery that takes its learner on a process of pain, emotional torment, and sentimental confusion. If you are seeking a process of personal growth, buyer beware. This avenue allows only the strongest to survive as it tests every piece of personal awareness and vitality.

Sarah said, "I have been through a lot in my life. We have been through a lot in our marriage. I have never been a stranger to pain. This pain, however, cuts to the core of me, of who we are, of our dreams." Oh, how I longed to expose something poetic that would dilute all the pain she was lamenting. But that would have been a mere bloviation, spoken just to make myself feel better.

The truth is, pain was a real experience for her. I am sure that it is for you also. It certainly became a place where I spent a lot of time.

We experience pain when we survive loss. We experience it when our expectations don't materialize into reality. Pain becomes the glasses through which we see the world far too easily.

Pain is a gateway to anger and rage.

Rage

Lydia and her husband, Kyle, had been married for years and had been infertile for many of them. Losing hope by the month, being robbed of joy after peeing on each stick, they reported their growing anger, bitterness, and rage toward anything and everything. Their feelings were often misguided; however, expressing those feelings felt very validating.

Lydia once told me, "Anger became my constant companion. It followed me everywhere and became the sense I experienced the world through. It was like an addiction I couldn't kick."

The couple became more resentful and contemptuous about life every time they had to leave their house. Everything was kindling the infuriating fire of rage inside of them, but this rage was detrimental as the only things affected by it were their own spirits. They were becoming hardened.

Deep-seated anger and rage, unless properly dealt with, become a cancer to the soul, robbing it of its potential for joy.

It is easy to feel anger in our society. Rage oftentimes seems more acceptable than sadness. If a person gets confronted or wrongfully accused, anger is seen as more respectable than tears. Anger and rage, however, are typically the gatekeepers for sadness and sorrow.

Sorrow

Loss of a dream. Loss of an expectation. Loss of hope. Loss of the family you pictured. Loss of a pregnancy. Any one of these elicits sorrow accompanied by an ugly cry. That is real-life pain.

Dictionary.com defines sorrow as "distress caused by loss, affliction, disappointment, etc.; grief, sadness, or regret."

Once, upon learning that my husband and I had experienced our own journey of infertility, a friend's husband asked, "Is my wife ever going to be happy again?" (In other words, "Is she always going to be this sad?")

He wanted what I could not give him. He wanted a time frame. He wanted a promise that happiness was around the corner. Sorrow can be so debilitating that the end is not always in sight. We may will it to be closer; however, it may be farther away than we think. We will explore grief and all its complexities more in chapter 4.

Disappointment

Rodney and Caroline lived in disappointment. Success driven all of their lives, they were driven to succeed at making the perfect family, too. When one month turned into two and then one year turned into two years, disappointment rooted itself in their hearts and took over their lives.

Caroline recalled, "I could do everything else right. Things came naturally to me. I got into the right college, was offered the right job, found the right guy. Now I could not do what was supposed to be a God-given ability. You bet I was disappointed."

Ask any person who has yet to leave the nest. He or she has a plan for life. Whether the plan is to be a teacher, doctor, millionaire, mother, traveler, investor, or beach bum, people have a plan. What about a five-year plan? We all have one, even if we haven't talked it over with those closest to us.

What happens when that dream doesn't come to fruition? What happens when all that you work toward does not become a reality? What happens when your expectation falls flat? Disappointment—that's what happens.

Fear

Fear is similar to its counterparts anxiety and worry. Fears says stay put. Fear says stay home. Fear says stay alone. Fear says, "Don't move forward."

Let me ask you a question about fear and worry: When have you given energy to a fear or worry and been able to successfully change the outcome of what you were concerned about? While you can worry about the egg and sperm making a successful meeting, can that worry will its success? You can worry about a treatment, but can you change the outcome with that worry? Absolutely not. It robs us of our present joy and peace. That is all it can do.

As we all know, fertility can also rob today, tomorrow, and yesterday of its joy. Adding fear to the mix certainly does not bode well for you if joy is the goal.

A friend said that during infertility, "An irrational fear overtook me. I was afraid to do anything and afraid that everything else in life would turn out as poorly as my fertility. Fear became overwhelming."

Apathy

Glenn and Carole recalled the years of trying and all the accompanying feelings. The highs and lows had produced an emotional whiplash that caused them slight posttraumatic stress. Months of caring, and caring a tad too much, led to the fear of caring. The fear of caring led to the overuse of defense mechanisms, which opened the door for apathy.

Apathy hit Glenn first; however, Carole felt that his emotional indifference gave her permission to feel halfhearted and stoic in her devotion to the child-making process. Apathy toward trying to conceive also became apathy about their marriage.

Together they began going through the motions. They were dispassionate and disinterested in a process and a cause that had once caused emotional turbulence.

Danger lives here, when the couple forgets what they are fighting for. Danger occurs when the apathy about conception becomes apathy toward each other and indifference toward life.

Where are you?

Sister, take a moment and look at the tangled ball of emotions. Where are you today? Rage? Pain? Rejection? Bitterness? Loss? Anxiety? Yearning? I wish I could wrap my arms around you and tell you that you are validated. You are not the first one to tread these murky waters, nor will you be the last. Feel the freedom to experience and walk through all those emotions, as uncomfortable as they may feel. Please, oh please, do not take up residence there. Walk through the feelings of bitterness, but if you set up camp there and live there for a while, it will begin to take a toll that will take work to get out of. If you are feeling rage, own it. Do not live there.

Depending on where I was throughout this emotional journey, you could have found me experiencing any one of these emotions.

Loneliness—I felt like no one else really understood what I was going through. Anger—I was mad that I was having to deal with such a hardship when it seemed mostly everyone in my life had little difficulty getting pregnant. Sadness/depression—when I would see other people with children or pregnant, it felt like I was punched in the stomach and like my heart was being squeezed and that I felt I might die if I didn't get pregnant. Hurt—I felt left out and not understood or supported by family and friends many times not because they didn't try but because they didn't understand how or what to say.

—Anna Marie

Many a morning—long after a healthy, functioning adult should have been out of bed—there I was, staring a hole through a perfectly good wall. Wondering. Hoping. Longing. Hiding, really. The day ahead held too many emotions that I wanted to hide from. It was a scary world outside of my bed. The first thing that was on my list was walking by our very empty nursery on the way to the bathroom. The idea of that walk was sometimes too much to bear. It felt like a slap in the face just to make it that far in the day.

Then came the day's actual to-do list. Typically it involved social interactions with people who didn't have broken uteruses, adding all the more pain to my reality. Doctor appointments, pregnancy symptoms I tried to will into my body, and waiting to hear from the nurse about HCG reports that weren't really supposed to come until tomorrow, all made my day feel like it was under a black cloud of impossibility.

Personally and professionally I was not a stranger to grief. However, I was completely ignorant, never before having given credit to how truly painful the process of infertility could be.

[I felt] anger, frustration, anxiety, fear, disappointment, and sadness, all around the process of waiting to see if we were pregnant, month after month of trying naturally and then using fertility meds with no success.

Anger and frustration around the fact that some people I know could get pregnant just by looking at their mate or people who would get pregnant with their boyfriends and have multiple kids (with or without the same partner or multiple fathers) and not be married and me feeling we were doing it "the right way." Also anger at God for me having to go through this process, having to have surgery, and knowing my body had endometriosis and polyps and wondering why, as I thought, God "did this to my body."

Anxiety around the fact that there was a possibility of us not getting pregnant ever or wondering if the fertility meds would work month after month.

—Kate

A precious friend sat across from me in my living room and explained her new reality to me. She and her husband had just crossed the year-two threshold of no baby. Not even a near-conception. Tears streamed down her face as she disclosed the innermost wounds in her heart that she felt were too ugly to admit. The pain she felt for being, in her mind, a broken woman was a constant lie she had yet to address emotionally. She felt like a failure as a wife and explained to me that she asked her husband to leave her so that he could find a healthy woman to bear his children. This, however, was not what she had wanted, but she interpreted the sentiment as love. Brokenness is the only way to describe the scene. Pain was evident as she uttered every word.

This, my friends, is a world all too hidden…a silent world where we join together, walk through it arm in arm, and proclaim that—despite the outcome—we will not be defeated.

A client whom I have been privileged to work with for a while is more profound and astute than he thinks he is. I love one-liners, quotes that you can't forget, and profound metaphors that teach. He frequently comes up with such little nuggets of truth.

While processing his own emotions, which he had allowed to linger for decades too long, he insightfully referred to those emotions as rotten fruit that he was carrying around in a backpack. He said that the more fruit he put in the backpack, the heavier the load became. The longer the fruit lingered, the more the aroma around him stank. The pack easily became awkward, unwieldy, and unmanageable.

Carrying an overstuffed, rancid backpack is no way to navigate any season, not to mention the emotional weight of this particular journey. It would be obtuse to believe that someone could experience such profound loss and have no rotten fruit accumulated over time. Shallow, also, is the assumption that someone has skillfully discarded all the fruit collected.

In a world that places high expectations on the appropriate filtration of emotions, hear my request. Allow yourself time and space to identify the fruit, process its impact on your story, and abandon it. Know it will find you again. Until then free your heart from its power.

In the depths of the emotional waves crashing around you, do not give yourself something else to weigh you down.

Find your freedom, and celebrate in it.

Personal Inventory

1. What emotions are you experiencing, and how much emotional space are they occupying in your heart and mind?
2. What emotions do you need to share with your spouse?
3. What is the rotten fruit that you need to throw out of your backpack so that it will no longer weigh you down?

CHAPTER 4

It Is OK to Grieve

I CANNOT TELL you the number of people who ruthlessly attempted to trivialize, minimize, and analyze our emotions during this process.

"I had a miscarriage once, and now I have two kids. So you'll be fine." Thanks, that's awesome help.

"It took me a couple of months. I totally know what you're going through."

"My stepsister's cousin, three times removed, has a friend who struggled with fertility. They adopted. I hope you don't have to do that."

People are relentless. Their attempts to empathize, bandage the pain, or ignorantly fill the silence are painful. Painful, right, ladies? It just plain hurts.

Their words challenge the validation to grieve. Our feelings of craziness make the lack of permission to grieve only worse, and this lack of permission intensifies our feelings of insanity.

Let's talk about the basics of grief.

Grief

Elisabeth Kübler-Ross is a psychiatrist who pioneered the understanding of grief with her innovative book *On Death and Dying: What the Dying Have to Teach Doctors, Nurses, Clergy, and Their Own Families*, which she wrote in 1969. She developed the five stages of grief that remain instrumental in the psychological and medical world.

The stages of grief are denial, anger, bargaining, depression, and acceptance.

DABDA—that's how I remembered it for the National Marital and Family Therapy Examination.

I've read Elisabeth Kübler-Ross's work. I know the stages of grief. I feel honored walking through grief with people professionally and in our ministry. It is a misunderstood process that no two people will experience the same way. I comprehend the process cerebrally.

In spite of that fact, no matter how much I try to intellectualize the process, the knowledge of what to expect doesn't make it easier to experience. It doesn't make walking this process any less painful, much to my chagrin.

Denial

If you are living in a world of defense mechanisms or mere survival, you are here, my friend.

"The ultrasound tech doesn't have an MD, so there's a possibility she's wrong."

"Maybe we were carrying twins, and there's still a good one in there."

"Maybe if I switched doctors, I would get pregnant."

"It's not that big of a deal. We've only been trying for two years. I know someone who tried for seven and then got pregnant. We'll be fine."

Denial. Even if your head knows the reality, your heart may still find itself securely in "denialville." Several times throughout our process, I would return to denial to get a breath of fresh air as I tried to convince myself that everything was still OK.

I knew it wasn't. But somehow, someway, I needed to survive another day, and I seemed to find my ability to do so here.

Anger

Many people become well acquainted with anger. We can synonymously call it *jealousy*. I am fairly sure it stems from the comparison game that we continue to torture our hearts with.

Anger is also fueled by the words we put in people's mouths. Anger is fueled by our sense of entitlement. Anger is fueled by spite.

Anger makes me want to run. Anger makes me want to act completely irrationally. Anger wants me to push everyone away. Anger makes people want to quit.

I am going to go so far as to say that anger is necessary to experience healing. Heed this warning, however. Experience anger. Go ahead. Experience it. Do not suppress it and deal with the pain of life in a self-harming way. Fight through it. Do not allow yourself to linger there too long. That, my friend, is a slippery slope.

Bargaining

"If I never _____ again, God, will you let me be pregnant?"

"If I get knocked up, I'll be kind to so-and-so from now on."

If you are stuck in the if-then game, you are bargaining.

We bargain. Plead. Negotiate in whatever way we can.

I think guilt was my traveling companion through this stage—irrational guilt but guilt nonetheless. It's a maze of if-onlys and what-if-I-hads that confused me to my core. Outsiders attempted to speak truth into the irrationality to no avail. Sometimes, unluckily for the truth speaker, it transports the bargainer into anger.

Trying to will pregnancy, egg retrieval, and the uterus and sperm into a healthy function became a full-time job.

Depression

Don't confuse this definition of depression with clinical depression; however, if you find that your symptoms of depression start to feel out of control, please give yourself (and your spouse) permission to seek professional counseling. These criteria are taken directly from the *Diagnostic and Statistical Manual of Mental Disorders: 5th Edition* (DSM-5).

⁘

Symptoms of Major Depressive Disorder, According to DSM-5

Over a two-week period, you need to have at least five of the following:

1. Depressed mood most of the day, almost every day
2. Markedly diminished interest or pleasure in all or almost all activities most of the day, nearly every day
3. Significant weight loss when not dieting or weight gain
4. Insomnia or hypersomnia nearly every day
5. Psychomotor agitation or retardation nearly every day
6. Fatigue or loss of energy nearly every day
7. Feelings of worthlessness or excessive inappropriate guilt nearly every day
8. Diminished ability to think or concentrate, or indecisiveness, nearly every day

9. Recurrent thoughts of death (not just fear of dying), recurrent suicidal ideation without a specific plan, or a suicide attempt or a specific plan for committing suicide (American Psychiatric Association 2013, 94–95).

These symptoms are not included here for purposes of self-diagnosis; rather, if you are experiencing several of the above symptoms, please make an appointment with a therapist or physician.

⟨⟩

Some days it's hard to get out of bed. Some moments you may cry and not be able to control it. Social isolation, check. Loss of motivation, check. Here the miscalculation that you're the only one who has ever experienced such a loss isolates the griever from the rest of humanity. Sometimes it even separates your desire from your motivation, as it feels like such an out-of-body experience. Here hope is paralyzed by the false belief that this process will never be over or that things will never be the same again.

The truth is, you won't be in this place forever, although the contrary certainly seems like the reality.

I grieved a bit initially, when we learned that IVF was the only option but honestly I'd done a lot of grieving early in our relationship when my husband became paralyzed. My decision to pursue a life with him required me to alter my idea of normal and this was just one aspect that I'd already begun to address from the beginning so three years later when we decided to try to have a kid, I had a little bit of a head start with regards to expectation and the idea that we might not be able to conceive naturally, or at all.

I did the most grieving when we were unable to have a second child that was honestly the hardest part, because once we got past having our first my expectation reverted back to my original—two kids a boy and a girl. It was hard to accept that we wouldn't realize that dream because it was just too expensive to continue. I experienced a very early miscarriage that was just very disappointing. A lot of time and money and emotional readiness go into an IVF cycle, so it just felt very disappointing. I cried and talked to my friends and my mom and that was what I needed to do for a little while but I also had my wonderful little boy to parent, so that didn't last very long. We shifted perspec-tive to a family of three and haven't looked back since!

—Susanne

Acceptance

Acceptance is the understanding that conception is not happening, that a viable pregnancy may not be your reality, and that you will be OK. Acceptance says that there is a new normal in your family, that your family picture looks different than you planned, but that there is a future in this new paradigm.

What is difficult is that couples and grievers get to the acceptance stage at different times and in different ways.

We all grieve differently.

Society does individuals a major disservice in the area of grief. We give people an arbitrary timetable to complete their grief. There is a sense of urgency to complete the grieving process within the week of the funeral because the rest of the world seems to be moving on without us. If we are honest, it does not always go the way we feel it should. Additionally, each person does not experience grief in the same way.

I remember when I was in college, and we were a family of five. It was in the early 2000s, and our brother was lying uncon-scious in a hospital bed after a motorcycle accident. His life was hanging in the balance. We were not sure if he was going to live, but we knew he would never walk out of there on his own. It only took moments to know that ICU bed would be his home for far longer than any of us were comfortable with. Grief, sadness, and fear penetrated the room like the stale air being circulated from the air vents.

My parents, older brother, and I grieved quite differently. My mom sought relationships to suffocate the place of fear, and she invited her community in to fill the waiting room. My dad, on the other hand, only wanted those waiting-room chairs filled with our family and wanted to exclude others from the intimacy of the situation. Our oldest brother, who works in the rescue community and knows quite a bit about medicine, was camping by my brother's bedside, asking the tough questions and monitoring his vitals. I was hiding in a closet. Praying. Seeking refuge from the pandemonium and despondency that lurked behind the door.

Here's the moral of the story: We were all grieving appropriately. No two were grieving the same, but based on individual needs, each was validated in how he or she was experiencing and expressing emotions.

I hate stories left incomplete, so let me tell you that my brother did survive. While he is wheelchair bound, he has not let the loss of feeling in his legs stop him for one moment. If you look up *inspiration* or *miracle* in the dictionary, you will see his picture.

Grief within the vicious cycle of infertility does not look all that different. One may want to talk about it endlessly, while the other might feel asphyxiated by the thought of talking. One partner may want to share the struggle publicly, while the other may interpret that as disrespect. One may cry, while one may avoid.

Let me just mention coping skills and ways of grief that are dangerous and to be avoided: addictions/impulsivity (drugs, alcohol, extramarital relationships, gambling, spending, etc.), avoidance of reality and support systems, anger that leads to behavioral changes, despondency, crime, and others. If you find that you or your spouse is grieving in such a dangerous way, please seek the help of a professional counselor in your area.

For me, grieving felt like the elephant in every room, consuming every last particle of air. Somehow my husband seemed to be able to compartmentalize a tad better. Stepping back and interpreting our paradigms of grief from a more macro view, it appears that we were both appropriate in our grief. At the time, though, he thought that I needed a break from the grief, as it mimicked symptoms of depression, and I thought that he needed to be more emotionally in touch with the process.

Please, for the sake of your marriage, be sensitive to your spouse and allow him or her to experience the unique cycle of grief.

Please, for your own sake, be sensitive to yourself and allow yourself to experience your own cycle of grief.

Healing will come. Not when you want it to come. Not when you expect it. It is possible to reach acceptance.

Personal Inventory

1. In what part of the grief cycle do you currently find yourself?
2. How do you need to pardon your spouse in his or her process of grief?
3. How will you know that you have found healing? What steps do you and your spouse need to take in order to achieve healing and/or acceptance?

CHAPTER 5

Sex Would Become a Job

I RECEIVED SOME sound advice before my husband and I got married.

I was at my bridal shower. The decorations were beautifully springy, the advice in abundance, and the merriment contagious. The young me was optimistically naïve about all things sex and marriage. All I knew was that our wedding was right around the corner and we were ready to begin our life together.

Much like when you're trying to conceive, everyone seems to have a story about marriage he or she feels compelled to share. They all tell stories about their own marriage or their sister's or their friend's or something they overheard when in line at Target. You know what I mean.

There is one piece of advice that seemed to stick with me, partially because of its validity and partly because of the sarcasm (my native language) that it was laced with.

Here were the instructions:

1. Find a new jar for every year of marriage and label it for that year.
2. Every time you have sex with your husband, put a coin in that year's jar.
3. At the time of your anniversary every year, empty the coins and take yourselves on a date.

She said that for the first few years, the coins would add up to enough money for a fancy date or romantic activity. By the fifth anniversary, she said, the coins would dwindle, and by year twenty, we would just scrape together enough money for a dinner for two at Burger King.

I dreaded that notion, and as most traditional new brides, I vowed to have enough intimacy in our relationship to equate to more than just a couple of hamburgers at Burger King.

However, the more I work with couples professionally, the more I know this advice to be true.

Here's the exception to the rule: *infertility*!

In the beginning it didn't change, but once years had passed it did. Dramatically. It became work instead of spontaneous. The fun, desire, and joy were mostly stripped away during periods of time. Our sex life became a calendar appointment, and once the window closed I became so stressed out that it was hard to even want sex any other time. It was most difficult when we weren't communicating well and the window of time would happen when I was ovulating and during times when I was feeling a bit more crazy about wanting to get pregnant. I'd force it, and it seemed almost dirty and so forced. It was terrible.

—Cameron

In the years a couple is trying to conceive, there would be a plethora of coins in the jar. The anniversary dinners would be extravagant. But even though there may be money for a nice dinner, the longer a couple tries to conceive to no avail, the more they find they have nothing to talk about—besides what has been consuming them since their last anniversary.

If a couple had high expectations for sex when they pledged their love to each other all those years ago, they can kiss those expectations good-bye if infertility takes up residence in their home. It sucks all the passion and romance from their marital bed.

Having sex on a schedule dictated by egg release can extinguish the romantic flame in any relationship.

Professionally we see this all the time. Married women walk into my office alone, longing for a baby while simultaneously wondering why their romantic connection with their husband has disappeared. Couples enter marital counseling, and the man wonders why his sole purpose has become the sperm donor for the baby they hope to one day make. A couple complains about sex becoming a job because they have to have sex when they don't feel like it. The ovulation stick tells them to, so they begrudgingly do the duty.

How romantic.

A young gal once told me that she was leaving on a trip for a week that happened to fall over ovulation week. "I woke him up at six in the morning I was leaving so that he could knock me up. There was no romance. We did it, and he fell right back to sleep. Off I went. It would have been more romantic to do it in a test tube."

You start the journey to conception romantically. You are united in your decision and connected in every way because the dream is about to become a reality. A couple's naïveté about the sexiness of making a baby when they start their journey becomes a big fat lie taunting them once they surpass the marker for the normal amount of time it should take to conceive.

Somehow along the arduous journey, it changes. Before you know it, the candles are burned out. There are no more rose petals (but a girl can dream, right?), and it's no longer something you want to make time for but something you *have* to make time for it. Time is limited, after all.

Please, oh please, do not feel shame if you are silently nodding along, wondering what happened to your love. Please do not buy into the lie that things will always be this way, that the romance in your relationship is permanently doomed or that you have a problem because the fire in your bedroom is only bright enough to see the ovulation stick.

Sister, this is an expected part of the process if a couple of months of negative pregnancy tests turn into several months or even years. It is more normal than what it probably feels to you. All of your mommy friends probably talk about their children who were conceived through the best sex of their lives. Mommy friends you envy may complain about being too tired for sex, while you would do anything to share in that amount of parental exhaustion.

Infertility is tough to empathize with if you haven't been there—despite the fact that each couple's journey is unique. If you throw the ever-so-ostracizing infertility talk in the middle of a lunch with girlfriends, you hear only crickets. No understanding. No compassion. Blank stares. You would crawl under the table if you couldn't feel gum under there.

You are OK, my friend. While a baby is worth fighting for, so is your marriage and so is mutually satisfying sex.

Obstacles to Sex

We all have our own respective obstacles to conception. For some, the act of sexual intercourse is that very obstacle. Gynecological pain, physical paralysis, medical complications, sexual aggravations, and allergies stand in the way of couples being able to conceive a child in an instinctive way. When such complexities pose complications, a couple's options seem limited.

Carlos and Rosie had known that from the words *I do* that everything in the bedroom was going to be complicated. From the outside, everything looked and worked perfectly. During the course of their premarital counseling, they both came to the realization that the bedroom—while possibly being a point of intimacy—carried the risk of complication, concern, and maybe pain.

Carlos had a medical diagnosis with a hereditary origin. He knew that his sperm were damaged and that they would most likely never fertilize an egg. In addition, due to an injury sustained in her youth, the nerves in Rosie's pelvis were damaged, causing extreme pain during penetration.

Together they had accepted that they would not conceive naturally due to his biological limitations. Sex was still difficult, however. The very act of physically expressing their love for each other was the source of her greatest pain. After an attempt at physical intimacy, he vacillated between guilt for causing the pain and rejection that he could not be with his wife physically.

The source of their emotional healing came when they connected with their local sex therapist. They were able to work through emotional blocks to sex, learn new ways to please each other, and learn how to communicate when their needs were not met. Intimacy between these two lovebirds, while it was not everything they had dreamed about, was a beautiful representation of who they were as a couple.

⌒⌒⌒

From Shannon

What a funny topic—not funny ha-ha but interestingly amusing. Few people become adults believing that there are obstacles to intercourse. Subconsciously most humans feel that the act of sex is a right and a perk of being part of the species. But when there has been emotional, physical, or mental abuse, it becomes a different story. In some severe posttraumatic-stress-disorder situations, the woman has to undergo anesthesia and artificial insemination because she cannot bear to have sex.

Other issues that can affect fertility include, but are not limited to, dyspareunia (painful intercourse), decreased libido, and, as strange as it seems, lack of time. In this busy world, individuals have different working hours or are traveling a lot for business and are not available to try and conceive every month. Medical conditions affecting both men and women's fertility are, fortunately, uncommon; however, if a couple is having trouble conceiving, anatomic variations should be ruled out, as well as major medical diseases. Medications can even affect libido and fertility. Antidepressants should not affect fertility, but they can decrease libido and contribute to feeling more and more like sex is just a means to a baby and not an intimate act to be cherished in and of itself.

Infertility is one of the most stressful situations a couple can encounter. Open communication with each other and your health-care provider is essential to maintaining a healthy relationship. Seeking help from a relationship counselor specializing in infertility can guide you along your journey as well. Treatments for these obstacles are neither quick nor simple. Usually a combination of medications, physical therapy, musculoskeletal manipulation, surgery, and psychological evaluation and therapy can be offered and explored. Every patient will react differently to different modes of therapy. You are an individual and should be treated as such. Be patient, and realize that your first treatment choices may not make you dramatically better or even help at all.

⁓

Fight for Good Sex

It is inevitable that things in the bedroom are going to change. Where sex was once fun, it is now a means to an end. You may have an app on your phone telling you when to get busy or a calendar that you both watch together, but that does not mean that you cannot still spice things up a little.

So it's sex night because the app says you're ovulating, but it can still be romantic.

I'm a woman who loves sex, honestly. I think maybe I crave it more often than my husband. But when we were trying to conceive, the emotional and spiritual connection that I would normally experience felt like it was missing. I felt as if it was more of an act of duty than an act of love at times. At one point, I just wanted to stop trying because I wanted the emotion back.

—Michelle

A man with whom I went to grad school appeared to me, a then-single girl, to have an amazing marriage with his wife. I asked him what the secret was, thinking he would say good communication or something Hallmarky like that. Instead his advice was this: twenty-four-hour foreplay. Duly noted, oh, wise man.

If you know your eggs are ready to be fertilized, start the foreplay in the morning with some sexy talk and get your spouse all hot and bothered for the evening's festivities. Dust the cobwebs off the old techniques you used when you were newlyweds. Be creative, be romantic, and have some fun. Worry about whether or not you are making a baby (or if you did make a baby) in the upcoming weeks when you're diligently watching for (overanalyzing) symptoms of pregnancy.

Go on a vacation. Get a room in a hotel. Get a sexy outfit. You know what he likes. You can still have fun-filled intimacy in the midst of heartache and delayed gratification.

Of course I am trying to make a heavy, *heavy* topic light. I know that it's not. These changes have, do, or will burden any couple in the throes of infertility.

Research shows that a vast majority of couples do not talk about their sexual relations—much to their detriment. Talk about it. In a loving and respectful way, make the covert overt. Get on the same page. Get a game plan, and get busy.

Personal Inventory

1. What toll has infertility taken on your sex life? In what way has it become like a job?
2. Discuss with your spouse what you can do to relight the fire in your sex life.

CHAPTER 6

It Could Be a Wedge in a Marriage

You get that life-shattering phone call in the middle of the night or face the reality that blasts your plans, and life around you seems like it was hit by a major earthquake, dislodging everything that previously held you together.

My job offers me a front-row seat to see how loss impacts marriage. Communication is gone. Intimacy is a thing of the past. Grief happens in different ways, extinguishing the unity candle that two people—once full of excitement for the future—lit on their wedding day.

My husband is the care pastor at our church, so we often see families and marriages crumble under the pressure of how to press on and how to press into each other yet another day after a loved one dies. Dilemmas over the distribution of money, the choice of a final resting place, or the decision about who gets to take care of Mom and Dad pierce the heart of the family, leaving its members raw, exposed, and broken.

Whoever said that marriage is work was right. Society gives that a negative connotation, however, demeaning the purity of marriage by saying marriage is like a job that many people hate. Let's step away from that view of marriage. Instead let's realize that both spouses must work to maintain intimacy, communication, and unity while struggling through whatever difficult circumstances may come. *That's work*. That's worthwhile, marriage-sustaining, intimacy-increasing work.

Our work started as the ultrasound tech turned off the monitor and I put the gown in the wastebasket. Somehow in just a few seconds, our life changed. Our baby's beating heart had stopped inexplicably, and it felt like mine was going to stop also. Hope was extinguished, while loss introduced itself in all its ugliness.

Words didn't need to be spoken about how difficult the road ahead would be. Leaving the room and facing the world seemed just as daunting as staying in the room to avoid reality.

Maybe your work started with the seventeenth consecutive negative pregnancy test.

Perhaps it started when that diagnosis punched you in the gut like a battering ram.

Maybe it was the day you looked in the mirror and wondered if you had enough to keep going.

Maybe it was the day your husband reached apathy and said he didn't want to keep trying.

You don't have to look far around you to see marriages falling—or that have fallen—apart because of loss and grief. Chances are, my friend, that your own marriage has probably faced some kind of similar circumstance. If you're hanging on, let me commend you. If you're fighting, you'll never regret it. If you've come out the other side, congratulations. Now cherish each other even more. If the pain of grief cost you your 'til-death-do-us-part, you have my deepest sympathies.

It has been rare that my husband and I have been on the same page when walking through our own grief and loss. All people deal with grief and loss differently; however, when you're experiencing infertility and miscarriage, it's often difficult for the man to relate. He doesn't feel the beautifully welcome nausea in the first trimester, nor can he empathize with the fear when those feelings all of a sudden go away. While he may be physically present with you in the process, he doesn't feel and experience the loss of the baby in the same way. He probably doesn't count days with such precision or have the roller coaster of emotions every month with high highs and low lows, depending on where you are in your cycle. It's hard to be on the same page, but even though you may find yourselves on different pages, don't forget that you are part of the same story.

If you're reading this and shuddering a silent, "Amen, sister," let me encourage you to talk to your husband and express to him what you're feeling. At the same time, forgive your husband for not understanding what it is that you're going through; you may be asking him to empathize with a process that he is not wired to understand.

Whenever you experience any kind of loss, healing in the marriage and unity in the process are possible. But it requires this word that we all try to avoid: *work*. Working to grow your marriage in the midst of your struggle will never leave you lonely or disappointed. It'll be the best job you ever do, and when two are working toward the same goal, the result is success.

The acknowledgment that *work* needs to be done in our marriages often comes like a late-night realization in college that your final project is due in six hours and you don't know what you're going to do it on. Your project partner was assigned half of the to-do list, but the two of you haven't even spoken about how your partner is holding up his or her end of the deal, let alone what you need to do.

[There was] lots of arguing, month after month, when we didn't get pregnant. I also felt the meds made me feel like I was crazy—like legit nuts because of my moodiness being on the meds. I didn't feel like myself which caused fighting because I was a different person when I was on the meds versus being off the meds. It made me feel bipolar. One minute I'd be OK, and then the next I'd be bawling, hysterical, or angry, and I'd be like, "What the heck is wrong with me?" I felt like I was ruining our marriage and like I dragged my husband into this process with me at times, and I thought he didn't deserve how I was treating him when I was on the meds. I felt like I was totally not the person he married.

—Rachelle

So you scramble. You throw that last-second Hail Mary pass to the end zone, hoping it'll go your way. You rush through the sections that are either easy, require little work, or are certain to get you some sort of recognition for your effort. Even though the project has been on your radar for the entire semester, finals week finally seems like the time to acknowledge its existence and do the work you should've been doing all along.

Don't put yourself in the position of trying to save your marriage with a last-second Hail Mary effort.

Professionally speaking, I love working with marriages. I love those rare occasions when two willing individuals come in to make themselves transparent—to take a magnifying glass to those broken areas of themselves or their marriage. I intentionally chose the word *rare*, as it just doesn't happen all that often. (The average couple wait too many years to engage in therapy.)

I appreciate the couples who are in a good place but just come in for a marital oil change every three thousand miles. Truthfully, therapists are usually the last stop on the way to the junkyard for a totaled marriage.

"We just didn't talk about anything."

"Our grief was different."

"If we had talked about it eight months ago, we wouldn't be here."

There were times when we could barely talk. I got so depressed and felt that he couldn't relate completely, and it made me withdraw and feel alone. I had a hard time com-municating my emotions because I was so distraught, and those times put our marriage on rockier ground than we'd ever experienced. However, there were also times that he would communicate understanding in ways that drew us together, and since experiencing it, we now have better communication and are much closer because of it all.

—Lauren

"He just never seemed to care."

"You never gave me a chance to care."

"Why did you talk to your mom/sister/coworker/friend instead of me?"

Work happens in the trenches, not on the way to the divorce lawyer. Work takes humility, brokenness, and the desire to look out for your spouse's interests above your own. Raw conversations may cost a lot; however, they are a lot cheaper than therapy or a divorce lawyer.

I remember when we were doing our premarital counseling. The couple who worked with us told us not only to put each other's needs above our own but also to *outserve* each other. This translates as, when you don't see eye to eye, fight to see your spouse's perspective. Don't wait to be asked to help; just help. When you disagree, keep the other's best interest in mind. When you're in the trenches, fight together to get out.

There have been so many times when my husband and I have been in different places in dealing with our own grief. That's not disrespectful to my husband to say so. *He doesn't have a uterus.* He can't understand. Even though he doesn't understand what I'm feeling, it's my job to educate him; even though he can't empathize, it's his job to meet me where I am, to the best of his ability. It's not just *my* struggles in those moments. We're still *one*, so the struggle is still *ours. Fight together!*

You're walking the same road, even if it's at different speeds.

Four Horsemen of the Apocalypse[2]

Doctors John and Julie Gottman are psychologists who reside and practice in Seattle, Washington. They run the Gottman Institute and have been doing research since before I took a breath on this earth. They are the marital gurus on whom I lean professionally and personally.

Through their research, they have concluded that there are four marriage killers—or what they call the "Four Horsemen of the Apocalypse."

THE FIRST OF THESE FOUR HORSEMEN IS CRITICISM.

Criticism takes a shot at your spouse. Instead of *complaining* about something that you see needs to be done or a need that is not being met, criticism goes for the jugular and condemns the person's character in addition to the need not being met.

Criticism: "Why are you so impatient with my emotions? You're so mean."

Complaint: "I feel like you are being impatient with my emotions. Can we talk more about it?"

Criticism: "Why do you always want to talk about making a baby? Isn't there anything else going on in life?"

Complaint: "I feel like we talk about conception a lot. Sometimes I need a break. Would you mind if we talked about something else?"

Clearly, with criticism, the person being critiqued is going to walk about feel hurt, defeated, defensive, or angry. If we are solution focused, which is the goal, criticism is something that we need to avoid like the plague.

---

2 If you have any interest in studying more about the Gottmans' research on marriages, I recommend you start with their book *The Seven Principles for Making Marriage Work.*

On the contrary, when we simply bring something to the table in the form of a complaint, you can see that this kind of communication brings the other person into the conversation, gives that person a voice, and opens the door for a solution and connection.

If we are honest, our humanity flirts with criticizing our spouses often. We know better than anyone how to hurt him or her. That's one of the results of intimacy and years together. However, in the midst of a battle—such as infertility—we need to work (there's that word again) to fight against all the raw emotions that may make us feel critical. We need to become solution focused with our spouses.

THE NEXT HORSEMAN IS DEFENSIVENESS.

You remember those days on the playground when someone took a jab at you and your rebuttal was, "Nuh-uh, you are."

Well, sometimes age does not mature every corner of our heart.

We still do this as couples.

"Honey, I am hurt because you _____." Now imagine a nuh-uh-you-did-that reply.

Whether we speak it audibly or not, we are all guilty of defensiveness. If you are saying no to that generalization, you are being defensive. "Nuh-uh, you are." I digress.

Defensiveness says, "I don't care what you are saying. It is wrong. I do not care. My opinion is better than yours. I am going to use all the artillery in my arsenal to show you how wrong you are. I am going to win at all cost."

When someone is defensive, the listener typically is not listening to what the speaker is trying to communicate. Rather he or she is thinking about a fancy counterargument in an effort to take the upper hand in the debate.

Defensiveness: "I know that's how you feel, but you are wrong. Let me tell you how it truly happened."

Defensiveness: "I know you are sad because we can't get pregnant. We're in the situation to begin with because you want to be a parent."

The antidote to defensiveness is to take responsibility for one's own actions. Own them. If you must defend them, do so humbly.

Now I have something corny to share. Ready? When I work with couples who are at a standstill in an argument or persistent arguments in their marriage, my charge to them is to be part of *Team Marriage.* Look at each squabble as if it involves three people: the husband, the wife, and the marriage. If either the husband or the wife wins the argument, then the marriage loses. If the marriage loses, ultimately both partners also lose.

If we are solution focused, then we are on the side of the marriage. This means that defensiveness—and the rest of the horsemen for that matter—has to take a back seat in the controversy or during communication at large.

Get rid of defensiveness. Be solution focused. Own it. Take responsibility. Be on Team Marriage.

As a woman, I just want to be heard. My girlfriends are so good at this. I had to teach my husband how to hear me better when we weren't conceiving. I had so many emotions, and he either wanted to fix them or got defensive. I stopped wanting to talk to him.

—Kathryn

THE THIRD HORSEMAN IS CONTEMPT.
When you think of contempt, think of extreme apathy. Malice. Mockery. Disregard. Ridicule.

None of those words promotes any warm, fuzzy feelings, nor will those words ever grace the front of a Hallmark card.

Drs. John and Julie Gottman say that in communication, a contemptuous spirit comes across in sarcasm, cynicism, eye rolling, sighs, demeaning humor, or name-calling. For obvious reasons, such a spirit ought to be averted.

A contemptuous spirit is damaging to a marriage.

Reconciliation is not the goal of a contemptuous spouse. Proving a point becomes the goal.

If problems are chronically unresolved, it is easy for contempt to creep its way in, fuel bitterness, and start to steal intimacy and positivity in a marriage.

When contempt has taken root, contemptuous spouses don't describe their own needs and wants; rather, they negatively describe their partner or antagonistically convey how they perceive their spouse. To counteract contempt, take a courteous approach and describe the problem rather than assertively crush the spirit of the person you once vowed to love for better and for worse.

FINALLY, THE FOURTH HORSEMAN IS STONEWALLING.
We have reached our final horseman. Isn't the Gottmans's research fascinating?

When people stonewall, they disengage. They have been berated, and they simply shut down. Turn off. Walk away. Slam the door. Done.

In the event of stonewalling, people are not only turning away from the argument, but they are also turning away from the marriage. A solution cannot be reached because one component of the partnership is absent.

To the person who is stonewalling, for the sake of your marriage, please, oh please, turn toward your spouse. Work on things together. Remember, hard work is done in the trenches. Intimacy is found in work. I have never met a couple, personally or professionally, who have regretted putting hard work into their marriage to resolve whatever impasse trapped them.

Throughout the course of infertility, it is so easy to drift apart. Hormones, griefs, and comments from the peanut gallery all try to divide those who are in the throes of adversity. Turn toward each other rather than against each other. If it seems like too big of an Everest to climb on your own, please seek help.

You will never regret it.

Your spouse is worth it.

Your marriage is worth it.

Personal Inventory

1. How well are you and your spouse talking about and coping with infertility together?
2. Has your communication style started to look like the four horsemen of the apocalypse from the Gottmans's research? How so?
3. How can you and your spouse better handle your grief together?

CHAPTER 7

It Would Be All-Consuming

I LOVE THE show *Friends.*

I will confess that I did not watch the show when it was telecast live. Blame it on the fact that we barely watched television growing up or the fact that my worth was determined by the amount of activities I was involved in. As a child or preteen, I could be found outside, playing on what my brothers convinced me were remains from an archaeological dig stemming from the days of our early Californian history. Color me fooled. They convinced me that the huge rock in the center of our driveway was an old Indian kitchen and that the rock overlooking the garage was where the chief sat. I felt so cool explaining this history to my friends. I guess this is the natural risk of being the caboose of the family.

Eventually I grew up, left home, and went to college in Los Angeles. One night I went with a group of friends to Hollywood to attend a live taping of *Friends.* After waiting for what seemed like forever (especially since I didn't care then), we were the first group that did not make it into the audience.

At the time I was relieved because I was hungry. Shame on me. Now that I am a fan, I greatly regret missing that event.

Since then in a way I cannot explain, I have accumulated all ten seasons. (Thank you, again, to all of those who have donated to my collection.) Much to my husband's chagrin, watching *Friends* is like having the radio on—to me. I don't need to pay attention to know what is going on. An episode of *Friends* plus a cup of coffee is a great way to implement self-care.

There is an episode where Monica and Rachel are sitting in Monica and Chandler's apartment. Rachel has just had her baby, Emma, and the two women are talking about all of Emma's newest accomplishments. They are discussing what percentile Emma has recently grown into and what her upcoming milestones are expected to be.

Sitting across from each other at the table in the famous purple apartment, Rachel looks at Monica and laments, "What did we used to talk about?" They sit, perplexed, with no idea of how they have reached this point in their lives.

This new life stage conversationally trumped everything they had believed was most important only months prior. This new reality had crept to the forefront of almost everything they did.

I recall driving to an anniversary dinner with my husband during our years of attempting to create life biologically and wondering what we would talk about at dinner. We had exhausted the subjects of conception, all things grief related, and our own plans of how to move forward. I sensed he had talked enough about past losses. I did not want to talk about our upcoming doctor's appointments, because despite the great care we received, appointments had just becoming depressing. What was there still to talk about?

"What did we used to talk about?" I wondered to myself.

I checked the app on my phone daily to see if I had jumped seven days closer to the pregnancy test in the last twenty-four hours. If there was a pie chart of what my mind focused on throughout a typical day, the chart would show that I was completely consumed with thoughts of infertility.

I constantly monitored symptoms of ovulation, conception, implantation, and menses. My friends would ask how I was doing, and I wanted to tell them where I was in my cycle, how many days until I peed on a stick again, my symptoms, or how I was feeling about it all.

Even though that's what I wanted to say, I did not share much. I always feared sharing too much. I didn't want my friends to look at me and say, "Cath, what did we used to talk about?" But during that season of life, trying to conceive was all encompassing. With every breath, I held on to the belief that I could make it another second. Sometimes I convinced myself. At other times, not so much.

I remember standing at a local convenience store. I was devastated after learning that a baby we had made no longer had a heartbeat. It was still occupying space in my womb and would forever occupy space in my heart. I was becoming a professional at managing the whole ordeal, but it did not make it any easier.

While I wanted to cry, I managed to keep the emotions roiling on the inside.

That was until the polite, unassuming checkout woman asked me how I was doing. Big mistake.

"Fine," I lied. "How are you?"

She went on to tell me about how she did not approve of the seasonal climate, how she needed a repair on her car, and how she still had more hours to work than she wanted but that she did not want to go home to her kids; therefore, being at work was tolerable.

I wanted to scream. If she would have got the wrath of decreasing hormones that all my willpower kept in, she would have heard, "Really? Really? You are telling me that life is hard? I have a dead baby in me, and it is not the first. I would do anything to go home to children. I cannot go to work because I have to discharge this pregnancy. I'm barren. Do you hear me? Barren! Stop your complaining."

Thank your lucky stars that I did not say that; otherwise, your tax dollars would have locked me up in jail that night.

Jenny and Ryan called my office to schedule some sessions. Infertility had crept into their home and robbed them of their emotional intimacy.

Between hormone-replacement therapies, forced sexual encounters, shots that he faithfully administered, incessant questions from the in-laws, and financial conversations to figure out how to afford it all, they had lost everything else.

The couple whom their friends enviously viewed as being the best of friends were putting on a facade. They continued to go on date nights and vacations. He sent flowers to her at work. Valentine's Day was lavish. Externally, the Hallmark channel could have made a romance special about their love affair.

The rooms of their home, however, were now filled with silence. They had exhausted the conversations about baby making. Their emotional intimacy had been reduced to knowing when to administer shots without having to say anything.

Jenny pleaded with me. "Teach us to talk again. Help us remember why we are together. We are working toward a family, but I fear once we get there, we won't have a marriage." They felt alone. Alone in their individual hearts. Alone in their marriage. Alone amid the rest of humanity.

It is easy to get to that place. It is dangerous to make that place the new normal.

In the midst of hardship, we forget how we started. Research shows that fondly being able to recall how your relationship began boosts the rates of success for getting back to a similar place. In the book, *The Seven Principles for Making Marriage Work*, John Gottman writes, "I have found over and over that couples who are deeply entrenched in a negative view of their spouse and their marriage often rewrite their past." He continues, "When I ask them about their early courtship, their wedding, their first year together, I can predict their chances of divorce, even if I'm not privy to their current feelings" (Gottman 1999, 42).

Talking for hours into the wee hours of the morning was easy when premarriage hormones were raging, and those hours have laid an excellent foundation for how to rekindle the fire you first lit years ago. Dr. Gottman adds, "Most couples enter marriage with high hopes and great expectations. In a happy marriage, couples tend to look back on their early days fondly" (p. 42).

Professionally, I have never worked with a couple who have regretted putting in the hard work to restore a relationship to its former glory. These couples stand at the base of Mount Change, wondering how they will ever scale this monstrosity in front of them. However, once progress has been made, I have never heard a couple regret it. The first step to reaching the highest peak of a mountain isn't hiking. It is putting on your shoes. The first step to repairing your marriage is just deciding you have something to fight for.

Similarly, I have never met an individual who has regretted putting in the hard work to find him- or herself again—to recover well-being. Society sometimes views self-care as selfish. On the contrary, self-care, when executed for the right reasons, gives the individual a more complete sense of self and a better desire to participate in the bigger picture.

Before my husband and I got married, I had only used a lawn mower a time or two. Those few times I had mowed a yard that was perhaps ten feet wide and twenty-five feet long. The mower did not even have a motor.

Even though I was inexperienced with said equipment, once we got married, I attempted to mow our now bigger (but not by much) yard. I figured out how to get the mower running and two hours later had accomplished the task, completely surprising my husband.

Here was an even bigger surprise—both to him and to me—I did not know that there was a lever you could hold on to in order to activate the self-propelling feature. I had been almost parallel to the ground, pushing that evil machine with all my body weight as it resisted me with its own. What should have taken about twenty-five minutes took two hours of my life that I will never get back.

While I am embarrassed to admit my ignorance, I am proud to admit that I found out that when I actually used the mower correctly, I really enjoyed it. We now have more property and a riding lawn mower that I frequently use.

Once winter fades and spring creeps in, I have to push my husband off the lawn mower because it is a happy place for me. I put on my headphones, blast music that no one else likes, and ride the mower extra slowly so that I can simultaneously work on my tan. It is my place. My job. It has become my self-care.

Once that hour is done, I am ready to rejoin the rest of humanity because I have had *my* time. Self-care for me is also watching *Friends*. Self-care for me is a cup of coffee while it rains. Self-care is a good song on the radio, turned up a little too loudly, while the windows are down and I am alone so that I am free to sing at the top of my lungs. Self-care is a soul-fulfilling conversation with my husband, my mom, or a dear girlfriend.

Self-care will look different for you. It is going to look different for your husband. Healthy self-care is good for your overall well-being, and when implemented respectfully, self-care is healthy for those around you. Healthy self-care for your marriage may be taking yourselves back to the roots of your marriage and doing something silly, romantic, or a tad immature like you would have done when you were just dating. Recreate the magic. Fight for each other. Reignite the romance.

It is when you are properly caring for yourself that big things feel less consuming.

Personal Inventory

1. What is infertility taking your focus away from?
2. What does self-care look like for you? How can you implement self-care?
3. How can you invest in your marriage and other relationships around you instead of focusing on fertility?

CHAPTER 8

It Would Be Really Lonely

PRETEND FOR A minute that you want to admit that you have seen the movie *Mean Girls.*

I'll go first. "Guilty, Your Honor."

There is a scene in the film where one of the characters is describing the school's cafeteria. The camera pans out to show a drawing of how the girls perceive the social divisions of the school.

There are several tables occupied by a variety of different school cliques. There are the geeks, techies, weirdos, dropouts, and, of course, the clique the audience love to hate (and covet simultaneously)—the plastics.

Characters walk into the cafeteria and know where they belong. They dare not venture where they do not fit in the hierarchy. Someone designated the spot. Even if they covet another clique, they ought not to go outside their social class. Perhaps a social promotion will ensue. One can only hope.

If there were cafeteria tables for your current social situation, you might feel a little like you were living in the scene described.

The first table hosts the newlywed women who are enjoying their date nights, having playful, uninterrupted sex, and enjoying spontaneous adventures on the weekends. Having recently secured their man, they have only hopes and dreams ahead of them on the horizon. Their naïveté is undeniable. Set before them are only their hopes and dreams of a family. I was there once; were you?

At one table you would find the young moms. Glowing in their exhaustion. Reveling in their stretch marks. Confident in their new clique. Oblivious to the group they left behind due to their seamless promotion to the new table. They have everything you have only dreamed of. They have experienced the joy of the mama-to-be parking when they registered for all the glorious mama-to-be paraphernalia. They have the maternity photo shots with the naked bellies. They had their moment with their gender-reveal party. They perhaps know what an episiotomy and an epidural feel like. They have the whole package. They are the maternal plastics.

Sitting at a table farther away are the moms of school-aged children. They have this mama thing down. They have survived the toddler years and are confident leaving their children in the care of another, unlike the previous grouping. They can go on date nights again and eagerly await autumn as they push their sweetie children back onto the school bus. Their stomachs have shrunk, and they may even long to try again for another child. If not, they are urging their husbands to schedule an appointment with their urologist to have the dreaded vasectomy—if only our husbands were so lucky to be faced with that decision.

Another table hosts the women who have recently launched or are ready to launch their children. They appreciate their mama role as they are about to graduate from the intensity of it. The children who belong to the moms at the other tables are currently being cared for by these women, who are stuck with I-remember-when-my-child-was-this-young bewilderment.

Last we find ourselves observing the wannabes' table. The infertile mamas sit there. Invisible. Quietly coveting. Insecurely processing. Blotting the corners of their eyes while the other women roar with laughter. You hope to be promoted one day. For now, however, you sit, head down, focusing on your food. Hoping that, like in high school, you don't start your period.

The divisions of the cafeteria are perhaps most observable from your table. All the people in the room are women. Scientifically speaking, all are the same. However, despite the life stage of the kiddos represented, one thing divides the women in the room. Some are moms. The others just aren't (yet).

A lot of my friends were getting pregnant, while we were not. One friend walked on egg-shells around me when talking about her newborn. That made me isolated even more. I bawled when friends told me they were pregnant, but I also told them through tears that my tears of heartache to have my own child didn't represent the joy I still felt for them. My heart was tender for a while, and it felt like any news of babies arriving ripped the wound back open. Funny thing is, I longed to be with the friends who had kids. I figured if I wasn't having my own, I would be the best auntie to other littles whom I loved so much

—Trisha

"I don't know how to talk to people anymore," she muttered as tears slid down her rosy cheeks. "It is like a muzzle. I feel like I don't know how to have a grown-up conversation that does not consist of my uterus or my husband's sperm or without calculating how close to my period I am."

All I could do was nod, head tilted to the side, eyes empathetic. She was so right.

"If I am at a baby shower, I feel like I have a sign stapled to my forehead saying, 'Please come rub my back and tell me it will be my turn one day,'" she said cynically. She could not have spoken any more sarcastically or more directly to the pain of loneliness she felt as a woman with an empty womb.

You cannot go into a department or big-box store without having to wander by the maternity clothing, the section for all things baby, or the nursery furniture. You have to covertly maneuver and ninja roll around that store if you actually want to leave feeling somewhat emotionally intact.

> The room that we have set aside for our first child is always difficult [to be in]. I go in there and daydream about a little one playing in there. Sometimes my car is a difficult place because I can picture a little one behind me yelling, singing, and kicking my seat. All the things that annoy moms are all things that I daydream about happening to me.
>
> —Annie

Attending family gatherings even brings up pain. On one hand, it feels like the safest place in the world to grieve; on the other hand, it leaves you completely exposed, because your family members are not strangers to what you are going through. The first Christmas morning of your journey, everyone expectantly anticipates the pitter-patter of another grandchild next Christmas and another stocking hung by the chimney with care. By the time the second Christmas rolls around, you get a hug in acknowledgment of the struggle. The subject is avoided like the plague by the third. You would avoid it, too, if it wasn't your uterus aching with the pain of what was missing.

> Honestly, I was jealous of all my friends (and sisters) who had kids. I was like, "Why them and not me, too? What did I do wrong?" A lot of my close friends aren't around me, so I don't see them much. So it wasn't like I avoided them. It was hard being around some family because they would ask questions like how we were doing. At times I wanted to be like, "How do you think we are/I am doing?" And other times I would be OK answering questions. I did get mad at my dad for saying, "Maybe you need to give up control."
>
> —Jasmine

You sit with the most precious of friends who innocently complain about the inconvenience of midnight feedings, their milk production, bags under their eyes, and the fact that they have no time for themselves. There were times when I just wanted to stomp around like a child and proclaim, "I would do anything for a midnight feeding. That would mean I have a child. I certainly would not complain about that gift. I would hold that baby so tightly and cherish every middle-of-the-night, sleepless moment." That would be a good way to ensure permanent loneliness, as that would be the last time you would be invited to a girls' Sunday brunch.

It is easy to penalize people who do not understand. Let's make a pact that we will choose to remember that it is someone's lack of experience in an area that creates misunderstanding or lack of empathy. It is not that people do not want to be relationally present. Be thankful for them that they have not suffered through infertility.

Loneliness creeps into the safest of places, into families, churches, lunch tables, and bedrooms. It creeps into marriages, workplaces, and the sisterhood.

Raquel told of the loneliness in her marriage. From every angle, it appeared that she and Sean were incredibly solid and united intimately.

They spoke fondly of how they met and told of a romance paralleled only by the black-and-white cinema greats. They appeared, even to those closest, to never fight. There was an overall level of remarkable respect. How might one feel lonely in such an accepting and loving relationship?

While they certainly were all of those things, loneliness had crept in for Raquel. Sean desired to be present in their journey of infertility. He went to all the necessary appointments; however, he had a way to compartmentalize that which she coveted. He had a way to intellectualize their situation, while she emoted all over it.

In addition, the reason for their infertility was not him. She was the one who carried the burden. The reason was unmistakably hers. Polycystic ovary syndrome and endometriosis occupied much of her pelvis. She felt pain during intercourse, which made her want to stay away from it, even though it was the means to an end. She felt like her husband could do better with another woman. She pushed him away despite his efforts to stay present, because no one could understand the pain she felt. While he felt the same pain, she still felt lonely.

> I didn't feel I had anyone I could completely relate to or who could understand the dark, hurt places of my heart. I feared talking too much to people, because they usually said things that were hurtful or implied that I somehow could change it if I tried different things. People always wanted to tell me stories they'd heard rather than just listen or com-fort me, so I began trying to keep conversations [on a] much more surface level. Whenever someone got pregnant, I had a very hard time being around her.
>
> —Cameron

Many days the fight seems to be against infertility. That is certainly the external fight that you are waging. Internally you experience the opposite—fighting the reality that the fight is against yourself, your spouse, or your marriage. Let me spur you on to continue fighting for yourself, your marriage, and your personal relationships.

If I am honest, I let being lonely sequester me into more loneliness. I projected my own emotions onto those whom I am confident sincerely cared. I pushed away those wanting to walk the road with me. What we need as women is relationships. What we need as infertile women is relationships.

I am not a runner. Let's get that straight right off the bat. I thought I could be once upon a time. My today-self laughs at that girl. The symbolism of running, however, is not lost on me.

I want you to picture a marathon—over twenty-six miles of pure torture, in my mind. Those who take on the challenge are rock stars. I stood at the finish line once and cheered on a former roommate. Those people, marathon finishers, are hard-core human beings. Strong. Resilient. Invincible!

There are three groups of people one needs for support in such a race—perhaps more, but remember, I am not a runner. So just go with me.

You need those who are ahead of you, setting the pace, inspiring you, and giving you a goal to attain. You know that if those people can make it to a certain marker, you can, too. We need those people to give us confidence.

Behind you are people who are following you. It is your job to inspire them. Cheer them on. Use your experience to help and guide them. I hope you see where I am going here. Give them the confidence to keep going.

Now imagine that those running alongside you are your teammates—those who know your process intimately. They hear your groans, stop with you when you need a break, and motivate you to keep going when the race just seems too long.

Throughout the race of infertility, let those further along than you are inspire you. Be an advocate to those who are a few paces behind you. Cheer them on. Encourage them as you would hope those ahead of you would do for you. Let them know that they are not as alone as they feel, even if you have to do so out of your own loneliness.

Finally, allow people into your pack to run alongside you, to push you along when you want to quit, and with whom you can share your most intimate feelings. Allow them in. Also enter when they allow you in. The most important person to let into this group is your spouse. Do not keep him or her on the outside—for your spouse's journey is your journey.

If you allow people in—even if they do not completely under-stand where you are in your race—you will find that maybe, just maybe, you are not as alone as you thought.

C. S. Lewis said, "Friendship, I have said, is born at that moment when one person says to another, 'What! You too? I thought that no one but myself...'" (Lewis 1971, 130).

Whom can you be that only one to?

Who can be that only one for you, my friend?

Personal Inventory

1. Who are those running the race ahead of you? What are you learning from them?
2. Who are the people behind you whom you are encouraging? How can you cheer them on?
3. Whom are you allowing to run beside you? How can you thank them? How can you reach out to them?

CHAPTER 9

———— ✦ ————

Fertile People Say Stupid Things

INFERTILITY ROBS YOU of your self-esteem. It sabotages your sex life. Steals joy. Promotes loneliness and isolation. That's all without the members of the peanut gallery opening their mouths.

Then they do. Sucking out more of your self-esteem. Killing more joy. Making you want to isolate even more.

"Are you ever going to have children?" If you only knew how hard we are trying. Don't you dare say anything about us being parents or about the joy of pregnancy! Don't share your story of childbirth or the nausea in your first trimester. Those things already suffocate my thoughts on a daily basis. I don't need to know what I am missing any more.

"Have you tried _____?" Yes, I have tried it all. I've stood on my head, lain with a pillow under me, rubbed a rabbit's foot, knocked on wood, picked a four-leaf clover, tried every position, and drunk every magic potion. Do not think for one minute you are suggesting something new to me.

"Do you remember the Smiths? They _____." Yes, I remember their story. I have tried to duplicate it. I am aware of the struggles of others—who have overcome and who are still stuck. Sharing another success or another failure with me is not going to change the shape of my uterus, fix the tail of his sperm, or make the embryo have more of a magnetic attachment. Thank you, though, for giving me more people to compare myself to.

"Would you consider _____?" Thank you for inserting yourself into the most sacred decision-making processes of our marriage. Please offer your suggestions and give us advice. In fact, we will set up a comment-card box outside our front door. Feel free to offer us any opinions. Before our decision, we would love to speak with you further about it in order to seek your approval.

"You just need to _____." Relax? Thanks. Be happy? I'll get on that. Turn around three times while pointing due east? Yes, I have even tried that. Trust me, I have done it all.

I realize that I laid the sarcasm on really thick. The peanut gallery is relentless, though, isn't it?

I will never forget the painful words spoken to me throughout our journey. They stick out in my mind like damaging reminders of where I have been and who has hurt me along the way. As much as I have tried, I seriously cannot forget some of the most painful things said or done, whether intentionally or unintentionally. Honestly, I know that I was an emotional basket case for a couple of years there in my late twenties; however, I am rational enough to know that people just say *crazy* things.

You know what I am talking about. As you read these words, I am confident that some of you are replaying the tapes in your head of the words that have damaged you to the core. Replaying the advice that you have received that is both maddening and that was thrown at you irresponsibly.

It was a snow-filled morning when my friend relayed her story to me. She laughed, as tears danced down her cheeks, while she recalled the painful encounter. She regretted the comfort level she had felt that had led her to tell an acquaintance about her recent struggle with miscarriage and the years of infertility that led them to that grief.

When my friend had finished speaking to her acquaintance, the other woman had looked at my friend, grabbed her hand as if to step into her place of brokenness, and said, "Well, God never gives us more than we can handle. Clearly that baby was more than you can handle, so God is going to try again." Miscarriage trivialized. Pain minimized. Heart shattered.

"Well, my God never makes mistakes," she said and excused herself from the exchange. Luckily her roars of laughter preceded mine, as I needed her permission to laugh, too. Sometimes people who haven't experienced your struggle just say silly things. You can add words other than *silly* into that sentence if you want. There are a lot of adjectives that are appropriate.

When I asked her what she felt at that moment, my friend recalled experiencing anger, bewilderment, hurt, loneliness, and the thought that she must be crazy. She stepped into the tangled ball of grief (chapter 3) all because of the pain a friend caused. She described wondering if this woman was correct, despite how asinine she felt the statement was. Her mental monologue ran like this: *Am I even cut out to be a mom? Am I not supposed to be a mom? Do I have what it takes? What if she's right?*

If only that woman had thought about the condition of her friend's heart, she would have seen a heart that was already wounded, exposed, and vulnerable. She would have seen that it needed a hug or a shoulder rather than more salt poured on it. If consideration had been given, she would have seen that her words were void of anything beneficial.

My friend took a risk in sharing her heart and fell flat. This was one more brick for her to put up around her heart to safeguard against such mistakes in the future. Enter more isolation and self-doubt.

Ignorant statements put a wedge in the middle of relationships. Painful statements put walls around our hearts. Uninformed opinions hurt to the core as they seem to minimize whatever the heart feels. Second-guessing endures and kindles the fire, which makes us doubt ourselves even more. It is damaging to the soul.

The truth is, it is difficult to truly empathize with an experience until we have walked the same road. We can try, but we cannot even scratch the surface of understanding. It's embarrassing for me to do a survey of past conversations I have had where I have told people in pain that I understood what it was they were experiencing.

I have done it wrong far too many times. As a woman, I have let people down. As a therapist, I do not always join people in their experiences adequately. On a human level, we try to understand, but sometimes we just cannot.

I know that. You know that. Nothing I said is a surprise.

It begs the question, though: Why on earth do we expect people to meet us perfectly in our experience? Are our lofty expectations of people setting them up for failure?

Why Do Our Spouses Say Silly Things?

What about when it is the person closest to us who hurts us?

Your husband is traveling the same road, experiencing the same circumstances, navigating around the same obstacles. Yet the lens through which he views those circumstances is different.

You are looking at infertility with pink glasses, shaped by hormones, maternal desires, feminine comparisons, and an empty womb.

He is looking at infertility with blue glasses, shaped by needing to provide for his woman, wanting to be a dad, wondering how he can do it all, asking himself if it is OK to experience emotions, and trying to solve all these problems on his own.

If I could count how many people told me (and still do), "As soon as you adopt, you will get pregnant," I think that the number would be somewhere near fifty. Even my doctor told me this. Don't tell me something you can't promise.

Not Pregnant

Something else that bugged me was when I saw someone whom I hadn't seen in years and she asked me, "How many kids do you have again?" I wanted to say, "Well, when I saw you I wasn't married and had no kids, so what made you think I had some now?"

—Laura

Roberto and Felicia felt stuck. They had been on this crazy train of infertility since before they were married. After meeting later in life, they decided that they wanted to try for children before their wedding date approached. When we met, they had just celebrated their third wedding anniversary. The snares of infertility had suffocated the joy of every month in between.

Once a couple who had prided themselves on communication, which they had fervently worked on in premarital counseling, they now tiptoed around each other so that they wouldn't detonate the land mines of misinterpretation surrounding them.

Since the time of their premarital counseling, they had been in counseling several more times. They had lost their ability to communicate, because the one was constantly offended by something the other had said.

If he said, "Honey, let's go on a vacation to get our minds off of infertility for a while," she heard, "I am tired of all of this. I want to quit. This is a waste of time."

If she said, "I really want you to come to this appointment with me," he heard that he was a disappointment to her in missing a few of the other appointments they had scheduled. He heard that he was letting her down.

It had become a constant tug-of-war of misunderstanding. Luckily their counselor was able to be a third-party mirror to help them reinterpret the reality of the situation. As it turns out, they were typically communicating the same things; however, they were hearing through their own experiences and their own set of emotions.

What one person may interpret as hope, the other may view as another irritating agitation. When one spouse is ready to move forward, the other may feel paralyzed by the notion.

While on different chapters of the story, one may inadvertently say the wrong things: Why is this such a big deal right now? Do we have to talk about this again? If you weren't so stressed, maybe this could work out. If this wasn't so important to you, we could use all this fertility money for something worthwhile.

While some of you may be cringing at these disrespectful and unreasonable statements, others are nodding along after hearing some similar sentiments from your spouse. Or perhaps you were the one to broadcast such words.

When my husband and his coworkers are in a meeting and bring up an off-the-wall idea that runs an equal risk of getting shot down or getting laughed at, they jokingly ask for the umbrella of grace. This suggests that they understand the stupidity of the proposal before the suggestion is uttered. They admit that they are probably wrong. But in order to find out for sure, they ask for the umbrella of grace, and then they tell their idea.

What if we offered the same umbrella of grace in our marriage? "I am going to ask you if you may be feeling something. I don't want to hurt you. But I want to be present with you, so I am going to ask for some forgiveness before I accidentally hurt you." Umbrella of grace?

What if we were free to extend grace and forgiveness to our spouses? What if during our greatest pain, we attempted to understand where they are coming from and give them the benefit of the doubt? What if we were free to excuse mistakes and missed attempts at empathy? What if every single time they said something hurtful, we pardoned them because we freely extended the umbrella of grace, even if they didn't ask for it?

Imagine what marriage could be then!

Personal Inventory

1. What are some painful things that have been said to you or your spouse?
2. How can you extend forgiveness to the sender of those painful messages?
3. How can you and your spouse extend the umbrella of grace to the peanut gallery? How can you extend the umbrella of grace to your spouse?

CHAPTER 10

I Would Become Resentful of Things I Used to Enjoy

As painful as Valentine's Day is to a single person, so are Mother's Day, Father's Day, baby showers, Tuesdays, holidays, and any celebratory event to an infertile couple. Please do not hear me minimizing the pain of singleness. It can be depressing, terribly lonely, and disheartening—as can infertility.

As the pages on a calendar turn, the pleasure of formerly enjoyed events seems to decrease. If you find yourself becoming a professional hider and avoider, you are in good company. I became a skilled expert at the bob and weave—eloquently bypassing all emotionally triggering events. But, my friend, let me warn you; isolation is also a symptom of depression. So while I appreciate the intent, please be cautious that this does not become symptomatic of something greater.

Several of the hats that I wear are not overly compatible with the avoidant lifestyle. The things that I felt I needed to do to comply with expectations I assumed people projected onto me and what I felt like I needed to do to maintain my own level of sanity were on opposite sides of my emotional capabilities.

I wanted to talk to people, but talking felt too risky sometimes.

I wanted to shop, but shopping meant I might have to experience something that I wanted to avoid.

I wanted to go on double dates, but I was torn between wanting to hear everything good going on in our friends' life and having to deal with what was not happening in ours.

I wanted to see our precious nephews open their Christmas presents; however, wondering if we would ever give them cousins was a pain I ferociously wanted to avoid.

I wanted to plan for the future, but that was debilitating. I wanted to know what the future held, but that was terrifying.

It was all too much. The only logical thing to do was to hide. Avoid. Run. Grow bitter. Become resentful. *Please read that in all its intended sarcastic glory.*

I hid. I did not want to see anyone or anything that would make me feel like less of a woman. Unfortunately, I lost relationships. I lost a lot. I am thankful for my therapist who helped me find my way and pulled me out of that lonely hole.

—Kate

If I were to poll each reader, we would find many more reasons for such avoidance. Triggers are everywhere.

During a walk to the park, you may encounter a pregnant woman trying to induce labor or a young mom trying to burn off the baby weight. It is too painful to even mention the feelings associated with walking by a play structure with all the adorable children you would like to kidnap (in a noncriminal way, of course) so that your nursery would no longer have a vacancy.

Walk into a giant box store. Wee little kiddos occupy the front seats of carts everywhere. Even the crying ones tug at your maternal heartstrings. The more you wander, the more likely you are to encounter the baby section. Do not even get me started. I cried while trying to speed walk by too many of them. Perhaps you dare walk into the section for the baby you pray for. Maybe you just tell yourself that you are going to peruse the selection for your niece or nephew. (Guilty, as charged, Your Honor.) Maybe you just take the long trek around to avoid it altogether.

Walking into your OB-GYN's office can even be a trigger. There are pregnancy magazines everywhere. Not to mention the beaming mamas-to-be, looking angelically pregnant with their growing bellies.

I remember fuming in Shannon's office one day because of the breast pumps that were being displayed. Of course they were there. Postpartum mamas walked into those doors more frequently than the wannabe mamas whose heartstrings were torn in half by them. Shannon's poor nurse was the target of the brunt of my pain. The pregnancy magazines, diagrams of birth, and postpartum-depression brochures glared at me. I remember wishing there was a separate waiting room for the not-yet mamas. That would have lessened the blow a little. However, I know it would have opened a whole other can of worms for those of us who would have occupied that room.

Baby showers are the worst. Despite your excitement for your darling friend or sister who is preparing to meet her baby, it does not negate the pain you are desperately trying to hide. You sit there, watching her open her gifts, hiding your tears, envying every inch of her stretch marks and perky, soon-to-be-saggy breasts, and wishing that you, too, could soon have midnight feedings and poopy diapers to change. You silently plan what you want your baby shower to be like; internally you know that you are going to inherit all of your friends' hand-me-downs, since yours will be the last baby to join your friend group's next generation. You are the first one to sneak out of the joyous event so that you can call your husband on the way home and vent your pain onto him.

Perhaps it's church—the place where you want to go, feel renewed, find peace, join community, and experience hope.

Others may be finding it there; however, you find loneliness, discontentment, and emptiness, and you feel you stick out like a sore thumb.

Mother's Day carries with it all sorts of joy for some and ugliness for others. Without even scratching the surface of the infertility world, the day is already hard for some. If your mother or significant maternal figure has gone too soon, the day is already excruciating. Maybe, just maybe, your mother is still alive, but she doesn't meet the definition of what you believe a mom should be. If given the opportunity, you will certainly do things quite differently. Better, actually.

You go to brunch or a family gathering celebrating maternal figures and secretly hope that your wish for the superpower of invisibility will come true. You equally celebrate all the women lucky enough to be mothers at the gathering, all the while wearing a tag that reads, "Hello, my name is Not Yet a Mom" or "Wannabe Mama" or "Broken Woman" or "I Want Out of Here."

As your infertile years add up, you may decide that participating in said events may just be too much for you. Be honest with yourself, and allow yourself to set boundaries for your own heart. Boundaries can be a life preserver for your emotional sanity. When implementing your boundaries, just make sure that you do so delicately. Outsiders may not understand the necessity of your boundaries.

I managed to make an appearance for two years of Mother's Day festivities. Fifty percent is not a passing grade, I realize, but it was the best I could do. At those two Mother's Day church services, I had to sneak out the door and decline a gift given to all the moms. Obviously the innocent man attempting to hand me the thoughtful gift to women did not know my story. He did not know all the courage it took to get out of bed that day. Little did he know what a trigger that little gift would be.

I managed to make it to two Mother's Day lunches and claimed illness for the following two. That seemed like a better option than collapsing into a puddle of my own emotions just after putting cheesy potatoes on my plate. No amount of compassion could have helped mop up my emotional mess.

Father's Day is similar in its festivities to Mother's Day, with simply a different focus. Just a month after the pain of surviving Mother's Day, you dredge it up all over again, but now the focus switches to what a great daddy your husband would be and how you failed him in every way. Just after you tell your heart to start beating again, you hold your breath to get through another day so that you can move on with the rest of your year.

Indubitably other occasions bring heartache. If you found yourself bobbing your head along as you read, you are in good company. The stories of painful situations overflow like the falling tears that find their way down your cheeks after each event.

Working at a school was difficult. Going to family gath-erings, especially reunions, was terribly painful. We stopped going to kids' birthday parties, and I stopped attending bridal showers.

—Amee

Let me quickly address the guilt or shame that you may feel about your newfound status as an avoider. The human body has an innate way to protect itself, and we systematically find ways to protect ourselves from the most primitive to the most sophisticated of situations.

There are, however, very healthy coping skills and unhealthy ones. Between those two camps is a very fine line. While I will not tell you what to do or how to judge what is healthy or unhealthy, my encouragement to you is to constantly take an honest inventory of what you are avoiding, why you are doing so, and what the ramifications are of attempting to survive something you wish you could hide from. Again what we are trying to avoid here is isolation and resentment, which can take up permanent residence, walling off your heart. Women typically crave community. Do not starve that need for yourself at the risk of emotion.

But if you do decide to encounter a difficult situation, then what?

Have you encountered this bizarre dichotomy? You want people to talk to you about your empty womb and all the accompanying emotions, and if they don't, it means they don't care. On the other hand, if they ask, it feels as though they are prying. Some days you may welcome the prying. If only they had a crystal ball, then they could get it right.

Maybe there are days when you want to bring up what you are experiencing and where you are in your cycle, but you also want to talk about something other than your babylessness. It feels impossible to get it right sometimes. It's a tender balance between not wanting to monopolize relationships with your depressing tales and processing all the emotions of this journey with those closest to you. This is what women do, however. You would contribute, too, if you were sure that you were still a woman.

Shopping and seeing maternity clothes or baby stuff seeing some commercials (babies, moms with babies, etc.) made me very sad. Also at times being alone would trigger [longing for] what I didn't have (kids).

—Michelle

I remember sitting with a dear friend, coffee cups in hands. (Coffee is our sweet spot.) She confided that she wasn't sure how to be a friend anymore. She said that her friends just didn't understand her anymore. They didn't understand her needs. They didn't understand who she had become.

Then she said, "But *I* don't even know who I am anymore. How can I expect others to know who I am?" Touché.

How can we expect people to anticipate what we need from the relationship, understand where we are in our emotional process, and know whether or not the elephant in the room wearing an *infertile* sandwich board needs to be discussed or not?

Communicate your needs and expectations in a humbly overt way so that those around you are not forced to read between the covert lines in an effort to predict how you are doing and what you need. This is especially important when it comes to your husband. The more you can be open about your emotional status, the more you can set up those closest to you for success. This provides you an extra layer of love and support, instead of setting them up for a guessing game that they are destined to fail.

Being a Student

It is my philosophy that in marriage, it is imperative that we are always a student of our spouses. Are we paying attention to things that are important to them? Of course we knew those things when we were dating, but once the seasons of marriage change, do we still know the little things that make our spouses tick? Most people in relationships, tested by time, know more about their spouses' schedule, the chores they have not completed, and the last time they were late to dinner rather than about their spouses' heart.

Being students of someone says that we are asking questions and learning. It means that we have a desire to know our spouses on a soul level. It means that there is two-way, overt communication so that spouses are simultaneously learning and being taught about the person they pledged their life to.

Imagine the ways that your spouse could enter into your story, carry you when you are broken, or hold the punching bag in place (as long as he or she is not the punching bag) when you are angriest.

I would imagine that those closest to you would also be honored to be your ally in your journey, but they may stay at a comfortable, quiet distance because they just don't know what you need.

Choose a couple of people outside of your marriage to whom you can teach about your heart. Gently instruct them in how to best care for you. Help them know what to say—especially what to avoid saying. If there is something you cannot attend for reasons you struggle to identify, help them to understand that you just know that it is going to be hard.

As an unknown author once said, "The best place in the world is in the arms of someone who will not only hold you at your best but will pick you up and hug you tight at your weakest moment."

Personal Inventory

1. How well are you walking the line between self-protection and self-isolation?
2. What do you need to do to move out of resentment into contentment?
3. Can you identify one safe person to help you out of your loneliness? Identify ways this person can help you.

CHAPTER 11

─── ⁓⦾⁓ ───

Pregnancy Doesn't Necessarily Mean a Baby

MIDDLE-SCHOOL YEARS ARE ruthless. If you made it through unscathed, all I can say is, "Well done."

Growth spurts happen at different times in middle school, and for some, those growing times cause real pain.

Friendships from elementary school change—as do body odor, attitudes, levels of entitlement, and stresses. There is a significant difference in maturation from student to student during the chasm between fifth and sixth grade.

Girls might have a tad of an identity crisis. What's it called again? Oh, yeah, puberty. Remember that? Terrible. I remember, as an awkward, little seventh grader, sitting at lunch with some girls I played basketball with. I looked around the circle and came to a terrible realization. Every girl around the circle had freshly shaved legs. Luckily I was wearing pants. Up until this point, I had not found the nerve to ask Mom if I could start shaving. That night I found my nerve because we had a game the next night, and there was no way I was going to wear shorts with Sasquatch legs.

Then people started to date. I slowly learned there were unwritten rules to the junior-high version of dating. Rule number one: "I will look in your direction a couple times during the day, and I promise to make eye contact with you in the cafeteria." Rule number two: "Soon I will sit shoulder to shoulder with you at recess." Rule number three: "Maybe if my mom isn't using the house phone [remember those?], then you can call. Not during dinner, though. We can talk on the phone but not during school." Ah, dating. One more rule: "You can't ask a person out directly. Your braver, more confident friend shall, of course, be the go-between until at least high school.

Once you started the junior-high version of dating, do you remember the song the kids would sing as you walked to class together? Sing it with me now: "First comes love. Then comes marriage. Then comes the baby in the baby carriage." But what if it doesn't?

Fast-forward to adulthood. You learned how to talk to boys. You got married, sealing the deal. You start trying to make future awkward junior highers of your own, and then you ask yourself, *What if there is no baby in the baby carriage?*

What if the stick reads *pregnant* once, but there is no baby to bring home?

Real life isn't all nursery-rhyme lyrics.

You make the appropriate preparations. You remove all residual effects from birth control out of your body in a timely fashion so that they will not prevent the making of a baby. You take your daily regimen of vitamins. You buy Costco packages of ovulation sticks, to tell you when to have sex. You even have sex on time. You do all the right things, in the right positions, just like everyone else, except it doesn't work.

In the off chance that the stick does turn pink, in the world of miscarriage at least, you know there is a possibility it just isn't going to end well. The devastating end to a pregnancy becomes the expectation. During our last two pregnancies, I didn't calculate my due date. Instead I calculated the date I needed to get past in order to give this little peanut a chance at breathing our smog-free Ohio air.

That first time the stick read *pregnant*, my husband got all lumberjacky, and I could not imagine the outcome being anything other than a baby. I was educated enough to know that some pregnancies terminate early, but like a naïve high schooler, I did not believe such badness would happen to me.

⸎

From Shannon

Twenty percent of all women in the United States who test positive for pregnancy will end up with a nonviable pregnancy. Although, according to the Mayo Clinic, the majority of miscarriages happen in the first seven weeks, a baby lost anytime up to twenty weeks is considered a miscarriage. After that time, the medical term labels losses as an *IUFD*, or intrauterine fetal death. We will not go into detail about the latter here.

Types of Miscarriage

Threatened: This term does not necessarily mean a patient will have a miscarriage. When a woman is experiencing symptoms such as vaginal bleeding and/or cramping that could result in miscarriage, she will usually be monitored through labs and/or ultrasounds.

Inevitable: This term is used when the symptoms of miscarriage progress so far that the miscarriage is certain.

Incomplete: The miscarriage process has started and is inevitable, but for some reason, the body is unable to naturally complete the process and the patient requires observation, medication, or surgery.

Complete: This is a miscarriage that has completed the process of resolving the pregnancy.

Missed: This term is used when a woman does not have symptoms of miscarriage, has testing done, and is found to have a nonviable intrauterine pregnancy (IUP).

Other Important Terms

Blighted Ovum: A pregnancy that is missing the actual baby or embryo. There are still signs of pregnancy and hormonal changes, but there will not be a completed pregnancy and delivery.

Ectopic: A pregnancy not in the proper location in the uterus. The baby can be found in the fallopian tubes—most commonly—or anywhere else in the pelvis. It is rare to have the ectopic pregnancy move out of the pelvic region and attach to the liver, but it has happened. The baby can also start growing in wrong areas of the uterus. These types of pregnancies can be dangerous, and women should always inform their doctor if there is pain or bleeding after a positive pregnancy test.

Diagnosis of a nonviable pregnancy is usually simple, through labs and ultrasound; however, sometimes multiple tests are required over a length of time. When a woman is waiting to find out if she is pregnant or not, this time can seem tortuous. We understand and will try to make the correct diagnosis as soon as it is medically evident. Patient treatment of a miscarriage can consist of observation, medications, or surgery. There are risks and benefits to all the options, and it is wise to discuss the options with the health-care provider. Investigating the reasons for miscarriage is not medically indicated until a woman has had three or more miscarriages in a row. Many physicians will offer a medical work-up after one or two miscarriages, depending on the circumstances.

As a side note, realize that the medical world uses the term *abortion* to describe the loss of an early pregnancy, whether it is elective or spontaneous. This can be a devastating term to an infertile woman or one going through a miscarriage. Understand that this is the language we must use on charting and coding; we are not trying to be uncaring or callous.

Pregnancies really do develop into real, earth-inhabiting human beings all the time—just not in my world. Sadly pregnancies do not end well for far too many women.

The second the stick reads *pregnant,* we dream. As much as we try and protect our emotions, we might still give our baby a nickname until we come up with an official name, write all the dates on our calendar, upload an app on our phone telling us what vegetable size junior is that week, imagine ballet recitals and soccer games, dream about how to tell our family and friends, and start browsing Pinterest for nursery themes. It's how a lot of women are geared.

Experiencing a miscarriage, to me, was like losing a part of myself. It was the part of me that felt like a woman, had hope, and had peace. I hate to admit that I am a different person now.

—Allyson

I resent the idea that we have to protect ourselves from feelings so absolutely beautiful and miraculous. However, defense mechanisms warn us against such hope. People thought I was crazy when I told them that hope felt paralyzing. I got tired of hoping. Hope became something that set me up for failure and pain. I wanted to know the truth. I wanted to know how the story was going to end. I wanted to protect myself from any more pain.

I remember visiting Shannon after each miscarriage. I was broken, sitting on crunchy paper on her exam table as she told me that one in four pregnancies ends in miscarriage. Despite my diagnosis of endometriosis, there was no reason (at that time) to believe we could not have a viable pregnancy.

Our second miscarriage happened after months of Clomid and ultrasounds to test for follicle maturation and after five weeks with this precious baby occupying my heart and womb. Shannon, with her empathetic style, just hugged me. "Sometimes there are just no explanations," she said. She spoke the truth. I, however, wanted answers.

At our third meeting for postpregnancy consultations, the hope was sucked out of the room. After the third miscarriage, the chance of a viable pregnancy vastly decreases. All three of us knew the magnitude of the meeting and the mountain we had to climb if our dreams had a chance to materialize. The small talk, sparkly salutations, and optimism had changed to pats on the back and it's-going-to-be-OKs.

It was not more than a few months before we were meeting again for the fourth time. That was it. Hope disappeared. Numb was the only thing I felt at that point. There were no tears at that appointment. By this time it felt as routine as getting an oil change. It was not a surprise when she told me that it was OK to stop trying. We could explore IVF, but our problem was not getting pregnant; it was carrying the pregnancy to full term.

I had two miscarriages before my daughter was born. The grief paralleled that of when I had to bury my grandparent. People minimized my pain, but it was so real. Why could I not carry a child? "Unexplained infertility" was my diagnosis. "Unexplained" did not help me one bit. I was so desperate for someone to explain the reason to me so that we could fix the problem, make a baby, and hold it one day. I just wanted to hold my baby. Is that too much to ask?

—Michelle

I felt like a failure as a mom. I could not keep my baby safe. I took prenatal vitamins religiously. I did progesterone suppositories faithfully. I did not consume carbohydrates, sugar, caffeine, or alcohol. I got plenty of sleep. I had one job that is uniquely mine as a woman, and I failed at it. That, at least, was the lie that I bought into.

By our fourth pregnancy, I was determined to love this baby and live well with it for as long as I was given. While I was desperate to hold him or her in my arms, I had come to grips with the fact that my womb might be the only thing that would ever hold my baby. If that was the case, I was going to maximize our time.

I went on walks and talked to the baby. People driving past me on the road probably thought I had a couple too many personalities.

As I drove, I explained to the baby what we were doing.

I told the baby what I was doing around the house, singing him or her songs while doing so.

I wished the baby good-night while rubbing my never-expanding belly.

If this was my shot at being his or her mom, then I was going to maximize every second of it.

You know how the story ends. Baby only got to hear about our adventures together for a few short weeks, but if it is true that babies can feel rejection in the mother's womb, then this baby felt nothing of the sort.

The only pictures we ever took of our four babies were of wee little circles with a strong heartbeat. Those babies were beautiful. I loved them with all the love I could extend to them. I dreamed big dreams for them. A lifetime of love was bestowed on them in those short weeks.

Sorting through Emotions

Gracie lost a baby at eleven weeks. She was a few short days away from the second-trimester breath of fresh air. Good-bye nausea. Good-bye paranoia. The viability date was in sight.

That's when the cramping started. Drops of blood did not concern her at first until they become gushes. A trip to the local emergency room determined that even though they had heard junior's heartbeat just five days earlier, it had since stopped. So did their world.

The grief and pain was intense. They had a terrible time reconciling to what had happened. Gracie felt like she had failed the baby, herself, and her husband. She questioned what kind of a woman could not protect the baby in her care.

Months later they found themselves pregnant again. Little Olivia was born eight months later. With a head full of hair and a nearly perfect Apgar score, Olivia was their dream come true and the healing to the pain they had experienced just a year earlier.

Everything seemed perfect until Gracie had to go back to work, and the pain of leaving Olivia with the babysitter was too great to bear. She became paralyzed by the what-if game. What if something happens to Olivia? What if the babysitter can't keep her safe? What if they get in an accident? What if she chokes? What if a criminal climbs into their third-story apartment window, slips through the bars on the windows, sneaks into Olivia's room, past their English bulldog, and kidnaps her, walking past the bellman downstairs?

It may sound irrational to some but not to a woman who has not been able to keep a baby safe in her very womb.

Women compare the pain of miscarriage to that of a death of someone they have known for more than just weeks. Only there is no funeral. No gravestone to visit. No closure. No public remembrance.

I had no idea what I needed after our first miscarriage. I recall telling my boss that I would take a day or two off. Little did I know what still needed to happen between that fateful ultrasound and the start of healing.

People offered meals, visits, a private memorial for our pregnancy, hugs, and encouragement. I thought I had it all under control, or at least that was what I tried to show on the outside. All the while I was breaking on the inside. I wish I would have let people love me. I wish I could go back and allow me to be present with those who tried to enter into my world. While trying to be too brave, I fear I pushed people away. While trying to be too brave, I know that I didn't speak my needs. Call it suppression. Call it stubbornness. I did myself a disservice. Do not do what I did.

Let me encourage you to experience the emotions rather than suppress them deeply. While suppressing these emotions may make it feel like they go away faster, suppressing them will almost guarantee that they will resurface. This may happen at the most unpractical and difficult moments, typically after others have already dealt with their pain from the miscarriage. Loneliness is frequently a companion to delayed grief.

I wrote in my journal often. Every pregnancy, I "buried" my babies there, with my words, my pain, my heart. I was able to openly grieve there. I would write letters to my babies on their due date. There I could acknowledge that they did exist; everyone else had forgotten, but I haven't. They were never allowed to be fully here with us. But they were mine, and I had plans for them. I sometimes get sad that no one remembers.

—Isabelle

Face the pain. Find a way to deal with the emotions in a healthy, safe, and effective way. Do not push your people too far away.

Find your healing.

Find your joy.

Find *you* again.

Personal Inventory

1. What emotions from Wright's *Tangled Ball of Emotions* (chapter 3) are you currently experiencing in relation to your miscarriage(s)?
2. Discuss with your spouse how both of you have changed since your loss, what you need from the other person, and how to meet those needs.
3. Whom can you allow into your story?

CHAPTER 12

Secondary Infertility Is a Joy Stealer

ROSE WAS FOUR years old when Tony and Robin decided that they wanted to have a second child. Their dearest Rose was a perfect mix of mischief, spunk, and love. Robin described her as the perfect child, confident that Rose would make the most excellent big sister.

Tony and Robin, excited by their decision to try again, presented Rose with a big-sister T-shirt in an attempt to preemptively engage her in the excitement of being an older sibling.

"The amount of attention she would get in about a year would be slighted, so we wanted her to feel like she was a part of it," Tony emphasized.

Rose was a product of just two months of trying, so why not tell her? By *trying*, I mean casual, romantic sex that anyone who is actually *trying* does not have. Their fertile cycles were their first two months off of birth-control pills—unmonitored by their physician—and did not include the meticulous counting of days. It seemed about as easy as going to a vending machine, putting in a dollar, and pushing the healthy-baby button. Nine months later their baby just popped out. Lucky them.

Not only did Tony and Robin tell Rose that they were going to try again, but they believed so unequivocally that another baby would be right around the corner that they also told their families and closest friends. History had proved that their sperm and egg had a magnetic attraction, so why not just tell the masses?

After a few months of trying, his family started to ask questions. A few months later, Rose tearfully asked when it was going to be her turn to become a big sister. By month eight Robin's sister announced she was pregnant and expressed hope that the two of them could be pregnant together. At month twelve Rose outgrew her shirt. During their doctor's appointment at month thirteen, Tony and Robin learned the term *secondary infertility.*

They were bewildered. Perplexed. Mystified. Tony wondered, "How can we be infertile? We have Rose. She is healthy. Conception was easy. What on earth is happening to us?"

Secondary infertility creeps into the vocabulary and the story lines of far-too-many unsuspecting couples. With one child (at least) already occupying their hearts and homes, many couples press forward toward fulfilling their ideal family picture only to find themselves stuck in the club of infertile couples. Hearts break. Dreams are temporarily put on hold. Pain takes over.

$$\infty$$

From Shannon

According to the National Infertility Association, secondary infertility is defined as the inability to become pregnant or carry a pregnancy to viability following the birth of one or more children not associated with infertility treatments. Thirty percent of all infertility rates are attributed to secondary infertility (Goldstein 2011).

Reasons for secondary infertility can include all the same reasons as primary infertility. The most common condition relates to advancing maternal age. As a woman gets older, her ovarian reserve is lowered, and she can experience an increase in miscarriages as well. Some previously fertile women will have changed partners, and together they as a couple might not be as fertile. Changes in medical health, new diseases or surgeries, and medications after a successful pregnancy can be all that is required to create infertility.

Methods of diagnosis and treatment are the same as those for primary infertility. You may want to start treatment sooner if you are older and have goals of family completion by a certain time.

⁕

In professionally assisting couples struggling with secondary infertility, I have observed guilt and shame. There is guilt in not being able to provide their child with a sibling. There is shame that they took the first experience for granted.

Matthew and Addy recalled their two successful births. Their family was complete. They lived as a complete family of four for seven years. After marrying and having both their children at a young age, they thought they knew what they wanted. Years later all their friends started having children, and now in their late twenties, they decided that maybe they wanted a third child. After all, it had been easy the first two times.

After much consideration, they embarked on trying for baby number three. Months later they were pregnant again. They beamed as they relayed the good news to their family and friends. Social media even took part in the occasion. Weeks later they had to relay the news that this baby had not made it.

This was a type of grief they had never experienced. Addy found it difficult to get out of bed. Her workout regimen failed. Their marriage suffered. Their two sons felt neglected because mom had no emotional energy in her reserve. She felt that when she miscarried, her ability to love again was lost.

Months later they found themselves on the path to healing. Their sex life began to flourish again, thankfully, as did their renewed passion to create another baby. Before long, Addy was expecting again.

Sadly, twelve weeks later—just prior to the second-trimester sigh of relief—she began to bleed. Her ultrasound revealed that their precious child no longer had a beating heart.

Addy threatened to never try again. Matthew was resentful. Their sons were confused. Their marriage was rocky. Their friends, from whom they had isolated themselves, were now birthing their healthy children. The couple stood confused and alone.

A cruel irony set in. While they already had two growing sons whom they loved wholeheartedly, Matthew and Addy, too, were now facing infertility. Once they had assumed that since they had two sons, a diagnosis of infertility would never plague them. Now like other previously optimistic couples, they were wrong.

Prior birthing success does not clear you of the potential for future problems. Even though Hollywood does not portray it, no couple is immune. All are at risk.

Is this the first time you are hearing about secondary infertility?

If so, that is not a surprise. Secondary infertility is discussed far less in society. While we discuss infertility infrequently, the attention given to secondary infertility is close to nil—unless, of course, you find yourself facing it.

When You Are Still a Parent

To compound the pain of secondary infertility, while you may be struggling on the inside, there is parenting to be done.

Somehow you must become a superwoman in order to magically manage all of your maternal duties as well as wade through the murky waters of infertility.

My grief made me selfish. I was all or nothing. When I couldn't have the child I couldn't make, I felt like I had nothing to give to my existing child. I struggled to do both simultaneously.

—Renee

Those treading such waters must implement an extra measure of care.

Do not take your support system for granted. Reach out if you need to. Let them help you, even if your defense systems want to push everyone away.

Show your child(ren) that while Mom and Dad are sad, they are pushing through. Modeling healthy coping skills will teach your child valuable lessons for the future. Gifts that you can impart to your child are a healthy marriage, individually healthy parents, and healthy coping skills.

Husbands and wives, push into each other. Do not push each other away. Co-parent together. Do marriage together. Overcommunicate your wants, needs, and emotions. Journey this season together. Listen to one another. Be an advocate for the other's needs.

Personal Inventory

1. If you have experienced secondary infertility, how has it changed you?
2. How has secondary infertility affected your family?
3. How can you work to make your family stronger despite the current infertility you now face?

CHAPTER 13

I'm Not a Failure If It Doesn't Work Out

IT HAD BEEN nine years since her last miscarriage. That did not stop the tears. One might assume that the experiences and joys that managed to sneak in those years would have mopped up the tears. No. The tears continued as she yelled about how unfair it all was.

"It is the simplest thing. Fall in love. Have sex. Make a baby. Have a baby."

Enter more tears.

"I failed. I just failed. I couldn't do what my body has the right to do. I couldn't do what animals can do. I am a failure."

She, like so many women, confronted strong feelings of failure.

An outsider looking in would not see a failure. She was an entrepreneur who had bought her first house when she was right out of college. She pursued the American dream before finding the love she had always been waiting for. Together they traveled to exotic, foreign places that I struggle to pronounce. She had designer everything. Her husband shared her passion for interior design—their house looked like the things that celebrities brag about in design magazines. They were weekend warriors—working hard during the week and bicycling the sum of my week's daily mileage to work on the weekends.

You would not look at her and think failure. For all intents and purposes, she looked complete. She appeared to have conquered it all.

Yet despite the career accolades, fancy accessories, and 401K, there was an emptiness inside, occupying her heart and her womb.

After one miscarriage, despite several attempts at IVF, they were never able to conceive again.

She recalled her daily routine of getting up every morning, walking to her vanity next to her walk-in closet (color me jealous), and—despite the money it took to adorn her appearance—seeing a failed woman. Failed because she could not do what is most primitive for her gender. She could do anything else that the world would deem successful, but she could not do the one thing that she would truly define as successful.

Paradigm Shift

What if we cannot change our circumstances? What if you are barren? What if you are that woman who feels broken? What if the biological chemistry between you and Mr. Perfect is toxic?

Then what? What are you going to do with your time as that broken, barren woman who could not utilize her feminine right to bear children?

There is a profound choice to make. It takes a moment-by-moment, daily decision to stand in front of the mirror and chose to see a *survivor* rather than a *failure*. To define yourself as *enough* rather than *failed*. To cling to the truth that your story isn't over yet, rather than to be stuck at the chapter that deems you not woman enough.

Is it possible that you are more than a sum of your brokenness and that the ability to move on is just over the next horizon, should you find motivation to continue walking?

If we cannot will our body to work appropriately, then we must will our mind, heart, and spirit to adapt in such a way that we are not penalized (even by ourselves) for our shortcomings.

J. R. R. Tolkien said, "All we have to decide is what to do with the time that is given to us" (Tolkien 2012, 112).

Time. It's a funny concept. At some point it is all going to end for each of us. Sometimes I ponder (don't call me morbid) what is going to matter when I am the one occupying the bed at the hospice center.

Am I going to recall that time I got so mad at the car that cut me off when I was running late? Am I going to care about the time I was inconvenienced? Will I ruminate on the things I did not get that I deserved? Am I going to wish that I had bought the other wrinkle cream or bought the dress that woman was wearing or that I should have tried bangs? I wonder if I am going to care that my body was too broken or that it took me months to conceive a child.

The truth is, I highly doubt I will think of any of those things. I don't want to lie there feeling indebted to my broken body. I do not want to still wallow in my failures. I do not want to waste time thinking about what I am owed.

I want to relish the fact that I was an overcomer. I want those who gather around me to speak of my strength in the midst of adversity and say that when I was knocked down, I got back up. I do not want to live my life like I failed. I want to know that despite hardships, I won.

So maybe looking like you have it all together isn't what is important. Maybe focusing on the failure isn't what is important. Maybe what is important is finding the joy in whatever is trying to steal the joy.

—Annie

It Is...You Are Not

Let me tell you something I feel strongly about: I don't want people to own or label themselves with what they struggle with. I completely understand why people take ownership; however, I want to protect people from the dangers of that mistake.

Look at the contrast between the following statements:

"I am depressed" in comparison to "I have depression."

"My son is autistic" versus "My son has autism."

"I am a failure" rather than "My uterus failed."

"I am an alcoholic" compared to "I have an addiction to alcohol."

The first is an adjective that is used to describe. A person is more than depressed. A person is more than a diagnosis. Individuals are more things than the adjectives we label them with. You are more than the struggles that define you. You are more than what you have overcome.

The alternative is claiming something that you struggle with—whether that be depression, autism, a body part that let you down, or a vice that you struggle with. It does not describe you, your character, or your worth. If you picture it as something that you are wrestling with rather than your personal identity, you strip it of its power over you. It may not hurt any less or change your circumstances; however, it lessens its impact on you personally.

The question becomes, how much influence do you want to give to what you are combating? Do you want to surrender your identity to it and let it describe you? Or do you want to call it what it is—the mountain you are climbing?

The choice is yours.

Not even knowing you, I want you to hear something. You are *not* a failure. You are not your circumstances. You are not less of a woman. You are not your struggle, even if its waves crash around you.

You have to give someone permission to make you feel less than. You have to allow someone to challenge who you are. That means the naysayers—those who feel entitled to an opinion about you or those you silently compare yourself to—do not get a vote. Do not give them the power of your self-perception. Be confident in who you are.

By all means, do not give yourself the permission to make you feel less than you are.

Personal Inventory

1. Have you bought into the lie that you are a failure if you are infertile?
2. How do you need to work toward redefining your circumstances?
3. What are you going to do with the time you have been given?

CHAPTER 14

—— ⌒⌒⌒ ——

Comparing Is a Waste of Time

I AM A crier.

I can admit it.

I cry when I am happy. I cry when others are happy. I cry during the last moments of *Full House* when Daddy Tanner is trying to make a sentimental, daddy-of-the-year point. I cry when people get reunited and when Ellen DeGeneres gifts someone an unexpected gift that only they deserve. Do not even get me started about military reunions or adoptions. Bring on the water works!

I love *love*, and I cry when it is displayed beautifully. This is why the movie *Love Actually* had me hook, line, and sinker. I watched the airport scenes repeatedly because I love watching people reunite. I love watching people express their love in the most beautiful of ways.

As I write, I am propped up in a corner of a local airport that serves as a huge midwestern hub. If you are a people watcher, let me recommend this little corner for you. I could sit here for days if my family was not going to be on the other side of this flight, waiting for me.

To the right, leaning against the wall, is an unassuming businessman working through what sounds like a deal. Perhaps coming from an interview, he connected with a loved one over the phone and claimed, "I know they want me. I don't know how it all fits, though."

Just down about another ten feet, there is a mom with a resting baby in the Bjorn and a toddler running around—wanting so badly to explore and exert his growing independence. If this were a playground and not a tile intersection for the masses, he would be in his happy place.

There is a line of busy travelers filing into the McDonald's line for a quick energy boost. The employees are handing out burgers, coffee, and fries at a rapid-fire pace.

Next to me is a beautiful woman with salt-and-pepper hair, who is talking with the female employee who has been assigned to push her wheelchair and make sure she makes it to her airplane on time. If only the wheelchair assistant would pay attention to her stories. The stories this woman is telling overflow with wisdom and years of life experience.

Down the walkway, groups of airplane personnel wait with their steamed suits and carefully packed suitcases—they are impeccably groomed for the hours of hospitality ahead of them.

Men are congregating at the sports bar over by the bathroom, discussing what they think of the bubble teams of March Madness, how they are going to fill out their bracket, and how much they are going to put down in Vegas for their Cinderella story.

I wish all the people would stop and tell me their stories. Where are they going today? Why? Who is going to meet them on the other side? Are they as put together as they seem?

Here is the thing about people watching or observation in general. One of two things often happens. Either you unnecessarily elevate another (subsequently making yourself feel less), or you unnecessarily elevate yourself (subsequently making yourself feel superior). In both scenarios, someone comes out ahead while another takes a hit.

I assume that all these people whom I have been observing have something I don't.

No one is cutting a business deal with me. No one flew me across the country to try and sign a contractual agreement with me. That gentleman must have professional savviness that I do not. Come to think of it, he probably has a bank account that I could only dream of, because I think his briefcase is made out of real alligator skin.

The woman with the children clearly shops at boutiques I could never afford and wears color schemes I could never pull off. Her wardrobe must put mine to shame, even though I haven't seen any other clothing article than what I am currently viewing. Plus she has recently had a baby, and her thighs don't even touch. So she has the woman thing down. Last, babies mean functional uterus. I will fail in that arena every single time.

The people eating at McDonald's have a higher metabolism than I do because I am fairly confident that if I put in my mouth what they are carrying away in those bags, I would have to buy bigger pants before my plane leaves. Just watching them walk by causes my waistband to expand a little.

The airline personnel have more hospitality skills than I ever will, have been to more destinations than I could dream of, and know how to pack a suitcase like an expert.

It is probably safe to assume that those betting on basketball have more money than I do. They also appear to have more free time than I do. They also appear to be extroverts. This little introvert is going to stay over here in my corner.

Sounds self-deprecating, doesn't it? This time I was self-deprecating on purpose, my dear friend. But we all do it. Am I right?

Any of these people may be internally crying tears of loneliness, may be traveling to empty homes, or may be scared to land because of whatever waits for them on the other side. I know nothing more than what meets the eye. I have not heard their stories and never will, and yet I can easily make myself feel worse about myself by the stories I tell myself.

We compare like it is our job, but the habit is something that leaves us emotionally bankrupt.

Webster's Dictionary definition of the word *comparison* is "the pointless act of making oneself feel worse by ignorantly viewing another in a grandiose light, often leading to depression, sadness, and shame."

OK, that is actually the Cathie Quillet definition of comparison. *Webster's* would have been much more sophisticated in its eloquence—comparison noted.

The point is, comparison leaves us nowhere good—especially as women. We instinctively assume that someone is better than we are by projecting our own story line onto another person, which is most likely categorically untrue. The result most often leads to our own self-worth ending up in the toilet, which forces us to try and put ourselves back together from the effects of something that has no basis in reality.

Warning: comparison and infertility are a detrimental, devastating combination.

Sally came into my office one day. The patient inventory she completed stated that she was experiencing increased feelings of anger. She was prepared to completely leave her social group of friends, all of whom she had been close with since high school.

Even though Sally felt furious, there had been no outward conflict between Sally and her friends, who had become more like sisters over the years. These other women knew nothing about the rage building in Sally's heart toward them. They had observed that Sally seemed a bit distant, but they assumed that she was probably really busy at work, which she had been many times before. If they had heard about Sally's anger toward them, they would have thought it misguided.

Sally, while feeling righteous in her anger, had misplaced feelings of sadness that had resulted from comparing her life with theirs. Comparison had dug this deep grave for her.

While she knew that one of her friends had experienced some tough stuff in her marriage, she deduced that they had more resilience in their marriage than she had in hers because they exuded joy now. They had the home that people flocked to, which—in Sally's interpretation—meant that people did not want to be at her house because she was less skilled as a hostess.

Another friend had a minivan full of well-behaved children. Sally didn't have children yet. She felt like she had surrendered her woman card somewhere because she hadn't had children yet (and because she did not even want a minivan, which—to her social circle—meant reaching maternal-superwoman status).

Another friend, another comparison, another inferred failure. Sally had spent so much time putting herself down through unnecessary comparison with others that she had abdicated much of her self-esteem.

Together we worked through Sally's misguided interpretations and definitions of femininity. Together we redefined the measuring stick she used to identify success. After dealing with some of the feelings she had inappropriately put in the mouths of her friends, she worked on identifying her own feelings and the way she felt about each particular friend who had reached a superior level of womanhood. Last, she spoke to friends on an individual basis and found that they had felt inferior to Sally in some areas and that they also had fallen victim to the comparison game.

Listen up, friend, you do not know the whole story. Do not pass judgment against yourself until you know the whole story. Even if you *do* know the story—I am telling you, woman to woman—do not pass judgment against yourself. There are too many other sources and people out there who are criticizing, judging, and itemizing. We cannot afford to do it to ourselves and to each other. No one can do *you* like *you* can. For the sake of your mental health, stop comparing, my friend.

The only person to whom you have to compare yourself is the person you see in the mirror. Do not let comparison rob you of your joy, your contentment, your relationships, or your marriage.

Something that many women have to do when they struggle in this area is to stay away from social media. Let's take a step back from social media for a second and truly examine how realistic its representation of a person's life is. While there are exceptions to the rule, not many people are vulnerable and transparent with the behind-the-scenes parts of their life. They post the best of themselves. They tweet the most eloquent remarks (typically) and Instagram the most joyful/beautiful/loving/sentimental/celebratory moments in their camera roll. Here's the question: are you comparing your life to their real life, or are you comparing your life to the only part of their life they are willing to share? The latter is not their reality, my friend.

Also for the sake of your mental health, please be careful not to define your present reality in the light of how you wish your life would be. That equation can lead you straight into the snares of depression and anxiety.

I had to let go of the comparisons that were strangling me. Otherwise I fear I would have completely lost myself.

—Anne

During our infertile years, I would get on social media, and I would just cry. Pregnancy announcements, newborn photo shoots, happy families vacationing together…I could not handle the pain. I wanted those story lines. I wanted to be out living life instead of coveting another. But there I sat—lost in the comparison game.

I had to say no to social media. You may need to also. If you are wondering if this is a trigger to your emotional pain, take a few days off and see what happens to your sanity. After all, if you do not protect your emotions, no one else is going to.

Comparisons and projected expectations are dangerous. Buyer beware. Guard your feminine heart. Do not buy into the cultural lie that you must achieve a certain milestone or gain something the world deems important in order to matter.

You are the only you. You are the only standard by which to compare yourself. Do not waste your life comparing things that are incomparable.

Personal Inventory

1. How is comparison compromising your sanity?
2. How can you take back your sanity by dismissing comparison from your self-talk?

CHAPTER 15

◦⌒◦⌒⌒◦

There Are Hormonal Changes with Fertility Medications

"I DON'T EVEN know who I am anymore. I feel like I am going crazy," she lamented. "I know I want a baby, but what kind of mom am I going to be if I don't even know who I am right now?"

Her husband had learned the art of silence as she broadcast her current emotional whereabouts. He was never quite sure of who she was going to be any time she walked in the door. He hoped for the woman he had once met, but he was always uncertain of how the artificial hormones were impacting her at the moment. During the dreaded days, he saw a woman he did not recognize.

Aware of the sacrifices her body was making, he longed to have his wife back.

One thing was certain: her emotional state was often fluctuating. She was happy. She was sad. She was apathetic. She was the whole tangled ball of emotions (see chapter 3) all wrapped into one moment. Most of all, she was confused.

Confusion had convoluted the purpose behind the madness. She had lost herself so much by this point that she was willing to throw it all away just to find herself. She was able to see clearly enough to know that she wanted their spare bedroom to be the nursery instead of her husband's music room. And that physical symbol helped her will herself into letting the process continue.

I was an emotional roller coaster, an emotional disaster, and a person my husband didn't know anymore. I felt bipolar; one minute I'd be good, and then the next I'd be a basket case. It was horrible, more so than when you are on your period with the hormonal changes.

—Sasha

Medicinal interventions in hopes of enhancing fertility promote a whole new level of intimacy in a relationship.

"I never thought that I would be giving my wife shots in the butt for a baby," he groaned. She laughed. Unfortunate circumstances had led to that moment. She pulled her pants down to uncover only the necessary section of her rear side. This moment of baby making did not yield a sexual experience but a medical one. It was after dinner, which meant shot time. A quick needle prick, and it was time for the dishes. Just like that.

Cycle Starters

If I could wish upon a star, I would wish that women's bodies could or would function how they were intended to. Then we wouldn't need any of the drugs in this chapter. Well, then we wouldn't have this whole book.

Since most of us in this club have dysfunctional girly regions, Clomid, Femara, and progesterone suppositories and shots are all necessary for certain conditions. These sassy little follicle-producing drugs get our girls flowing and ready to meet the sperm of their dreams. Ideally our little miniegg will successfully mature and make its way down to our healthy (fingers crossed) fallopian tube to happily ever after. Ideally. That is the drug's purpose, at least.

Six cycles was the magic number for Sydney and Tyson. That is how long their insurance would approve her to take Clomid. Six cycles, and her body had to learn how to function like a grown-up.

In six cycles, his little manly men had to take their maiden voyage to find their match. Six cycles. No pressure, right?

Cycle one failed. *That's OK—five more!* she thought. *Crap. We have to get this all worked out in five months, and we have already been trying for three years.*

No pressure.

Cycle two started. It entailed one pill, days of trying, an ultrasound to confirm that the follicle was ready for the exchange, and progesterone suppositories from sex to period or pregnancy test. All systems were go. Spirits were high until her pregnancy-test date was marked off the calendar. Sydney had started her period yet again. Hope diminished.

Blast, only four more cycles.

Up and down, up and down. Her hope went up, but her HCG didn't. Down went their hope.

By cycle number five, they were hopeless. Defeated. The pregnancy test that she had bought for their Clomid endeavors never even made it out of the closet this time. Wearily they trudged forward, reluctant to care.

Number five released a perfect follicle, which matched a perfect sperm, which produced a perfect baby boy, whom they should have named Clomid. Without the help that the medicinal intervention had given them, they would never have had the baby of their dreams.

While not all stories end on such a positive note, it is nice to celebrate the ones that do!

IVF Cocktail

Embarking on IVF treatment oftentimes brings a prospect of hope that a couple may have lost while taking a stab at natural conception. Hope is sometimes scary, however, because hope means that there is the potential to be disappointed. Disappointment means more grief and more loneliness.

It's easy to be emotional and confused even before artificial hormones enter your body.

Then you enter the roller-coaster ride of waiting for doctors' appointments and follow-up phone calls from the nurse. Upon intervention, you have to wait for your levels to do what they are supposed to—grieving if they react inappropriately and celebrating if they respond well.

This is all happening while you try to maneuver through mood swings and anxiety about the unknown.

∾⌇∾⌇∾

Symptoms of Generalized Anxiety Disorder, According to DSM-5

A. Excessive anxiety and worry (apprehensive expectation), occurring more days than not for at least six months, about a number of events or activities.

B. The individual finds it difficult to control worry.

C. The anxiety and worry are associated with three (or more) of the following six symptoms (with at least some symptoms present for more days than not for the past six months):

1) Restlessness or feeling keyed up or on edge
2) Being easily fatigued
3) Difficulty concentrating or mind going blank
4) Irritability
5) Muscle tension
6) Sleep disturbance (difficulty falling or staying asleep or restless, unsatisfying sleep)

D. The anxiety, worry, or physical symptoms cause clinically significant distress or impairment in social, occupational, or other important areas of functioning.

E. The disturbance is not attributable to the physiological effects of a substance (e.g., a drug of abuse, a medication) or another medical condition (e.g., hyperthyroidism).

F. The disturbance is not better explained by another mental disorder (American Psychiatric Association 2013, 122–23).

These are included not for purposes of self-diagnosis; rather, if you are experiencing several of the above symptoms, please make an appointment with a therapist or physician.

⁓

For Mason and Marcy, IVF was their only shot at having a biological family. For reasons dictated by family history and heredity, they skipped all the natural attempts at trying to conceive and went straight to their neighborhood reproductive endocrinologist. While Mason wished he could have skipped the room with the cup and that his wife could have avoided all the pokes and prods, they knew that this was their only chance.

Like two gleeful teenagers, they proceeded with all that was required. She did the blood work, the hormones, the ovulation stimulation, and the resting. They witnessed conception in the petri dish. They cried as they watched the life of their little son or daughter begin. Implantation, progesterone, rest, hope and more rest. Days later her HCG level showed signs of success. They were going to be parents. While not every story has a happy ending, those that do ought to be celebrated!

Artificial Menopause

Hello! What's with these symptoms? Hot flashes, night sweats, weight gain, facial hair (what!), mood swings, depressive episodes, insomnia, panic episodes, bouts of anxiety, and anger. To quote the ever inspiring and motivating *Dumb & Dumber*, "Mmmm, that sounds good. I'll have that."

Lupron was not kind to me. (Please note that not everyone's experience will be as dreadful as mine. Remember, my biological makeup does not mix well with hormones).

I knew to expect hot flashes, night sweats, mood swings, and irritability. It is quite different to *experience* them; I'll tell you that. Within a matter of days, the estrogen (which our bodies *naturally* produce) is unnaturally sucked out of your body as if a dam broke and a tidal surge sucked it away.

The dam broke for sure, and I had nothing left.

Nothing.

Picture a frail elderly person in a rocking chair in a corner of a nursing home. She is but a shell of herself, rocking rhythmically back and forth, staring out the window, and making imaginary friends with the birds. No old lady in this scenario—the one in the rocking chair is me.

I sat.

I stared.

I watched the birds.

Somewhere inside, I knew that I was still myself; however, I didn't have the energy to find me.

I was but a shell of who I had been a mere two weeks prior. I knew that this wasn't really me. Thankfully it was a temporary change.

The sweet pharmacist lady, Theresa, called one day to confirm I wanted to refill my prescription. Sure, unassuming saleswoman of poison, please send me more of the mood-altering, life-paralyzing, toxic mess of a drug. I am, indeed, a masochist and find complete pleasure in damaging my body. Please send that right over.

Boy, was menopause draining. I felt like I needed to write a formal apology to my mother for giving her so much grief during her (what felt like) decade-long battle with menopause. Sometimes I saw my mother in the mirror as I struggled through the same symptoms I gave her a hard time for. *Oops! Lesson learned!*

As quickly as the side effects appeared, they departed. My body was none the wiser. I was supposed to be on Lupron for six months. Shannon and I agreed after three months that the benefit did not outweigh the side effects.

Lupron was a godsend to me. I had been experiencing a lot of symptoms that needed medicinal intervention. It saved me from those symptoms.

—Michelle

If you are going to take this, or any other drug for that matter, please find a physician whom you trust, who is an advocate for your body, who is aware of your family history, and who is willing to talk with you as you need. Having that person in Shannon made me so much more comfortable throughout the journey. I was confident that she was alert to symptomatology and side effects and able to judge whether or not the balance of the two was appropriate or too damaging.

Truth

For every story that tells of the negative side effects and craziness, there are women everywhere who daily survive assisted reproduction without so much as a hot flash, extended waistline, or emotional imbalance. I am eternally jealous of those who make it through any medicine unscathed by a side effect. They have to write all those terrible warnings on the labels because of people like me. For your hypervigilance because of people like me, I apologize.

The experiences reported in this chapter are here to help normalize your journey if you are feeling a little bit crazy. They are not intended to scare you away from the miracle of childbirth that is often the finish line of such treatment. Those cherished babes will make every shot in the tush, mood swing, and extra pound worth it.

Surviving Hormones

We have discussed this previously; however, let me remind you of the necessity of self-care. When we do not feel like ourselves, it is easy to speak as though we are inebriated—having verbal diarrhea. Sorry for the visual, but in the context of communication under the influence of hormones, it makes perfect sense.

Keep in mind that your spouse, coworkers, family, barista, and the driver who just stole your parking spot are not under the same kind of curse that you are. They are completely unassuming and going about their regularly scheduled programming. Sure, that may frustrate you a bit, but thank your lucky stars that not everyone is hormonal like you.

Turning Toward the Spouse

As a result of their years of research, Drs. John and Julie Gottman founded the idea of turning toward the spouse.

Dr. John Gottman says, "In marriage people periodically make what I call 'bids' for their partner's attention, affection, humor, or support. People either turn toward one another after these bids or they turn away. Turning toward is the basis of emotional connection, romance, passion, and a good sex life" (Gottman 1999, 80).

We make daily bids for our spouses' attention as we seek to be noticed, pull our spouses into conversations with us, or make repair attempts.

"Honey, when you're done with the newspaper, can you please help me take care of the leaves outside?"

That is a bid for attention that gives the spouse a chance to turn toward the bidder or away.

Turning away: A long silence. A shrug of the shoulder. "Whatever."

Turning toward: "I will be done in about five minutes. I will meet you outside."

When the spouse on the receiving end *turns toward* the bidding spouse, the very act welcomes constructive, intimacy-building feedback.

With a *turning toward* response, the bidder is more likely to make a bid again.

How about when the wife says, "Babe, I am really struggling with this latest rounds of hormones"?

Turning away: "What else is new?" "Shocking!" "You don't say."

Turning toward: "I know, love. What can I do for you?" "What do you need from me?"

Think of such communication as a bank account. To move the money around in a bank account, you have two options: withdrawal or deposit. Now think of your spouse as having an emotional bank account. If you turn toward the bids for attention, you are making a healthy deposit in your spouse's emotional bank account. However, if you are consistently turning away from his or her bids, you are making withdrawals and depleting your spouse of emotion.

Here are three things that can compound or deplete the sanctity and purity of one's emotional bank account: marriage, infertility, and hormonal treatments. Marriage has the potential to be risky enough. If you throw years of infertility on top of that, the roller coaster of deposits and withdrawals can compromise your emotional bank account's executive balance. Then (drum roll, please) you add hormones to the mix. The emotional bank account becomes more sensitive and exposed, sometimes not fully able to interpret a withdrawal or deposit or trust a deposit's validity.

Take care of each other's emotional bank account always. After all, if you and your spouse are both functioning with full emotional bank accounts, you have more freedom to continue to pour into your spouse. If you are both functioning out of depleted bank accounts, you will more likely work to take from your spouse, which will often leave you both depleted.

As the childhood-television hero Fred Rogers profoundly said, "Love isn't a state of perfect caring. It is an active noun like 'struggle.' To love someone is to strive to accept that person exactly the way he or she is, right here and now" (Rogers 2003, 30).

When your marriage is being tested—either by internal or external forces—be increasingly diligent to err on the side of deposits rather than accumulate withdrawals.

A word to the wise: when there are hormones on board, the more deposits, the merrier. I don't have to tell you where withdrawals will land you!

Personal Inventory

1. How can you turn toward your spouse rather than allow hormones to push you away?
2. How can you better communicate what the hormones are putting you through with those closest to you?
3. How can you and your spouse better make deposits (rather than withdrawals) in your emotional bank accounts?

CHAPTER 16

It Can Cost a Lot of Money

TRAVIS AND JENN had been married close to a decade by the time our mutual friends introduced us. She was from a rural area, and he was a city boy. They met in college and were like two long-lost loves with paths destined to intersect one spring morning.

Jenn saw Travis kneel down and talk to the little boy in front of him while they were standing in line at a local coffee shop. In that moment, he caught her attention and her heart. When she told her friends about him, she boasted about what a great father she knew he would be.

Their love affair was intense. Not much time passed before they knew that a trip down the church aisle was imminent. Their friends emphatically supported them, and so did their respective families.

College graduation. Marriage. Wedded bliss. A new home. The stuff real-life fairy tales are made of.

Our paths crossed years later because we had one thing in common: infertility. That ugly, heartbreaking road plagued us both. No words needed to be spoken when we realized why we had been introduced. A crooked smirk with an empathetic nod of the head was enough to bond us on this unfortunate road.

Let's be real. Isn't it an unexpected blessing when you find someone familiar with the journey? While you want to hug and wish the pain away, there is something comforting—like finding a long-lost friend—when you meet a fellow infertile-club member.

Not Pregnant

We created a strict budget when we started thinking about IVF and all of the testing prior. We cut out dates. We cut out trips to the bar with friends. We eliminated summer vacations. We eliminated gift giving. I guess you could say we eliminated anything that we enjoyed.

—Laura

Travis and Jenn had spent years pursuing their careers and saving for their dream home that would one day securely hold the family that they planned to create.

Now their love and their pocketbooks both showed signs of fatigue. The trials of infertility had put their love to the test, while the strain of fertility medications, tests, trials, inseminations, and everything in between drained their savings.

Jenn had loved growing up in a small, rural town with three siblings. And her desire to homeschool and raise a small village motivated every decision. Her family was known as being an inclusive, little, self-sustaining community of its own. Her siblings were her peer group. The cherished memories were plentiful.

Travis, from a single-child home, enjoyed his career but wanted more family than he'd had growing up. He had been lonely during his childhood. He was often alone with his thoughts. His companion was his imagination. He wanted more. He wanted socialization. He longed for excitement—perhaps a sleepover or a vacation. There had to be more to life than loneliness.

There we stood. She appeared weary. His shoulders drooped from the pain of their journey. The light in their eyes had dimmed, robbed by the grief they had encountered.

I asked where they were in their journey and how they were emotionally navigating it all. With all the emotion depleted from his jaded smile, Travis looked at Jenn and solemnly said, "All we do is fight about money." She agreed. While they had met a lot of life goals, they felt they were failing at the one they had been fighting for all along.

Both of them seemed to crumble in shame to admit that their love had reached this point. There were only bags under the eyes of their soul. They were weary, and so was their love.

Even without infertility, financial struggles inside a marital relationship are known to drive a catastrophic wedge between spouses, lamentably leading to divorce all too often. When infertility is thrown into the mix—along with the emotional toll it brings—it is no wonder that this is such a colossal dispute.

The American Society of Reproductive Medicine states that "the average cost of an IVF cycle in the United States is $12,400"[3]. That is without the cost of medicine. That is without taking into consideration multiple trips to the reproductive endocrinologist. That is without considering time off from work. This is with the hope that the first implantation will be successful. This sum does not take into account the emotional and physical expenditure.

The procedure alone is the price of the used minivan you hope to need one day. That dollar amount is a third of the price of a traditional domestic adoption. It is no wonder that the very price tag of such an endeavor is maddening and divisive.

The stress of such an insurmountable debt is a burden for many. Those numbers are enough to get some couples to turn around, reevaluate their choices, and find an alternative plan.

Others—who dare proceed along the journey of tests for him, tests for her, hormone replacements, egg retrievals, fertilizations, artificial menopause, and ultrasounds—embark on their last hope of a biological child. Now accompanying those hopes are the bills in the mail and tough financial conversations.

---

3 For further information go to: http://www.reproductivefacts.org/detail.aspx?id=3023.

Every bill from the IVF clinic was a reminder of what we did not have. However, every bill from the IVF clinic was a glimmer of hope that we were closer to a baby than ever. Every time we paid the bill I had to remind myself that it could all be worth it in the end.

—Shayna

As Travis, Jenn, and I spoke further that afternoon, they personalized the struggle more. He had been willing to stop many times, thinking about their retirement plan. A place on the coast of southern Florida had been calling their name for years. She, however, was reluctant to stop because she feared the years prior to retirement would be desolate without the opportunity of raising children of her own.

Travis wanted to protect them from debt while also protecting them from emotional bankruptcy and grief. Jenn was ready to give it all to make her dreams come true.

Countless financial debates and wisdom seeking about how to proceed ruined date nights, dinner parties, and most days of the week. The wedge was agonizing and cutting deep. It seemed that almost daily one of them would bring another cost-cutting option to the table. She was ready to get rid of his Major League Baseball cable package in order to save a few dollars. His brilliant idea was to cut out her monthly massage and pedicure. While their ideas were good, they were divisive.

The chasm between financial freedom and the birth of a child was too wide to cross most days. On occasion, they saw eye to eye. Those days were growing increasingly infrequent, however.

Months passed, and they decided to plow through the impending financial strain and jumped into the IVF club. There is always more time to make money, they decided. However, due to her age, there was not much more time to pursue baby making.

If IVF is successful, the money spent is well worth it. The dollar signs become a thing of the past, and the monthly money sent to the clinic is mailed with a smile and thankfulness.

If IVF is unsuccessful, each dollar owed compounds the grief and painful emotions that have been collecting for years. Payments are written with reluctance, bitterness, and an imaginary passive-aggressive letter that never gets written.

Sadly, Travis and Jenn's story is not unique. Professionally, Shannon and I work closely with many delicate souls embracing the reality that reproductive endocrinology is their best shot for expanding their family. They reach this quandary already frazzled from the years of trying for a baby biologically. Taking temperatures, trying different positions, pregnancy tests, and diagnoses now give way to hormone replacements, pokes, prods, petri dishes, frozen embryos, and large dollar sums.

If you are there, remain committed to your connection with your spouse. Be diligent in communication. Do not forget that your marriage came first and your marriage deserves to be strong at the end. Remember to fight *together*. Be devoted to each other, your individual needs, and the needs of your marriage. You are both going to have to sacrifice a lot for both of your dreams to come true.

Active Listening

When couples have polarizing arguments, it is really easy to focus on your own point. While your spouse is talking, you are busy thinking about refining your rebuttal and finding the most eloquent way to win the argument. That's the operative word: *win*.

The problem with this style of communicating is that while both parties have a chance to speak, neither person has the opportunity to be heard. Like a dog chasing its own tail, you end up in the same place that you started. The only thing accomplished is a rise in blood pressure, excellent elocution, and the feeling of pride. What is not accomplished, however, is the ability to restate your partner's point, because you were busy thinking about your own point while he or she was communicating. No one is heard. Nothing beneficial is accomplished.

When people are actively listening, they are void of distractions. They are not looking at their phone, not paying attention to the television, not thinking of their own agenda, and not wondering what to make for dinner or if make-up sex is going to bookend the argument. They certainly are not thinking of how they are going to absolutely annihilate their spouse with the next point that they are about to make. They are paying complete attention to what the communicator intends to communicate, both verbally and nonverbally.

Active listening says that you pay so much attention to the speaker that you are able to regurgitate his or her points. Active listening says that you pay attention to voice inflection and can reflect back the points that seem the most important to the speaker.

While actively listening, give subtle signs to communicate that you are paying attention. Saying "Uh-huh" or "Tell me more" encourages the person to keep sharing with you as the speaker knows that he or she is being heard and valued.

I realize this is stereotypical psychobabble; however, therapists are known for doing this because it works and elicits further communication. Asking probing questions about how what the speaker is saying makes him or her feel or nudging the person to say more will allow the speaker to share more of his or her heart with you.

While listening, avoid the four horsemen of the apocalypse from the Gottmans's research, which we discussed in chapter 6.

During conversations about money, both spouses are going to bring ideas into marriage from their family of origin and lessons they have learned individually, as well as spousal expectations. Each person has different priorities in terms of spending and saving. Sometimes couples have similar views, but more often than not, they have polarizing opinions and methodologies that create conflict.

While coming to agreements on money, especially during the season of infertility, make sure that you hear each other while communicating. Practice active listening strategies so that both partners feel heard, their emotions attended to, and their points valued.

Then and only then can you come to a conclusion together.

Personal Inventory

1. Personally, how can you improve your active listening?
2. In what ways can you and your spouse become more united in the area of finances?
3. Is there an expense that you can temporarily surrender to alleviate the financial strain?

CHAPTER 17

A Hysterectomy Is Survivable

I REMEMBER THE first time Shannon said that miserable word *hysterectomy*. I nodded like I heard it, but somewhere in my spirit, I suffocated the reality that it was indeed an option.

I ignored the notion that it was something that I needed to honestly contemplate at the age of thirty. It was, after all, something that older, postmenopausal women did, right? Someone please tell me I am right! These women no longer needed a uterus. There was no longer an option of them filling their womb with life. They had experienced their monthly visitor for too many years, so ridding them of a few organs would be a nonissue. Right? Come on!

Chalk this up to an issue that you don't fully contemplate until it smacks you upside the head.

There I sat.

"Hysterectomy," she said, "is your best option to defeat the pain."

I had already tried everything—and I mean everything. How on earth did we get to this point? Just four years before, I had walked down the aisle toward my best friend with plans of adding to our family two years later. Now permanently ridding myself of those dreams was my best option for a pain-free life? I felt like I had a case of emotional whiplash.

I certainly had a lot to think about. Let's be honest about that. This was *not* going to be a quick answer. Stubborn old me was going to try and suck every last day out of this uterus before I surrendered it to the medical-waste department at the hospital where I had become a frequent flier.

I felt like I was being forced to surrender my woman card. "Here you go. You can have my uterus. My ovaries. My fallopian tubes, sure take those, too. While you're at it, you can have my femininity. Anything else you want?"

I had to emotionally process what still made me a woman. Sure, it was a bizarre eschatological question to be asking at such a moment, but I wanted to make sure that I had cleared up this semantic debate before taking such a plunge. It may sound crazy, but who are we to judge when someone is faced with something so personal?

My husband was ready to take it all out yesterday. Every time I winced in pain, he was ready to anesthetize me at home, call Shannon, and have her rid me of my torment. He was ready, but my stubbornness stood in the way. Months before I could, he had closed the door on the hopes of a biological child. He knew the odds were stacked against us and had made peace with our reality. I was not too far behind him, but I needed to make my own peace at my own pace.

Throughout this whole journey, we owe ourselves this at least: peace. Throughout the plethora of decisions, opinions, and theories, seek your own peace—however you find it. You are entitled to it. Seek it out. Own it. Can I get an *amen*?

I am someone who needs closure. If I am moving to a new town, I have to symbolically say good-bye to some significant locations and all the people who made my old town a home for me. If I am ending a vacation, I need to make peace with the amount of stuff I have completed and/or seen, in the event we don't make it back. I dread something being its last.

I remember going to Alcatraz with my mom and some friends of hers when I was a wee, little traveler. We all took pictures in front of the sign by ourselves. My mom did not. She didn't care. It wasn't important to her. I cared enough for both of us. I lay in bed that night and cried, dreading that mom would never make it back to Alcatraz Island to complete my picture-taking need for her. I did not get the closure that I needed.

Call me crazy, already. I give you permission to laugh. I dreaded missing my period after a hysterectomy; I would never again be entitled to this feminine experience. (Now is the time to laugh if you didn't pick up on that. My prehysterectomy self was completely confident that I was going to miss the monthly misery.)

I had a complicated relationship with Aunt Flo. Before she visited for the first time, I had willed puberty to start so that I could finally have a period.

From then until seventeen years later when I had a hysterectomy, I cursed its devilish name, hated its monthly arrival, and dreaded the pain accompanying it. However, for some reason, my need-for-closure self wanted to be assured that I would not miss it when it disappeared forever. I needed everything I could get out of it, even though it did not accomplish all it was meant to do.

Having a period was a normal part of life. It was going to cease, and I needed to have closure.

Once upon a time, I was a tomboy. I joke that I didn't become a girl until high school. I wore boxers under my overalls (you are welcome for that visual) and long gym shorts with T-shirts and was constantly seen with either a volleyball or soccer ball. Those were the days, I tell you. I ran everywhere and spent my time practicing, especially in the house, where I was not supposed to. Sorry, Mom.

Somehow I grew up. Years passed, and somewhere along the line, I lost the majority of my athleticism, drive, and coordination.

For the first six years of our marriage, my husband was the youth pastor at our church. One day we old people challenged the students to a game of kickball in the gym. Remembering my glory days when I could win a race—or even hop on one foot at a time—I did not even bother to stretch. Rookie mistake.

I was on second base. Another old-timer kicked the ball, and I proceeded—full sprint ahead—to third base. I was running like I was competing against Usain Bolt. (You know, that guy with all the gold medals?)

It was somewhere between second and third that someone moved the floor out from under me. I'd like to believe that I was running so fast that I began to fly. But if I'm truthful, my legs just didn't move as fast as my dignity.

There I lay on the floor, laughing hysterically while my pride spilled out around me. My husband just looked at me and shook his head. Luckily none of the students noticed that there was *supposed* to be a runner heading toward third, so no one threw the ball. That's right. I was safe! I made it. No shreds of honor or athleticism left, but I made it.

I knew that day that my tomboy, jock-like existence was completely behind me. (Well, that was the day I was willing to admit it, at least.) It was time to turn a corner, admit my age, and admit that I wasn't as cool and sporty as I once was.

At some point you just admit it: enough is enough.

This is where I needed to get with my uterus! I knew that the glory days of my uterus were behind me, too. Hopes and dreams of it being a young, well-functioning machine were behind me. There was no opportunity for it to resurrect itself. Everyone else on the team knew that it was past its prime. I just needed to admit it.

Once I could admit it, I could find the peace I needed.

One ordinary day I stumbled upon it: the peace, that is. No, I didn't stumble on the gym floor again. I told my husband I was ready. I had done the necessary work emotionally. I had found contentedness being barren. No longer was it a scarlet letter I had to wear. It was not my identity. It was something that I had experienced at some point in time.

With little emotion in my heart, I called Shannon to schedule my appointment. I spoke with as little sentiment as I would use to order my coffee at Starbucks.

Shannon did her due diligence every time I saw her after that and made sure that I knew what I was doing. Made sure that I would not regret my decision. Made sure that I was confident that I did not need more time.

Fast forward to the day of my surgery. There I lay, ready to surrender my uterus and an ovary. I kept one ovary due to my age and my desire to postpone menopause as long as I can.

Waking up from the surgery, I did not care about the outcome, as long as she had got it all. As long as Shannon had not found anything life threatening during the procedure, I was fine. During prior surgeries, I had been eager to regain consciousness and to understand what she had found and what it meant for future baby-making endeavors. This time I didn't care. It was finished.

No more ovulation sticks.

No more negative pregnancy tests and the subsequent emotional roller coaster.

No more miscarriages.

No more trying.

It was over. The struggle was complete.

It was time for my husband and me to move on. Together. To whatever that meant.

Talk about a paradigm shift. We walked out of the hospital the next afternoon, ready to start anew. And that, my friends, is exactly what we did.

One more thing. It's been two years, and I have never once missed having a period. I know you were curious!

Personal Inventory

1. If having a hysterectomy is an option, what emotions are you experiencing about it?
2. With whom can you share those emotions?

CHAPTER 18

It Is OK to Stop and Move On

To QUIT OR not to quit, that is the question.

Meet the elephant in the room. How long do we have to do this? When will we know to stop? How long do we have to put ourselves through this? People around you may even be contemplating this for you: how long are they going to continue do this to themselves?

Karyn and Dale were eight years into their infertility struggle. Approximately every eight months, the stick turned pink. They were elated but grew to know how the story ended. Every taste of optimism tricked them into hope. Hope dwindled after a few more negative pregnancy tests. They were left alone, wondering what the purpose of it all was. Wondering if the story would ever change. Wondering why she could not seem to carry a baby into the second trimester. Wondering if it would ever be their turn.

They knew that the choice to stop was theirs and theirs alone. They lamented about the struggle and knew what they needed to do to make the madness stop; however, stopping seemed cruel. Stopping meant that their childhood hopes and dreams were terminated. Stopping meant premature capitulation, as she was indeed able to conceive. What if there was another treatment that would surface soon that would help her womb be more accommodating to life? The what-if game was like molasses to her healing.

The conversation of how long to keep trying haunted us. The dilemma seemed to be everywhere we were. Whether people actually were thinking it or not, I felt like it was painted on everyone's face. We quit for my sanity. He supported. Sometimes I wonder if we made the right choice. Our choice is now permanent, so I guess we'll never know. I just have to live with that choice now.

—Grace

You hear magical stories where couples give birth to a baby after seven miscarriages and eleven years of trying.

Some couples don't have the same sort of stamina, perseverance, or luck.

Some do.

In the mid-1960s, a youthfully enthusiastic couple fell in love in a sailing club sponsored by their local university where they both attended. It was not long before they knew they were the real deal.

These crazy kids got engaged, and months later they walked down the aisle to forever, pledging their hopes and dreams to each other, promising to love each other through *better and worse.*

Better came immediately as they honeymooned, bought a house, and added a dog to their family.

He was an engineer, and she was a home-economics teacher. These two, young in love, wanted one more thing: a baby.

In the summer of 1971, their dream came true. They had their first baby boy, and they were elated.

This young lad grew and became a big brother in the fall of 1974.

Worse came not long after. They wanted a third child. After struggling with a miscarriage between son one and two, they were fearful to continue trying despite their two healthy children.

In 1978, they were excited to welcome their third child. What they did not know throughout the mom's entire pregnancy was that their sweet child, still in utero, was not compatible with life outside the womb. Their precious son lived long enough to be baptized and make it to their local children's hospital. He lived long enough to be named Christian. Five and a half hours after his birth, he was back in the arms of his creator. His parents never got to hold him. Christian never got to feel the love of his parents outside the womb. He passed away, alone, in an NICU.

These two grieving parents were forced to go back home and tell their two little boys that they would not be bringing home their little brother.

Their hopes and dreams for their family of five were now threatened by the bassinet that would not welcome a baby home. Sadness overwhelmed them. Grief was now the fifth member, constantly occupying their once-happy home.

They were at a crossroad of whether or not Christian would round out their family of five or if they wanted to try again.

Grief lasted months—years, rather.

Many people stand at that crossroad where grief and dreams collide, desiring a family but fearing being let down again. And again.

This couple's viewpoints differed. She—the dreamer whose maternal arms longed to hold more babies—wanted to keep pushing for another child. He, the realistic engineer, thought that they should quit while they were ahead with their two healthy children.

Tears. Conversations. More tears. More talking.

They decided to try again for child number four.

She was able to conceive once again and endured late pregnancy in the heat of a Southern California summer. Optimism, pessimism, and the not-too-distant reality of a baby lost confused their joy about their upcoming arrival.

Much to their surprise, the mom had a baby girl in the summer of 1981. A girl. Such, such joy. And confusion, really. These were presonogram days, and so when the doctor announced that it was a girl, the exhausted mama, said, "Shut up. Check again!"

Healthy. A family of five.

That little bundle of unexpected healing was me.

The teacher, the engineer, and those three older brothers are my people.

I am so glad that my parents decided to keep trying.

Every November my precious mom and dad celebrate those beloved hours of Christian's life. Every November they wonder what his life would have looked like. Every November I wonder why she and Dad had to experience such pain. Every December there are no new answers.

Here's what I know: my mom and dad look back and are happy that they did not quit.

I know of many other success stories. We have some precious people in our life who could only conceive through the miracle of IVF. And conceive they did. The life of their treasured child is a blessing to our family.

Another couple in our community tried to no avail for years, and then with the help of science and medicine, they miraculously just gave birth to their third darling little bundle of love. Their family looks just the way they had always prayed for it to look.

Yet here's another not-too-surprising truth: not every story ends with a child at the end.

Our story didn't turn out how we had originally planned all those years ago. Three diagnoses and pain only a horse tranquilizer could quench ruined our hopes for a biological child.

A friend and her husband stood at the precipice of not being able to add biological children to their family, and they decided to foster kids whose parents could not keep them.

Another couple found themselves in the predicament of whether to chase the dream of conception or to move to Europe and start a different life. They refocused the trajectory of their lives and decided to put all their energy into working at an orphanage. They discontinued their efforts to build a biological family and embraced the children in the shelter.

Another couple decided that they would adopt some dogs rather than continue the fight to have biological children.

I will never forget when we finally reached the point in our journey where we knew it was coming to an end. Our first appointment with our reproductive endocrinologist went fairly well. He was the perfect combination of relational and brilliant.

He convinced us that he was fairly sure what the problem was. It wasn't me. It was the embryos. In a nutshell, he believed that the eggs I was creating weren't viable and, therefore, could only continue growing for so long. He gave us a treatment strategy that left us believing a successful pregnancy wasn't far off. He was going to order blood work, which he said would confirm his hypothesis, and then we'd be good to go.

I got my blood work done a few days later, and within the next week, we had our results.

"Your blood work came back normal, Mrs. Quillet." Awesome news if I were trying to rule out a potentially dangerous diagnosis. Instead what I was hoping for was something minor to be wrong so that we could treat it and be on our merry way.

"So what does that mean?"

"It means that we've ruled out everything. There is nothing wrong. The doctor said that he doesn't need to see you again. Good luck to you."

Hope was gone. The tests results meant that I/we had to go into every pregnancy blind.

The nurse did say that I should continue to walk daily and eliminate carbs from my diet, which the doctor had instructed when we saw him. I had already begun this regimen, so it seemed easy to continue.

I asked, "Is the need for me to continue exercising and eliminating carbs substantiated by my insulin levels?"

"No. Your insulin level is perfect and within normal limits."

"So why the diet and exercise?"

"Well, the doctor thinks that it's your only shot. We can give you medicine to help you ovulate, but it won't help you keep a pregnancy."

I managed to spit out a muttered, "Good-bye." That's it? It was at that moment that we knew we needed to shift our focus.

Of our four pregnancies, we conceived two of them sans any medical help. There was no method to the madness. There were no medical answers. We were at a dead end. We never did get an answer to why we never had a healthy pregnancy and birth. Sometimes there are just no answers.

In my case, my pain necessitated that we discontinue our journey by way of hysterectomy. Despite the diagnoses and surgeries, we exited the process with little more information than that it just did not work out for us.

At some point if infertility still weaves itself into your story, you may face that same choice.

Peace is necessary. Unity of mind within your relationship is paramount. Do not proceed one step forward or backward without having harmony in your home.

Experience all the emotions related to grief before you make the decision. By this point in your journey, you have certainly heard that you should not make any impulsive decisions while you are emotional. Please heed that advice when standing at this crossroad.

Allow both spouses, or all the members of the family if you are experiencing secondary infertility, to feel all the emotions before making a decision.

With clear heads and peaceful hearts, set out to make the decision together.

I'm surprised that as I type these words, they no longer elicit a response. That is peace. According to Elisabeth Kübler-Ross, that is acceptance. It feels like freedom.

How you get to freedom or what you do afterward is up to you. My hope for you, sweet sister, is that you find your freedom. But, please, give yourself (and your husband) peace in the process.

Naturally I am going to champion my profession; however, if you and your spouse are at a stalemate over life-changing decision, let me encourage you to seek therapy. That very word has a negative connotation in society. But seeking therapy does not necessarily mean that you cannot handle it on your own or that you, your spouse, or your marriage has a problem. Rather a third party may be an excellent support system or sounding board as you make this decision. (I'll get off my soapbox now!)

Personal Inventory

1. Take an honest inventory of where you and your spouse are regarding whether you want to continue or quit your journey.
2. What would reaching *acceptance* look like for you? To your spouse?

CHAPTER 19

How to Move On

THIS JOURNEY, AS with any, has to end somehow. While each story will be written differently for each couple, it will end one of two ways: with offspring or without.

If this road has yielded children for you, then congratulations, my friend. Happy dream come true to you! May the journey ahead be void of tantrums, middle-of-the-night tears, sibling rivalries, poor choices, and years of intensive therapy.

If you are still moving forward or nearing the admission that biological children may not be something that you are blessed with, lean in, dearest. Here is a big hug for you, accompanied by a shoulder, should you need a place to cry.

For women in the second category, I ponder which is worse: the complexity of personal choice dictating that the road is over or the physician's professional opinion that hope may be gone. Perhaps they are both equally evil.

The question becomes, how do we move on? How on earth do we pick ourselves up from this dreadful experience—an experience that I hope one day stops hurting so badly and that I hope one day I just completely forget?

The answer is that we do so one step at a time—letting go of the past and being ready to embrace what lies ahead.

Moving On

Little did the thirteen-year-old boy know, but I was watching from afar. He was in his own world, while I merely observed. He wanted a pop (*soda* or *Coke* for all you non-Ohioans) from the vending machine, and perhaps I had a lesson to learn. Years later the lesson continues to teach me...

For years my husband oversaw the youth ministry at our church. Wednesday nights were the big event nights. For one hour a week, the church was full of hormone overdrive, pubescent stink, and a whole lot of energy.

Down from the room the teens occupied was a row of vending machines. Before the event began, students flocked over in droves to get yet another kick of caffeine, which was really beneficial (sarcasm on) for the hour of listening ahead.

This spring evening I watched the teen, dollar in hand, walk to the vending machines. His sweaty post-dodgeball body walked straight over to the row of neon machines that were beckoning him to buy caffeine goodness.

He perused his options. It did not take him long to decide what he wanted and put in his dollar.

Then he pushed his selection.

He waited.

Nothing.

Then as most of us would, he pushed his selection again. And again nothing (except for a small chuckle from me). There was no one around him at this point except for me, and he was oblivious to that fact. The allure of the caffeine must have been too overwhelming.

He proceeded to shake the machine to no avail. Shaking turned into shoving with a little more force.

I thought that he had given up as he walked to the other side of the hallway. Then this little junior higher turned around, eyed his opponent, planted his foot, and charged at the vending machine like a bull who'd just had a red flag waved in front of his face.

He sprinted toward the machine, and about a foot before he reached it, he sprang from the ground and crashed all his not-quite-five-foot flying momentum into the unassuming machine.

Nothing. Again.

He had been robbed. He had responsibly contributed his part to the equation. He had waited longer than he had hoped. Momentarily he was overcome with emotion. He walked away from the failed transaction with a holy vengeance ready to express his emotion to someone. Anyone.

He had been shortchanged, and he thought he deserved more.

There I was—at that time in the middle of our journey with infertility—empathizing with his anger. While my pull was not toward a caffeinated beverage (at my age, I can't have caffeine past 2:30 p.m.), I desperately wanted a baby.

I had educated myself sufficiently. I had done my part. We'd had sex when we were supposed to. I had been patient for as long as I could. I had felt shortchanged. Cheated. I was owed. If there was something to beat on as an expression of my anger, I am sure I would have.

There is a crossroad that inevitably comes if your womb has not yet been blissfully filled with all of your hopes and dreams. Some couples have the ability to continue on until the health risks associated with older parents approach. I always hear those miracle stories, such as, "We tried for ten years and had five mis-carriages, and then it worked. We have three children now. It just wasn't the right time, I guess." In my book, those stories are absolutely remarkable. I held on to hope for well past the point I should have surrendered my uterus. Hope is a funny thing.

Then reality sinks in. This reality says that for your sanity, you ought to just throw in the towel so that you can have real life again. Move on so that you can navigate through the pain and hopefully find happiness again. Sometimes the end of a journey can be the beginning of another. Unfortunately the door has to be closed behind you in order for you to move forward into the next chapter.

Here's where the peanut gallery is going to come into play again. Unless you have a health concern or something externally obvious that initiates the closing of this chapter, people are going to offer their opinions. And we know how much we love their opinions.

People are going to want the best for you, so they are going to offer their unsolicited advice in an attempt to protect you from more pain.

They are going to offer you advice about what they would do and about what their friend's sister's ex-brother-in-law's college roommate did.

Let me tell you a secret: when it comes to this decision, they do not get a vote. They may try to cast it, but do not let it matter. You may hear their opinion or even take it to heart. The final decision, however, comes down to *only* what the two of you want—or the three of you, if consulting with your medical professional is in your best interest.

Sally and Evan listened to the peanut gallery. Friends attempted to give them unsolicited advice. They were practically all friends from the womb, so if anyone knew them, it was their friends. In addition, their friends had walked similar roads, so they felt entitled to share their own opinions.

Sally's best girlfriend and her husband had wanted to stop trying for a long time. Finally they felt like the time was right. They stopped actively trying. While they did not do anything to stop a pregnancy, the days of intentionally trying were behind them.

The next month it happened. Three years of trying and nothing. They stopped, and nine months later little Amanda was born. Wouldn't you know it.

Their friends were convinced from that point forward that a couple should not stop. They had almost given up on their dreams. What if they had started birth control again? What if she had got the IUD that she had considered? What if? The results of all those what-ifs would have the same: no Amanda.

These friends talked to Sally and Evan all the time. Their friends' mantra of "Don't stop" was constantly ringing in their ears like tinnitus, even though both of them were ready to close the door on these dreams and find a new dream together. They had found peace in that decision. However, those who felt they had an opinion they had to share made the couple's newly forged peace murky.

At the end of the day, only you and your spouse are responsible for making these decisions. Rely on each other for this. Don't lean on parents or friends unless you both feel comfortable doing so together. Sift through the advice together. Do not use it as leverage or ammunition against the other person.

What we are trying to avoid is bitterness and long-lasting contempt. Do you remember from the Gottmans's research how desperately we need to avoid contempt? Work together to avoid it like the plague.

Actively listen to each other. Do not listen with your own agenda. Hear your spouse, his or her heart, and all that your loved one seeks to communicate to you.

When everything gets hard, turn to each other instead of turning away. Turning away is easy and society's cop-out. Turn to each other in order to preserve the intimacy of your marriage and to avoid resentment.

Work toward the healing of yourselves individually as well as the healing of your marriage.

Healing

Do you remember how it felt to twirl around when you were little? I loved to spin in my prepubescent years. (Now I'd be vomiting for days. I hate admitting that.)

I would stand safely in the middle of a room so as not to fall on any of the household furniture or disturb Mom's trinkets. If you were a serious spinner, you put your arms out to the side.

Then I would spin and twirl until the floral, '80s-print skirt no longer fell to my sides but twirled out around me...twirl until giggles filled my lips and giddiness extended to my fingertips...twirl until I couldn't twirl anymore and the momentum knocked me to my knees.

Exhilaration.

Twirling can happen in the company of friends who are fellow twirlers, with a familial audience, or just alone.

Then it happens.

You fall, and as a kid, it bewilders you. Why is the room still spinning? The truth is, it doesn't matter. Why? Because the sensation makes you collapse to your side as you spill out more giggles and creates motivation for you to stand and do it all yet again.

The most important part of the game is that you get back up again.

What about now? What if your room is still spinning? You have been suffocated by infertility for far too long, and your life has been orbiting so quickly around the pain that you haven't had a chance to stop. I want to tell you that healing can come.

What if it is too difficult to stand back up? Take your time. Find your people. Lean on your friends. Enlist the help of your spouse. It may take longer than you want. Remember, there is no timetable for grief. Let me kindly remind you again, healing can come.

What if you are too dizzy? Things will calm down. The pain will decrease. Whatever caused this pain will someday be something that you experienced *in the past tense*. Healing can come.

What if you feel like spinning again? Go for it, girlfriend. Stand back up. Be confident. Healing can come.

You have the right to focus on your healing. It is not selfish if you need some time. It is self-care. You are allowed to heal at your own pace. Continue to move forward, navigating all your emotions. You are validated in taking your time.

There is beauty in two people trying to find healing in their brokenness. This quest is love.

Let me challenge you, as you pursue your healing, to find the beauty and the uniqueness in your journey.

As I look back on the years of our struggle, I can see the beauty in some of the ugliest moments. I don't want to share the specifics here due to the beauty in the broken; however, I find some intimacy in sharing those moments with my husband. They are some of the most painful and ugly parts of my existence. Yet my husband and I chose to lean into the hard together. There we were, alone with our grief...experiencing the hard and the raw together.

While I wish that all of it would have gone another way, to some extent I would not change it. Why? It grew us in ways that I never knew we needed to grow. Perhaps that growth would not have come another way. For me, those moments are beautiful. Beautifully intimate. Beautiful in their brokenness.

Find the beauty in your story. While it will not redeem it all, it is sure to lessen the blow if you can find the growth and the healing throughout.

Personal Inventory

1. How connected are you and your spouse about how to proceed with your journey?
2. How will you know when this chapter of your relationship has come to an end?
3. How are you both finding healing individually and in your relationship?

CHAPTER 20

Our Adoption Story

I DO NOT have a green thumb. I barely know the difference between annuals and perennials. I am not the girl who has a favorite flower or who needed a specific flower in my wedding bouquet. I know what I like when I look at it. Arrangements of roses are gorgeous for both the eyes and the nose. Tulips are pretty, too. There are other flowers I like; I just do not know what they are called. That about exhausts my knowledge of flowers.

I have a dear friend and former roommate who is a florist near San Francisco. This girl has an eye for beauty that comes in the form of flowers. It is remarkable to see the arrangements she puts together. The colors, textures, fruits (yup, she is that creative), and other elements she puts in the arrangements are absolutely awe-inspiring to me. I wish she would have done the flowers for our wedding, but it was too important for her to be standing up with me. I am glad that people like her were put on this earth. She makes things beautiful.

I could only dream of having that kind of talent and vision.

We have an area in our front yard that we left unmaintained for our first few years in the house. It was pretty when we moved in, but after a few years, my missing green thumb meant that it was not aesthetically pleasing. Where was my girlfriend when I needed her? Oh, yeah, California!

When family came over, they would spend a minute or two fixing the parts that we had let go because I could not tell the difference between a weed and the intended plant.

Recently I was sitting by the window that looks out over this garden. I use the word *garden* loosely, as it's more like a plot intended for a garden. At this point in the year, it's even less of a garden and more of a hodgepodge of dead leaves, soggy mulch, and brown weeds.

I sat and pondered what needed to be done once the earth defrosted. I began to think of what types of bulbs I wanted to put in the ground this spring. Since I know little about flowers, I got stuck pondering a bulb. The purpose of a bulb. The process it goes through.

No offense to the bulb, but it's not very attractive in the beginning. It gets buried alive. Alone, in a single hole. No one puts a bulb in a vase on the table. It has not reached its potential yet. This is only the beginning. Its purpose is great, however, even from the beginning—even when you can't identify what it's going to become. Its beauty has yet to be discovered. But just wait; you're in for a treat. Just wait until spring, and you will see its full potential.

Patience is necessary, though, if you're going to experience the beauty. It takes some nurturing and fortitude. It takes endurance—which applies both to the bulb and to the one waiting for the end result.

But then there is some hope. Some green begins to peek out from the earth. The one waiting feels restored hope.

Now it's time for more water. More cultivating. More investment. You're almost there. The wait is almost over. The finish line is close.

We can't have the beauty without the process. There are no blooms without the bulb. The flowers that adorn our home, that we put in our hair, and that we give as gifts would not be possible without the bulb that was hidden below the earth's surface.

Throughout our journey, I loved the metaphor and symbolism of spring. Spring bursts forth after the desolate winter. Death takes place. There is a lull in the majesty of creation. (Well, it takes a different form of beauty if you like snow and ice!) But regardless of the length of winter, spring always comes. It may not come as soon as you want; but it has never missed its cue. The buds always bloom. Life always comes back. The landscape is always repainted with brilliant greens, amazing color, and abundant life.

The process of waiting is hard. Sometimes we, as impatient humans, focus on the birds that peck the growing flowers, the insects that devour, the potential that is never fulfilled, or the length of the wait. It defeats us, makes us angry, and causes a hardening of our heart.

As I look back at those periods of life when I have hated the wait, hindsight reveals the beauty and the purpose of it. Looking back, I fail to see wasted moments. Perhaps there are moments I wasted, but I can certainly identify moments where there was movement around me, impacting me and preparing me.

There is great advantage to hindsight. Now I can see that during our whole fertility journey, I was crippled by my inability to see the full picture. My thoughts were consumed with vacillating waves of hope and despair. I began to hate the word *hope*. This *hope* guaranteed that we would have kids that looked like us. Hope told me that my paralyzed brother would walk again. Hope told us that pregnancy would not end with an early-term miscarriage. In the process of life, hope became too risky.

I remember praying throughout the journey that God would just allow me to get pregnant and make it stick. "Just let Tyler knock me up, and hold Baby in there for forty weeks. Please and thank you."

I had it all planned. Our family picture—once our family was complete—would feature my husband and me along with two (or three) children who looked like a perfectly adorable mixture of both of us. It was going to be darling.

Little did I know, or little was I willing to admit, that the picture was changing. Winter was holding on, but our spring was around the corner.

Throughout the journey, my picture-perfect photograph of the American dream family started dwindling until my mental image was just the two of us. Things began to change inside me. Like the bulb in our front yard at night, I finally felt that the darkness was being pushed back. I knew that something new was happening; it was just too premature to know what was going on. For some reason, this was also the first time in the process when I was content with taking my hands off the wheel.

My prayer changed from "Get me pregnant, and make it stick" to "God, what do you want our family to look like?" For the first time, I was open. Freedom began to set in.

For some reason, both my husband and I simultaneously—but unbeknown to the other—started having dreams of international adoption. As a little girl, I had always struggled with the idea that I was born into safe, white affluence when too many other children around the world struggled to find dinner, warmth, or a nurturing hug. Selfishly, I have to admit, this burden to care for other lonely children was asphyxiated by my own stubborn desire to make our own children. Once I opened myself up to something bigger than myself, my heart was broken in the best of ways.

Eventually, while talking about what to do next, we agreed that both of our hearts were being moved toward international adoption. From there, we decided that we would pray about the idea, learn about the experiences of others who had adopted before, and talked through all of our fears. We were nearing the end of the road in terms of our own fertility. We agreed that if more doors in the fertility realm closed, then we were ready to open the doors for adoption.

I will never forget that frosty January morning when we were sitting in our reproductive endocrinologist's waiting room. My HCG levels from our most recent miscarriage had not yet gone down to zero. My heart was broken down by the process while, for the first time, it was being simultaneously reenergized.

My phone buzzed, notifying me that an e-mail had come through. It was our adoption agency. Upon reading the opening line, I looked at my husband with tears in my eyes. "We passed the first step of the process."

He was completely caught off guard. This step in the process was supposed to take four weeks. It had taken only forty-eight hours. We could not keep up with the adoption agency, which was a gigantic paradigm shift after four years of beating our heads against a wall trying to make our family naturally. Now with a complete change of plans, we were struggling to keep up with what was happening around us. The bulb was beginning to blossom, and it was beautiful!

That day we also received news from our reproductive endocrinologist that hope was seemingly lost on the biological front. While we could continue trying, there was no real way for a baby to attach to my uterus because of all the damage that had occurred. IVF was not an option since we did not have a problem with conception, and there would be no place to implant the baby due to scar tissue.

You would think we would be devastated. Instead while one door was closing, another was swinging wide open, and we were running through it.

We struggled to keep up with the adoption process for a good eighteen months.

Sixteen months after we embarked on our adoption journey our dear adoption consultant called my husband's phone. He was on a hospital visit when he took the call, and I would love to have seen the look on the faces of the people he was visiting. I am sure he turned a ghostly shade of white. He put his hand on the patient's father's shoulder, told him that we had just got the call we'd been waiting for, and drove straight to my office.

What a surprise it was to see his beaming smile, swollen eyes, and tear-stained cheeks. It was just like the moment in the delivery room I had dreamed of for four years when Shannon would hand Tyler our firstborn. I had longed for that moment; it was here in a way I could never have planned for or imagined.

We called our consultant back.

"I have two boys for you."

I cry even typing those words. That phone call made me a mom. There were two boys an ocean away who were now waiting to become our children.

My response was a little like my mom's after she had me and told the doctor to "shut up and check again" when he announced that I was a girl.

I asked our consultant if it was a joke and if she was telling me the truth. After four years of negative pregnancy tests, dead ends, and heartache, I was becoming a mom. My husband's prayer to become a daddy had finally been answered. It was beautiful. The ground had broken, and spring was bursting forth in all its radiant glory.

Let's get one thing straight, though. In no way did that phone call erase all the pain. It was not the total cure for my broken heart. I still had some things to work through. While we now had the anticipation of flying around the world to meet our two boys, I simultaneously longed to take our four other babies with us.

Those four babies whom we had lost still occupied much of the territory in our hearts. They are whom we had wrapped our hopes and dreams around. Now, however, our hearts had grown even more to welcome these children into our hopes and dreams. They were going to be our family. They are our family.

Our family picture had certainly changed. There are now two of the most handsome, brown-complexioned boys who have our complete hearts, standing in that picture with us.

What? You Aren't Called to Adoption?

Writing this, I am fully aware that not every story of infertility will end in adoption. If you are experiencing trouble in this realm, I am certainly not suggesting you look into adoption as a quick fix to filling that empty nursery. If your heart is remotely open to adoption or foster care, please do yourself a favor and at least look into it.

I remember sitting in graduate school listening to a classmate do a presentation on adoption. She told both the benefits and the risks of adoption. All I heard were the risks. At that moment, I pseudopromised myself that I would never put my family through all that potential heartache. I have shaken my head many times at that younger version of me. Let's look at this predicament honestly. The risk of adoption is far less than the risk *not* to adopt. If we choose to protect our family from the risks of adoption, we are setting up an orphan for the risks of life without a family. While it may be difficult to bring a child who does not share your DNA into your family, the pain of knowing what may happen to that child without the gift of adoption is much, much greater.

People always tell my husband and me how lucky they think our children are to finally have parents. While this is certainly true, our response is that our reality is quite the contrary. We, in fact, are the lucky ones. These brown fingers interlaced with ours, the sloppy kisses, the questions about their adoption, and the ups, downs, and everything in between are all a complete honor and joy to us because these children are ours. It is our beautiful story of redemption.

Regardless of how your story ends, I want you to know there is a possibility for joy and peace at the end. That is not a bandage for your emotions.

It is the truth, my friend.

Personal Inventory

1. Have you considered pursuing adoption?
2. Have you and your spouse discussed adoption?
3. If you are on the same page about pursuing adoption, what are the next steps you need to pursue?

CHAPTER 21

There Can Be Happiness at the End of It All

MAXWELL AND AMEE were married for thirty years and had been parents for half of that time. A decade of trying to naturally conceive, plus multiple miscarriages, delayed their dream of being parents. Never mind their hope of being younger parents.

Both were educators, helping teach a decade worth of future adults and praying that one day they, too, would have children running through the halls of their local elementary school. Their dreams were large. Their home was, too, since they had bought one large enough to accommodate all the children they planned to have.

Not only did infertility ruin their hopes of having children in their early twenties, but also secondary infertility stole their dreams of filling that home with children. Their son, Douglas, was the only one to sit in their classrooms and avoid eye contact while he was in the hall with his friends.

There had been fifteen years of joy with Douglas. While Maxwell and Amee were happy with life, the what-could-have-beens crept into their hearts too often. When Douglas took his first steps into his kindergarten classroom, Amee grieved that this would be the only time she would have this experience.

Then her heart began to mend.

When Douglas made his first attempt at T-ball, Maxwell could not have been more elated. His proud-daddy grin was unmistakable—that was, until he realized that this would be the one and only first T-ball season he would witness.

But soon his spirit rebounded again.

Years passed, and Douglas found his first crush. He was in fourth grade, and he was smitten. Maxwell and Amee, being the conscientious parents they were, sat him down and talked about how to treat a girl and how in fourth grade, dating wasn't the most necessary thing for him to be focused on. Then they grieved together that they did not have a daughter to have a similar conversation with.

After a few weeks, the wounds healed up again.

Like my parents, who still celebrate Christian's birthday in November, Maxwell and Amee are still straddling the fence of grief. One foot is firmly planted in the here and now, while the other foot slips on the what-could-have-beens.

Life moves on; however, I do not want to give the illusion that once you find acceptance in the stages of grief, you leave the grief behind you—never to walk through it again.

I found acceptance years ago. Two sweet little African boys helped heal my heart. I have to admit, though, that the tears have flowed many times while writing this book. A few weeks ago, a friend announced she was pregnant. My healed heart swelled with yearning for my own womb to be full. Momentarily I thought about trying again, until I realized that I am without the necessary organs to do so.

Grief spilled out in a way that was different than but mirrored my former experience. The hankering for biological children was back. It did not take long for estrogen to take over. I longed. I grieved. Yet such a process only takes moments now rather than the weeks it took just a few years ago.

Once thing I know for sure is that I have found happiness—most days, at least. Sometimes the thoughts and the feelings creep back in. But I have worked too hard to get out of that prison, and I am not going back in.

Todd and Amber had wanted kids since they had met when they themselves were mere kids. Flirting in seventh grade turned into something a little more serious their freshmen year of high school. Different universities tested their commitment, but they remained faithful to each other.

They were married the spring after graduation and had hopes for a honeymoon baby. By their ten-year anniversary, their family still consisted of just the two of them.

Ovarian cancer, four years into marriage, had robbed Amber not only of her hair but also of her ability to have children. They publicly said they were at peace because at least Amber was alive. Knowing them as well as we did, I knew that while those words rang true, they were also devastated they never got to birth Todd Jr.

Todd was already the fourth Todd in his family line. It was up to him to continue the family legacy. Unfortunately the name will die with him.

Like Maxwell and Amee, Todd and Amber have found a new happiness. This is not the story they discussed through hours of phone conversations in their separate dorm rooms, but the paradigm has shifted. The story line altered. New characters and plot twists gave them a run for their money.

Amber said, "I will never understand why things happened the way that they did. I had two choices while I was getting chemo: fight or die. Now I have two choices again: fight for joy or let barrenness rob me of any opportunity to be happy. I daily fight for joy."

That is it, my friends. Fight for joy. In this life, it is not going to be handed to any one of us on a silver platter. If someone does offer you the silver platter, you come find me!

I love this quote by Max Lucado: "The key is this: Meet today's problems with today's strength. Don't start tackling tomorrow's problems until tomorrow. You do not have tomorrow's strength yet. You simply have enough for today" (Lucado 2001, 63).

I never fully understood the one-day-at-a-time mantra of those fighting cancer until my beloved mama was diagnosed. I was in my early twenties and did not quite understand the magnitude of what she was enduring at the time.

> I was stuck in an ugly place for a long time. I was convinced I would never find my way out. I assumed that I would always resent pregnant women, avoid all children, and hide from happiness. I was wrong. We even started to enjoy sex again. I am still awestruck sometimes when I admit that we are truly OK. It's not just something we try and convince people of anymore. We truly are OK. We have no children, and we are happy. That seems crazy to write. I say that from a complete place of emotional and mental healthiness.
>
> —Sarah

I was afraid of finding out information, but I wanted to know. I wanted to know the end of the story *now*, while we were in the first chapter. That way I would have my shield and arsenal ready for the combat ahead. I would be prepared. I would know how to divide my strength.

Mom, in all her bravery and courage, was the one calming my nerves while she fought her own health battle. She reminded me to take one day at a time. "Don't worry about tomorrow, honey. All we have is today."

She was right. (I wish I could go back and tell my high-school self how wise she truly is).

Today was the only guaranteed day she had to fight.

She had all the strength she needed for *today*.

Worrying about tomorrow, next Thursday, and three years from now did not benefit us at all.

Being present was where we found our happiness, our contentment, and our peace.

Infertility is not going to be the last battle any of us face. Sorry to be the bearer of bad news. There is more to come. If you look back to any already-closed difficult chapter of your life, you may have once thought you would never make it through, but you did.

Likewise you will make it through infertility even if the road ahead is long. The pilgrimage is going to be arduous, painstaking, confusing, and often maddening.

While I can't put a pretty bow on the whole journey and tell you that at the end of this road you will be galloping on a unicorn through a field of lilies and leprechauns, I want you to hear something: you are going to be OK. You will! I assure you. I cannot tell you when. I cannot guarantee how it will go. I cannot tell you how wholeness will be ushered in.

While your story may not have been written as you would have chosen to author it, it is *your* story for your one life. It may be different than you had hoped, but it is where you are. Live fully where you are.

It took me a while to be able to start processing the fact that I was dealing with infertility. I often thought, "Really? Is this happening?" None of what happened was part of our plan. I can sit here today and say, looking back on the last few years (of infertility and miscarriage), that I wouldn't change a thing. It was hard; it is hard, but we live in a painful world. I am not someone special who would be immune from that. Now, that being said, there are days when I look at women who are expecting and think, "Damn you and your working uterus!" I grieve a little every time my husband and I are lying in bed and it hits me that we will never lie there sharing a moment of pure joy, watching my belly move, knowing the living being in there is from us. I wanted that so badly.

—Isabelle

Thankfulness

In hindsight, I have found thankfulness. Hear me out; I dislike this story having to be any of ours. But if I choose to be happy, I find I must be happy...

Happy with the lessons. Thankful for the lessons.

Thankful. Thankfulness seeps from my soul as a giant paradox most days.

Thankfulness has hoped for redemption from years past that will manifest in dreams resolved.

Thankfulness sometimes turns into shattered hopes but then flows into streams of joy.

Thankfulness is brokenness. Broken *but* redeemed.

Thankfulness isn't always a prettily wrapped presentation of togetherness but is instead a messy composition of trust.

Thankfulness is real. Thankfulness is authentic. Thankfulness doesn't mean that our desires are met but that we're content in the journey.

Regardless of dreams gone awry or hope fizzled, I am thankful. Thankful for where I find us in the story. Thankful for brokenness that is finding its way to redemption. Thankful for tears that have turned into hope and promise.

It feels strange to find myself thankful for where we've been. As I've said before, this isn't how I would have pictured this story. I imagine you would say the same about whatever journey you've been on that has led you to pick up this book. If we take the blinders off and try to frame our story in the big picture, what I see most days seems to solicit a certain amount of gratitude. I refuse not to be thankful. I'm not the author of the story; I'm a mere tourist, thankful to find myself within the story I'm in.

Even when my soul is restless, I will choose thankfulness.

In my doubt, I will choose gratitude.

In my unbelief, I lean into belief.

When I would rather pen the story myself, I will put my pen down.

I will find thankfulness, regardless.

I will try.

Will you?

Personal Inventory

1. Are you able to feel moments of thankfulness?
2. In what areas do you struggle with thankfulness?
3. How can you integrate thankfulness more into your life?

Appendix A
A Note from Cathie's Husband

I can recall the moment like it was yesterday—actually more like this morning. The overwhelming joy and anticipation of our first child quickly turned into fear as things just didn't feel right for Cathie. I remember walking into that ultrasound room with an equal amount of excitement and pessimism. Certainly nothing could be wrong, as we had just recently seen our baby on the monitor and heard the heartbeat, right? I'll never forget that sound when we first heard our baby's heartbeat, the sound of life. Amazing!

That particular day, though, as the nurse began to place the wand on Cathie's stomach, my heart sank while I still felt excited, hoping to hear that sound again. It never came. All the nurse could mutter was, "I'm sorry," and she quickly exited the room. A long season of trying brought us to a momentary season of joy that was quickly replaced by this new season of despair that we had just entered. Little did we know, we were just getting started. A longer season of grief, discouragement, heartbreak, loneliness, fear, anger, fatigue, and loss was about to begin.

Husbands and wives, I'd like to use this little slice of **Not Pregnant** to encourage you, challenge you, speak truth to you, and to, I hope, be of some comfort to you...all from a male perspective.

More than anything else, I want you to know that I'm sorry. My heart breaks for you. It really does. Wherever you are on your journey of not being pregnant, I want you to know that we're grieving with you. Grief over constant not-pregnant sticks, grief over the loss of your baby, and grief over the broken expectations and what-ifs. For whatever reason your heart hurts, I'm so sorry for what you've had to endure.

Please allow me a minute or two of your time.

To the Men

Here's what I want you to do. Are you taking notes? Fix her emotions. Fix the situation. Bottle up your own emotions. Keep her at arm's length because you don't know what to do with her feelings. Get angry with your circumstances. Run away from it all because it's hard. Ready? Break!

Just kidding! Seriously, I hope you didn't stop reading there. I also hope none of you just got fired up and burst out of the room like you were running out of the tunnel to play a football game—testosterone through the roof, ready to take on the challenge! Please come back. Keep reading. I was only kidding...

The unfortunate thing about what I just wrote, men, is that these are typically our default settings. We're big and strong and tough, and we can fix anything. So we take matters into our own hands and try to fix this. We keep our emotions to ourselves; as we bottle them up, they fester, and that stuff never comes out looking pretty. We get angry. Anger comes from an unmet expectation, and as people seeking to have a child, there is an expectation.

Let's break it down into a math equation. (I failed math in high school, but this seems really simple.) Husband + Wife + Sex = Baby. Let me break that down further, and I promise there are no pictures to go with this. If a husband and wife have unprotected sex, then there is an expectation that she will become pregnant, and they will have a baby. The expectation is real because that's how it's supposed to be. Right? Well, if you're reading this book, I'm assuming that's probably not the case. And so your expectation has been unmet.

For men, especially, this often results in anger. I'm confident that's where this difficult season of life has left many of you. And yet for others, you don't know how to respond to your wife, to the circumstances, and to the emotions you are feeling, and so you retreat. You don't want to face this reality, and if you're honest, you don't know *how* to face this reality. Unfortunately retreating has left your wife feeling alone, vulnerable, and desiring your comforting words and arms wrapped around her. I may be a little weird here, but I oftentimes found myself angrily retreating. I let all my anger fester, and I retreated from not only my wife but also from many of my closest relationships because I didn't want to talk about it; I didn't know how to deal with it. Good thing my wife is a therapist, so I could get some free help in dealing with that stuff!

Men, let's be honest. Most of us aren't good at this. For me, personally, I *think* I can fix anything—from the dishwasher that's currently been broken for months (I swear I'll get it back up and running) to difficult circumstances that have my wife reeling, as a man, I think I can fix it all. I can't, though, and quite frankly I shouldn't. Cathie doesn't need me to fix the circumstances. She needs me to love her through them. She doesn't need me to get angry about difficult stuff. She needs me to hold her while she cries. She doesn't need me to retreat because I don't know what to say or do. She needs me to be present, listen to her heart, and lead her by pointing her toward the truth.

And for most of us, one way we can bless our wives mightily is by sharing some of our feelings with them. "I'm fine" just doesn't cut it, fellas. Let her know if you're pained by this season of life. Share your fears if she asks you. Do you feel heartbroken or discouraged? Pessimistic about or paralyzed by what the future may hold? Are you grieving? Then have those conversations with your wife. Pray for wisdom in when to share these things with her, but be present and have open communication regarding the state of your heart as you endure this season of life together.

Now I get it. I come from a family of stuffers who stuffed our emotions. From extreme joy to deep sorrow, you just kind of keep those things to yourself and stay even-keeled (or, as some call it, boring). Because of this, there hadn't been deep conversations that went below the surface, because if we had gone below surface conversation, we might have had to share our heart. This isn't a slam on my family at all. I love them and have a great relationship with them. However, I don't come from a family that often gets into intimate, heartfelt conversations.

I've come a long way over the years, but if I'm honest, I know that my natural bent is to not go to a place where I show the depths of my heart. I still have a tendency to bottle up my emotions and let them fester. The thing I've found to be most helpful is to pour my emotions, my circumstances, and my heart out to God. If this is a desire of yours and you want to know more about how to do this, check out my boss, friend, and mentor Matt Boyers's book *Consuming Christ: Broken and Poured Out for You.* You won't be disappointed!

Men, we tend to keep our emotions to ourselves when facing difficulty, but I found that in our darkest seasons, this did not bless Cathie at all. At times it made her feel like I didn't care. Like I didn't care that we had just lost another baby. Like I didn't care that our world was flipped upside down. I did. I cared a lot. I was crushed. But I found myself bottling that stuff up and retreating when all she wanted me to do was sit and cry with her, grieve with her, and feel helpless and broken with her.

Men, let me encourage you in this. Share what is in your heart with your wife. Talk with her. Be present with her. Just hold her. (Sometimes that's all she wants.) If you don't know what she wants, ask her. In those times of another not-pregnant stick, in those times where you no longer hear the heartbeat, in those times when you hear your doctor say, "I'm sorry," in those times when it feels like there is no hope—in those times, she often feels broken, unlovable, and unable to do what a woman was created to do. So in those times, be present and love the heck out of your wife. You'll never regret doing this. You'll always regret the response of retreating.

I know that it's not our natural reaction to comfort. I want to encourage you to step out of your comfort zone to be a comfort to your wife. Maybe you've never really done this, and it's going to catch her off guard. I can guarantee you that she'll love it. And as we often say around our office when it comes to marriage, "It's not about points, but they don't hurt!" You're going to score *major* points with your wife for comforting and loving her the way she desires. And if she is able physically, you are probably going to get a very happy return, if you know what I mean! Again it's not about points. It's not—not at all. It's about loving your wife and shoring up your marriage. But points don't hurt.

Men, I don't know if you've read this whole book or if your wife just threw it at you and said, "Here, this part of the book is for you; read it." Earlier in the book, Cathie mentioned our friends who led our premarital counseling, and she described the encouragement they gave us to outserve each other. They did not mean that we should do this in a ledger sort of way: "She made me dinner tonight, so I should repay her by doing dishes" or "I cleaned the bathroom today, so he'd better mow the lawn." This would be bad. Very bad. Nothing good comes out of a ledger where we keep track of each other's acts of service. Instead make it a game without keeping track of the score. Seek to outserve your spouse without seeking anything in return. Go over and above, surprise her, do it without her noticing. Men, you'll score points here! *Remember*, though it's not about points, they don't hurt!

Guys, in these seasons of infertility and grief, your wife needs you. I want to challenge you to step up to the plate if you haven't already. If your wife is anything like mine, she's hurting physically, hurting emotionally, and reeling spiritually; she's tired, emotional, and at times irrational. Serve her. Without asking what needs to be done, do it. Dishes, laundry, kids, errands, do what needs to be done. Even if she is capable of doing these tasks, you are communicating that you notice her, that you love her, and that you desire to serve her. She may not notice, may not say thank you, and may even tell you that you did it wrong. It doesn't matter. Love and serve her unconditionally. Give 100 percent to your marriage, even if you do not get what you feel entitled to in return.

Fellas, this is a tough place that we are in. Yes, as husband and wife, there is unity and oneness. You live through infertility together. You have the miscarriage together. You wait together. You do appointments together. You cry together. You hurt together. But when it comes down to it, it's her body feeling the way it does. She's dealing with this in ways that we, as men, will never understand. And so show her grace (which is undeserved kindness).

She's hurting physically in ways you can't imagine. She's struggling with her identity and purpose in ways we men never consider. She's irrational about things because, well, she's a woman. (We love you, ladies!) Love her well through it.

I know that many men don't do this, but I'd encourage you to attend every possible OB-GYN appointment that you can. This communicates that you care, obviously, but it also gives you more insight as to what is going on instead of making her rehash everything she learned at the visit. I can't tell you how good it was for me to be at those appointments with Cathie when we met with Shannon. Shannon was a huge help to me in understanding Cathie's condition and the ways in which I could best serve and support her.

You also will have opportunities to sit by the tub holding her hand while she tries to soak up some level of comfort from the hot water; give her a massage when her body aches, and take time off from work to be with her as her body experiences those miserable days of miscarriage. It is in the midst of these difficult times when she needs to hear, all the more, "This is not your fault, and I love you unconditionally."

This is a journey that none of us would ever ask to be on. This is a journey that, if you are like me, never crossed my mind that I'd end up on until we started it. You don't grow up thinking about getting married and battling infertility and grieving the loss of your babies. So not only is this new but I'm sure most of you were caught completely off guard and don't know how to handle it. Stay unified with your wife. She's your teammate. She's your helpmate. She's your partner in crime. She's yours and you are hers, and you are doing this together. It's hard, I know, but in time, there comes a joy in the fact that you get to do the hard stuff together. I never wanted to endure these horribly difficult things, but I couldn't have asked for a better teammate to live it with, hand in hand. Make sure your wife knows you think the same thing about her.

To the Women

There's not much left to be said that Cathie and Shannon haven't already offered you; however, from the perspective of a man, can I just quickly share with you some ways you can help your husband in this season?

Our culture does an excellent job of painting husbands in a bad light. Fat, drunk, stupid, incompetent, insensitive, lazy, and rude. If you just read that and thought immediately of your husband, please do not tell him that. Think of husbands from *The Simpsons, Everybody Loves Raymond, Family Guy, Modern Family, Peppa Pig* (our kids' favorite), and countless other shows. Idiots. All of them. They show little-to-no love to their wife, and they are insensitive and out of touch when it comes to their wife's needs.

You have an opportunity to help your husband break that stereotype. This takes work on your part though. Please don't think I'm saying that we are insensitive and stupid and that you need to fix us. (We could all use a little help, though.) I'm confident that many husbands are doing a great job of leading, pursuing, loving, serving, and comforting their wives in the midst of difficult circumstances and beyond. However, there are a lot of things that you can do to help us go from doing well to thriving as husbands.

1. **Overcommunicate your needs.** Not in an overbearing way and not with a raised voice. Let us know how we can serve you. Give us opportunities to serve you. If you notice that something needs to be done, don't assume we notice. (We are men, after all; plus we can't read your mind.)

2. **Be gracious when we try to fix it.** Let us know that you simply need some words of affirmation or a hug instead. Cathie did a great job of this by starting out saying, "Honey, I don't need you to fix this, but here's how I'm feeling…" That immediately reminded me not to try and fix things; she just needed a hug and for me to be present with her.

3. **Be mindful of his heart.** He may not be sharing his feelings, but be aware that even if he isn't, he's hurting, anxious, and grieving. Tell him that you'd like to know how he's feeling in the midst of this season as well. This means giving him an opportunity to speak. And when he does, listen. Accept that his feelings may not mirror your own. Appreciate his efforts.

4. **Give him grace when he doesn't seem to be affected.** He is. I promise you that he is. Don't be upset with him if he doesn't cry when you cry or get angry when you get

angry or see eye to eye with you on what steps to take next. Your body and all you are experiencing, unfortunately, remind you of this stuff 24-7. He doesn't have that same gut-wrenching reminder that is always present with you. We all process things differently, so give us grace when we process in other ways.

5. **Simply say, "Will you hold me?"** I'm not sure there were many things in our difficult season that were more healing, more unifying, and more incredible than when we just cuddled. I'm confident enough as a man to admit that I enjoy snuggling with my wife! Seriously, though, there were so many times when I didn't know what to do for Cathie and just wanted to fix it, and she would simply say, "Will you hold me?" Men oftentimes aren't going to initiate this. (I'm sorry; I don't understand us, either.) But we certainly aren't going to pass up the opportunity to cuddle with you. Give us that opportunity. There's a lot of good that comes from this kind of physical intimacy.

Women, you have a lot on your plate here. I'm proud of you. Don't give up. As a man, I'll admit that I still have no idea of the full scope of all that you endure. I watched firsthand what Cathie went through. She explained what she was experiencing, and Shannon told me exactly what Cathie would endure. And even after living through it all firsthand over the course of years, I'm still quite clueless. Not because I didn't care or wasn't attuned to the situation but because it's just a different ball game when you're the one in the woman's body.

As men, we're never quite going to get it. But I do know this. It's hard. This is really, really hard. We are praying for you as you endure, as you take next steps, and as we, as couples, walk hand in hand together to face what is yet to come.

As Cathie has mentioned, I'm a pastor at our church. Cathie and I have walked alongside those who are grieving in a multitude of ways. We've faced our own infertility issues, anxiously endured surgeries, lost four babies, heard heartbeats and then didn't hear them, and cried more tears than I care to count. I've lost family members, friends, students, and those I worship with and live life with. I've battled through some serious seasons of grief.

I say all this to get to this one point that has encouraged me greatly over the years, and I believe it can encourage you as well moving forward. In the book of Lamentations, Jeremiah is grieved. He has lost everything and everyone.

As someone who has placed my trust in Jesus, I have found so much peace and healing from Lamentations 3. Don't know or believe the Bible? That's OK. Can I simply encourage you to keep reading, though? The preacher in me needs to speak a little truth quickly, and Cathie didn't trust me with more than this little section (kidding…kinda). So at least humor me, and give me a chance.

Break down the word *lamentations*, and you see the word *lament*. What does it mean to lament? Lamenting merely means to cry out in sadness, sorrow or pain. I'd say that about sums up most of our feelings when it comes to this topic of infertility. Let's dig a little deeper, though. In the Hebrew language, the word used for the name of the book of Lamentations is *Eikah*. Oh, you don't know Hebrew? Me, either! (I may be writing a chapter in a book right now, but trust me, I'm not that smart.) I find it curiously interesting that *Eikah* means *how*.

Does that word sound familiar? "*How* is this happening?" "*How* did we get to this place?" "*How* am I going to move forward?" "*How* could God allow this?" "*How* is our story going to end?" "*How* do I do this?" "*How* am I ever going to find peace?"

How? It's a small word—with a *lot* behind it, huh? At some point, I imagine, we've all had that moment of disbelief when we slowly shake our head and ask, "How?"

In the third chapter of Lamentations, Jeremiah is grieving heavily. He spends the first sixteen verses talking about how God has afflicted him. He goes on to talk about his lack of peace and the fact that he's even forgotten what happiness is. He says that the thought of his suffering is bitter beyond words. Have you been there? Are you currently there? Maybe you feel like you've been stuck there?

But he changes his thinking. He turns to God. And so can you. Jeremiah says,

> I will never forget this awful time, as I grieve over my loss. Yet I still dare to hope when I remember this: The faithful love of the LORD never ends! His mercies never cease. Great is his faithfulness; his mercies begin afresh each morning. I say to myself, "The LORD is my inheritance; therefore, I will hope in him! (Lam. 3:20–24, NLT).

Your time of grieving is a time that you'll never forget. Some of you are thinking back on those tough seasons. Others are in the throes of that season. Know that this season will always be with you in some way. You won't grieve this deeply forever, but you also aren't going to forget about it. I'm not going to preach to you here, but I want to share a simple truth with you: in your grief, God hears you, and he'll respond to you. He's faithful like that. Oh, and he loves you a lot, so your season of grief also grieves his heart. This heavy stuff you're facing isn't the way the world was created to be. Try turning to God in this season, and see how he responds. Cathie and I have done this, and we'll shout from the rooftops to tell you that God has given us much peace as we've trusted him through it all. You and I both know you'd love to experience peace in your heart right about now.

It's been a joy to allow our story to be redeemed so that others may be encouraged by it. We pray that your story would be redeemed as well!

Appendix B
Interviews from a Male Perspective

Quotes from husbands who have struggled with infertility

1. Would it have made a difference to you whether the cause of infertility was related to your health or your wife's?
For my situation, I figured it was going to be my issue because of my accident. I'd rather take the blame than my wife.
—Brian

It did not. It wasn't that it was somebody's problem, because that never allows resolution. It doesn't matter the reason why. The fact was we weren't able to have children, and nobody should shoulder blame for something like that when it is completely out of [our] control. I'd have loved to have taken that problem from her and made it my own so that she didn't have to carry that burden though.
—Jake

Not necessarily. It was painful. No one was at fault; the problem wasn't hers or mine. It was ours. But I remember when we started investigating what the barriers were, we started with my test. Besides all the awkwardness that went into that, I do remember thinking, "What if it's me? What if I 'can't deliver'?" I remember wondering how I would deal with that. If anything, having to entertain some of those thoughts helped me empathize a bit whenever I sensed she might be falling into thinking it was *her* issue.
—Trevor

Yes, it would have broken my heart either way, but if I would have been the infertile one, I would have been completely devastated.
—Jayson

It was my fault. It made a huge deal. Would it have made a difference if it were her? Maybe. I've dealt with the reason (of why it was
my fault) for years, and I'm tired of it. I didn't want to pay money
for a kid because it was my fault. I was pissed I had to do it.

—Hunter

2. Do men think of infertility differently if the cause is a male factor versus a female factor? How so?

I do. Infertility attacks the heart of what it means to be a man. If
it is the man's issue, he seems to feel like he is less of a man. As
I have learned more about the process, it happens to men more
than we realize. There are so many aspects of a woman's body
that you can test and make changes to. Men are really just a one-
trick pony, and you can only really change the sperm.

—Brian

I didn't. I can't speak for others; I'm not sure.

—Jake

I really don't know. I don't think I do.

—Trevor

Not really, we would just feel terrible if it was our fault.

—Jayson

I think it's an individual factor. It's up to the person. What it came
down to for me was doing it for my wife. The motivation to do it
was for my wife. It took me a while to put all my stuff aside. If it
would have been my wife and I was normal, I don't know how I
would have looked at it. I had to stop being selfish about my stuff
to give her what she wanted.

—Hunter

3. Did you attend doctor visits with your spouse? Why or why not?

I attended all doctor visits when it was appropriate. I did not take part in any of her blood tests and ultrasounds when we were going through IVF. I wanted to be part of the process as much as I could.

—Brian

Absolutely. If it had any importance at all, there was never a question. In the same way that we never looked at a pregnancy test without each other, we didn't do this stuff alone. We're one, unified, together, and that doesn't change when one of us has a more personal doctor's appointment. This was our journey together, so we did this together as a team. And more than anything, why would I allow the person I love more than anyone else in the world to do a stressful doctor visit alone? We do this stuff together!

—Jake

Yes, all of them. It was an *us* issue. It was *our* longing/desire. I cannot *fathom* either of us trying to do it alone. And eventually, having found our way into Creighton, that was one of the things that was stressed. Though she was doing most of the tracking work and other things, I found ways to share it. I thanked her for going through the endless process of adding a step to her daily bathroom routines. I was the one who eventually gave her the progesterone shots throughout the process. As *awful* and *gut-wrenching* as the up-and-down roller coaster of those couple [of] years was, we indeed did grow closer together. It could have easily torn us apart, but it was a strengthening season of our marriage and our shared faith/reliance on Christ. Ultimately it was a season of placing God's intentions, without knowing how those

would work out, in front of our desires—as biblical and reasonable as those seemed.

—Trevor

Yes, because marriage is a *we* thing, not a *me* thing.

—Jayson

I went to the important ones. I was there to support. I was curious
and wanted to be a part of it. Sometimes I had to miss because
of work.

—Hunter

4. What were some of the emotions you experienced?

Frustration—I didn't want to be forced to make it so clinical.
Sadness—I didn't even get a chance to have a child naturally.
Joy—I was able to have a child even though it seemed like the
cards are stacked against me.

—Brian

Ugh. This could take a while. (The emotions were many.) We had
days when we felt both overjoyed and in despair. We would go
from optimistic, excited, at peace, relaxed, and feeling certain…
and not too long after that, feeling annoyed, powerless, pessimistic, scared, and completely heartbroken.

For me, personally, I was a roller coaster of emotion, and if I'm
completely honest, my heart hardened a lot during that season. I
became irritable, angry, and felt a bitterness I never had before. I
was angry with people who had what we couldn't. I was enraged
by those who took for granted what we could never have. I felt
crushed when insensitive words were spoken, and I had to keep
a smile on my face when I really wanted to punch them. It was a
season of grief that I didn't know existed. I didn't understand the

emotions that could go along with such circumstances. I'm not an overly emotional person, but that was a season that brought them all out in me.

—Jake

All of them: anger, frustration, excitement of expectation, disappointment, weariness, apathy, numbness, etc. Desperation and helplessness were two of the most reoccurring, and the fatigue... the fatigue of persevering through the process—the communication process—talking about it when she wanted to and I didn't or refraining when she seemed to have reached her limit. The fatigue of just trying: sex wasn't fun; it was a duty. It was on the clock. It was scheduled; it was awful. And frankly, we are healthy sexually, but I still feel like that season has forever affected our sexual relationship/rhythm. I remember feeling like I could finally empathize with women. The guys' joke was always, "Well, it must be fun practicing." No, no it wasn't. It got old, fast. And you felt like a selfish idiot thinking, "I don't want to have sex. You just want me for my body...in particular, my penis." I felt like a stud dog or stud horse: just deposit your semen and go. It was awful...which didn't help at all.

—Trevor

Anger: infertility made me angry all the time. Sadness: I felt terrible watching my wife struggle with this. It makes you feel helpless.

—Jayson

From being angry to feeling sorry for myself, fighting the system to feeling sorry for my wife and why my issues were causing her to not get what she wanted in life. There was heartbreak when things didn't take [off].

—Hunter

5. How was your emotional process different than your wife's?

My end of it all was short and sweet. I gave the doctor my sample, and I was mostly done. My wife's journey was much longer and in depth.

—Brian

I process everything inwardly. She's a verbal processor. More than her wanting to process it verbally herself, she desired to hear my heart. I didn't do a good job of sharing my heart with her during this season. I think there was so much emotion that I not only didn't want to share it, but I knew if I did, I would fall apart...and as a man, I didn't want to fall apart in front of my wife. I wanted to be strong. Not justifying my actions there...But as a man, I felt the need to stay strong, put on a good mask, and be the rock that she could lean on.

Because I kept it in and I didn't pour it out to the Lord well, either, that junk festered in me and just made me miserable. I wish I had processed that season differently, but it definitely helped me move forward in making sure that I—number one—poured that stuff out on Jesus, and—number two—let my wife in on the state of my heart.

—Jake

I'm sure it was quite different. She's a woman; I am a man. It had to be different. But honestly I'm not sure how. I think we went through a lot of the same emotions. What was different was not which emotions but who was experiencing what emotion when and how long or how intensely. On top of dealing with our own emotions personally, we had to be acutely attentive and aware of how the other person was feeling. Praise Jesus, each of us would say his grace allowed us to be attuned to each other while nursing our own individual pain and struggles.

—Trevor

Wife: emotional at all times. Me: I keep myself and my emotions internalized, which is not necessarily a good thing at all.

—Jayson

I was keeping everything inside. She lets everything out. She wore it on her sleeve, and I was guarded until I couldn't be anymore.

—Hunter

6. Did you consider leaving your wife if she couldn't have a child? Why or why not?
No. It is all about our relationship. Having a child would have been icing on the cake.

—Brian

Never once. I didn't marry her to bear children. I married her because I love her and wanted to spend the rest of my life with her. Circumstances aren't going to change that.

—Jake

Hell, no. But it did leave us prayerfully wondering, "Lord, are you keeping us mobile? Is this a timing issue trying to prompt us to relocate to do mission work internationally? Are you wanting us to explore adoption? We don't want to adopt, just to get what we want. But if you're moving us that way, OK." It's a crazy, crazy process that gets you questioning, wondering, and trying to find explanations for all kinds of things that simply can't be explained—medically, spiritually, or otherwise. But, no, divorce would be cruel, sinful, and the epitome of selfish[ness]. This was *our* struggle, *our* desire, *our* journey. About the only thing that wasn't questioned was the *our* of it all.

—Trevor

No, never. She is my wife, always.

—Jayson

7. Did you feel adequately informed about infertility during the process?
Yes. Going through IVF, we got to know much more about fertility than any class.

—Brian

I did. We had an incredible doctor. (Thanks, Shannon!) She walked this journey with us and couldn't have helped us along more. We understood what was going on (even though we didn't like it), and she made sure to always keep lines of communication open. We were blessed!

—Jake

No, and I'm not sure I would have wanted to be. The things we valued and our rationale for thinking through our options and processing the whole struggle seemed so different than people's opinions or approaches to fertility—be it the medical community, friends, family, or whatever. The only thing I wish I would have known from the get-go is that most, from the medical side, seem to approach it as a problem of probability: "Well, if we do this, there'd be this percentage of success." Or, "If we started here, we might be able to jump the percentage." It felt like no one could get to the heart of the medical issue; it was just a probability to achieve what we all wanted. And for us, the end didn't necessarily justify or define the means.

—Trevor

Yes, we were kept up to speed on everything.

—Jayson

8. If you had to go back and do the infertility process again, how would you do it differently?
I would do it again. Not much I would want to change, except for the cost.

—Brian

Pray more. Talk about it more. Ask Jesus to change my heart more. Allow more people in. I put up walls and became quite angry. This was toward family, friends, coworkers, and God himself. I'm thankful for his faithfulness to us through the journey and how he provided for us in ways we could have never imagined. He was with us through it all, and I think I so often got caught up in the pain/anger of it all that I kept my focus there instead of on him, especially when I needed him most.

—Jake

I'm not sure we would change a thing. Granted our season of struggle was only two to three years. So one could say we got what we wanted in the end. But we struggled with both sons. And yet we received much more than two sons from the process: an incredible appreciation for and perspective on having sons and incredible love and support from family and friends. (Sure, some was awful, but I think most of it was well intentioned.) Greater growth with each other. Deeper faith. And the list goes on, and frankly looking at it feels trite or cliché. But it's profound and impossible to articulate all that grew out of that struggle.

—Trevor

After we found out that we were "normal," I would prefer if we had stopped using meds.

—Jayson

I thought it actually brought us closer together. The process of shots actually brought us closer together. It obviously brought conflicts, as you would assume it would.

—Hunter

9. How did you see infertility affect your marriage?
We have always had a really great, open relationship (not the swinging type of open), and we were able to process everything together. We hit highs and hit some lows, but we were always on the same page.

—Brian

Truly, over that time, I think it drew us closer together. We went to battle together, fought as a team, and came out beaten and bruised but closer than ever. At the same time, I think there were emotional wounds from that season that forced us to put up some walls, and unfortunately I think we put some walls up toward each other—not on purpose, but we just became hardened and closed off for a time, and we did that to each other, unfortunately.

—Jake

Not a ton more to say here. It tested it and proved it genuine.

—Trevor

Positive: made the moment of finding out we were pregnant that much sweeter. Negative: everything else. Fighting constantly. Tension was high. Sex felt like a job. We could never feel like we were on the same page. Do remember, this was a two-year process.

—Jayson

Check yourself and make sure you're ready for it—all the self-induced embarrassments and insecurities—because the money leaves your pocket (for IVF) really fast. Make sure you and your wife are on the same page. Make sure you are doing it all for the right reasons. Make sure you're in a good place before you get going and have asked the tough questions because it is an emotional roller coaster. You don't want to bring the kid into a divorce.

—Hunter

10. If you could advise another man going through the process of infertility, what would you say?
You have to be open and honest about the process. There is no fault to be placed on you or the wife. Work through all of it together.

—Brian

Run to Jesus. Pour out those questions, hurts, and afflictions on him, and let him give your heart peace. Also find another man whom you can talk to and who can encourage you daily. Don't shut down, don't put up walls, and certainly don't keep your wife at arm's length. Your wife is going through more than you will ever be able to imagine. Love her. Comfort her. Hold her. Pray for her. Listen to her. Be silent with her. Just be.

—Jake

Drop any tough-guy image or expectations. Cry with your wife. Talk to other guys. Vent your anger and frustration vertically [pray], but don't be afraid to invite your wife in joining you to vent vertically. People mean well but speak awful, flippant, idiotic things. Don't take it personally, and don't let your own pain and junk justify awful, flippant, or idiotic responses from yourself.

—Trevor

Pray and be patient and emotionally available to your wife. Nothing means more than your support.

—Jayson

11. What was it like as a man to not be able to fix the problem for your wife?

It was more of a problem that I couldn't fix—my own problem.

—Brian

Incredibly hard. I tried *really* hard to fix this. Even in the midst of realizing I couldn't, I was just stupid enough that I kept trying. "Maybe if I say this, it will make her feel better. Or maybe if I do this, it will fix everything." *Wrong*! You can't fix this, no matter how handy you may be. But you can give a *lot* of healing to your wife by simply loving the heck out of her. Fight the temptation to try and fix it. It's our natural bent, men…but don't fall for it…We don't have the power to fix this one. But God will give you the words, actions, and energy to continue pouring out love on your wife. That's what she really needs.

—Jake

Humbling and helpful. And because it truly was *our* problem and not *her* problem, I couldn't try fixing too much. I joined her in longing for a fix—longing for a solution. But unlike all the other stupid times I tried to fix things, I frankly didn't have the solution to fix this. And I'm *so* thankful that we both had the same hesitations, reservations, and eventually conviction in regard to not using some of the fixes offered or recommended by others.

—Trevor

The worst thing I have experienced. I am a fixer. It was like torture.

—Jayson

I didn't care. Hear me out. I had told her from the beginning of our dating relationship that I might not be able to have kids. She knew about my problems. It was a problem neither of us could fix.

I got my support from the bottle. I would caution anyone deciding to use that as a coping skill. I did need to share my feelings. If you don't have someone to talk to, pay someone for therapy, so be careful when drinking your emotions. How is that for a public-service announcement?

—Hunter

Appendix C
How to Support Those Who Are Infertile

Advice given by men and women who have survived infertility

What is some advice that you would give to someone trying to support an infertile couple?

"Ask them what they need without assuming you know, even if you yourself have experienced infertility."

"Don't be afraid to show up. Be present with them."

"If they have lost a pregnancy (especially if they have named the baby), don't be afraid to acknowledge important milestones. Use the name they chose to refer to the baby. I got flowers on the due date of a baby I had miscarried, and I will never forget what that meant to me."

"Don't be afraid of awkward questions. Questions accompanied by a genuine listening ear is one of the best gifts you can give. I think too often we are afraid of bringing it up because we don't want to add to the pain. Ninety-nine percent of the time, it's on that couple's mind, and even if you ask the 1 percent, they aren't going to mind being asked genuine questions in love. Don't be paralyzed by awkwardness."

"I would say that it's very important to really listen to the couple. Sometimes they may want to relate or need validation or help, but other times they may just want to be heard—without the offer of advice or sympathy—and would appreciate a sense of normalcy...not to feel like their life is completely defined by infertility."

"Don't tell them stories about other people. Just listen. Tell them you love them. Tell them you're praying for them. Tell them you can't understand and you're sorry for what they're going through. Tell them you don't know what to say rather than filling the time with empty words that may do more harm than silence. Hug them. Sit in silence with them. Ask them if there's anything you can do for them. Invite them out for distractions, and don't bring it up. Don't ever ask if they are pregnant yet."

"Accept whatever fertility decisions they make; it's their decision to make, and unless they ask your opinion, don't give it."

"Be patient with them. Be there with them."

"Honor the boundaries they set forth for themselves or their marriage."

"Be teachable, and let them tell you how to help them."

"Don't give them your two cents about how to conceive a baby."

"Don't tell them your religious or political views on medicinal interventions."

"Don't make false promises or give false hope with all the other success stories you have heard about or experienced. Someone else's success doesn't guarantee mine. We all have different stories—some with the outcome we want, some not."

Appendix D
Final Thoughts from Dr. Sutherland

Stop! Breathe! Remember that your situation does not define who you are. Some women feel like their femininity or womanhood is called into question when there are infertility issues. This is a medical issue just like people would think of heart disease, cancer, diabetes, and so on. Your infertility is not a question of who you are as a woman—as long as you don't let it.

There are so many pathways in our life. Some we handle well, and some we don't. Don't let this experience change you for the worse. Don't miss out on the rest of life while you are on this journey. Grow from it. Be better; be stronger.

Life becomes so hectic, especially with instant information of the media and Internet. You can get caught up in a false reality. Continue to do fun things, live your life, and don't shut people out for fear of being hurt.

All of us hurt as some point in our lives. We don't know other people's stories, but these hurts make us who we are. It's up to you how you will be affected and how you relate to other people. When there are so few things we can be in control of, embrace the one thing you can control: your attitude.

References

2012. *Holy Bible,* New Living Translation. Carol Streams, Illinois: Tyndall House Foundation.

American Psychiatric Association. 2013. Desk Reference to the Diagnostic Criteria from the DSM-5. Washington, DC: American Psychiatric Association.

Boyers, Matt. 2014. *Consuming Christ: Broken and Poured Out for You.* Archbold, OH: Matthew Boyers.

Goldstein, Jerald S. 2011. http://www.resolve.org/about-infertility/medical-conditions/secondary-infertility-evaluation-and-treatment.html.

Gottman, John M. 1999. *The Seven Principles for Making Marriage Work: A Practical Guide from the Country's Foremost Relationship Expert.* New York: Three Rivers Press.

Kübler-Ross, Elisabeth. 1969. *On Death and Dying: What the Dying Have to Teach Doctors, Nurses, Clergy, and Their Own Families.* New York: Macmillan Publishing Company, Inc.

Lewis, C. S. 1971. *The Four Loves.* Boston, MA: Houghton Mifflin Harcourt.

Lucado, Max. 2001. *Traveling Light: Releasing the Burdens You Were Never Intended to Bear.* Nashville, TN: Thomas Nelson.

Rogers, Fred. 2003. *The World According to Mister Rogers: Important Things to Remember.* New York: Hyperion ebook.

Tolkien, J. R. R. 2012. *The Fellowship of the Ring*. Boston, MA: Houghton Mifflin Harcourt.

Wright, H. Norman. 2003. *The New Guide to Crisis and Trauma Counseling: A Practical Guide for Ministers, Counselors and Lay Counselors*. Ventura, CA: Regal Books.

About the Authors

Cathie Quillet is an independent marriage and family therapist, practicing in northwest Ohio. With eight years of wedded bliss under their belts, Cathie and her husband love all things family and community. If there is a free moment, Cathie can be caught relaxing with a cup of coffee and spending time with her three men.

Dr. Shannon Sutherland is an osteopathic obstetrician-gynecologist in northwest Ohio. Shannon moved around the East Coast before calling Toledo home. She is passionate about women's health and helping couples complete their family.

Made in the USA
Monee, IL
30 June 2022

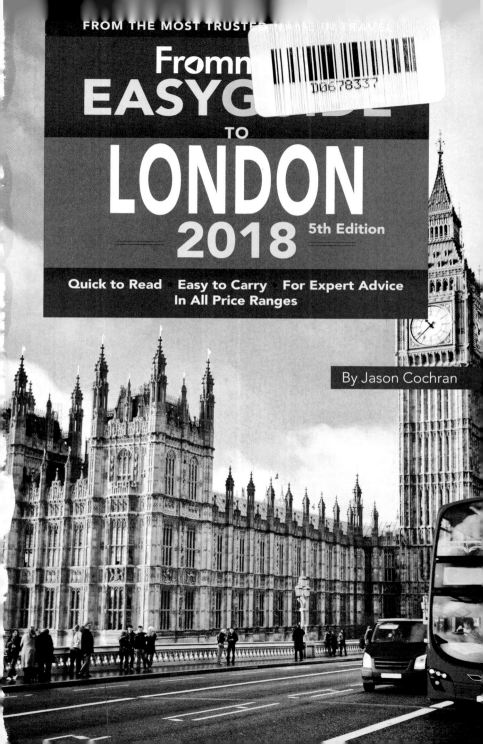

Frommer's
EASYGUIDE
TO
LONDON
2018 5th Edition

**Quick to Read   Easy to Carry   For Expert Advice
In All Price Ranges**

By Jason Cochran

The neo-Gothic Tower Bridge spans the
Thames near the Tower of London.

FROMMER'S STAR RATINGS SYSTEM

Every hotel, restaurant, and attraction listed in this guide has been ranked for quality and
value. Here's what the stars mean:

 Recommended
Highly Recommended
A must! Don't miss!

AN IMPORTANT NOTE

The world is a dynamic place. Hotels change ownership, restaurants hike their prices, museums alter their opening hours, and buses and trains change their routings. And all of this can
occur in the several months after our authors have visited, inspected, and written about
these hotels, restaurants, museums, and transportation services. Though we have made val-
iant efforts to keep all our information fresh and up-to-date, some few changes can inevitably occur in the periods before a revised edition of this guidebook is published. So please
bear with us if a tiny number of the details in this book have changed. Please also note that
we have no responsibility or liability for any inaccuracy or errors or omissions, or for inconvenience, loss, damage, or expenses suffered by anyone as a result of assertions in this guide.

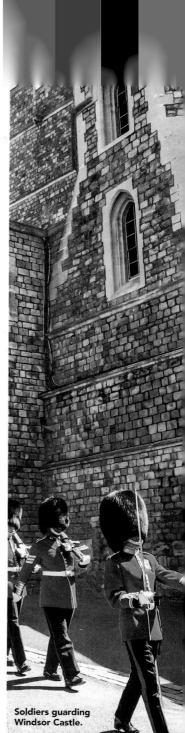

Soldiers guarding
Windsor Castle.

A LOOK AT LONDON

Throw away any preconceived images you may have of a gray, button-downed, or reserved London. The weather may occasionally be soggy, but London is a Technicolor cornucopia of tantalizing things to do and see. From the eye-popping contemporary art at the Tate Modern to the jumble of upscale shopping arcades near Piccadilly Circus, from the bird's-eye views over the Thames from the London Eye to the bursting picnic hampers spread out in the green grass of Regent's Park—London dazzles wherever you look. Whether you explore the city by foot, boat, tube, or bus, expect a bright mixture of architecture, creativity, and culture to meet you around every turn.

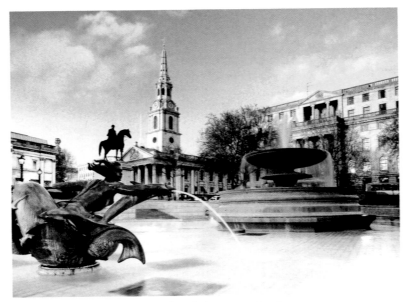

Trafalgar Square has always been one of London's great meeting places.

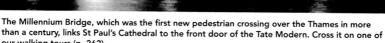

LONDON ATTRACTIONS

The Millennium Bridge, which was the first new pedestrian crossing over the Thames in more than a century, links St Paul's Cathedral to the front door of the Tate Modern. Cross it on one of our walking tours (p. 262).

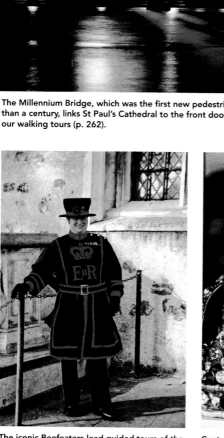

The iconic Beefeaters lead guided tours of the Tower of London (p. 164).

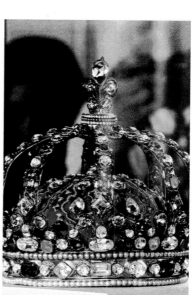

Centuries of imperial wealth are on display in the vaults of the Crown Jewels at the Tower of London.

V

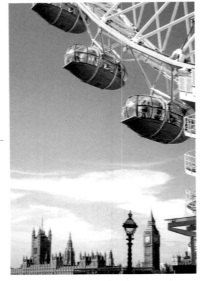

Taking a slow spin over the Thames on the London Eye (p. 154).

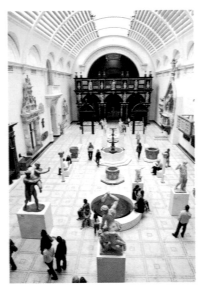

The popular Victoria & Albert Museum (p. 148) honors the most beautiful decorative objects in the world.

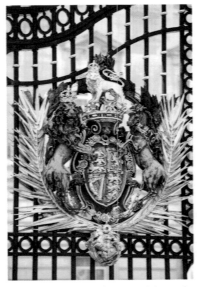

The lion and the chained unicorn of the royal coat of arms of the United Kingdom.

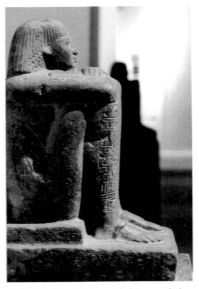

Antiquities from all of recorded time pack the huge British Museum (p. 113), Britain's most popular tourist attraction.

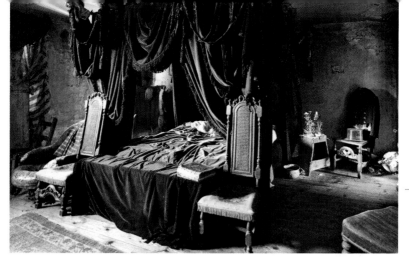

A visit to the Dennis Severs House (p. 170) feels like traveling through time to 19th-century London.

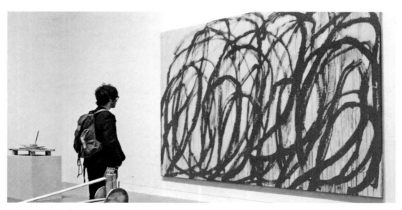

ABOVE: **Tate Modern (p. 155), a superlative contemporary-art collection in a rehabbed power plant, is one of London's cultural landmarks.** BELOW: **The Palm House at the Royal Botanic Gardens (p. 180) is one of the most important iron-and-glass Victorian buildings in the world.**

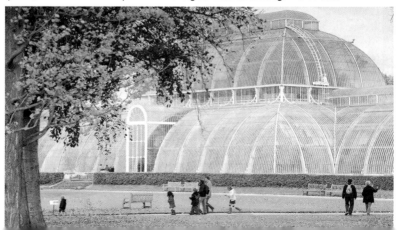

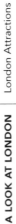

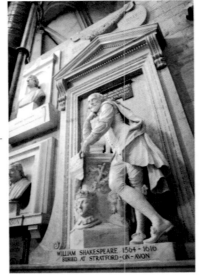

The country's greatest artists, writers, and performers are buried or memorialized at Westminster Abbey's Poet's Corner (p. 136).

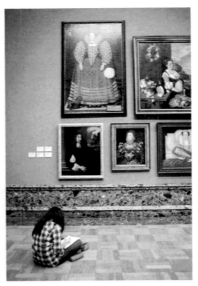

Tate Britain (p. 132) collects the best of the country's paintings and sculpture—and it's free to visit.

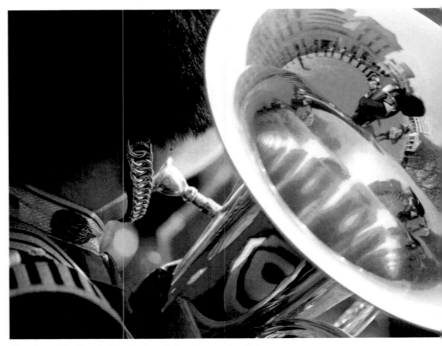

Changing of the Guard at Buckingham Palace is a popular photo op.

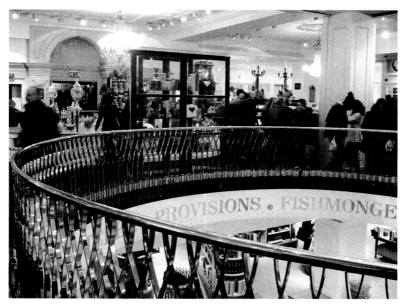

You can't say you know London if you haven't taken the Tube, the world's first underground railway. Its first segments opened in 1863, and each stop has a unique design.

Fortnum & Mason (p. 203) is an opulent department store for gourmet foods, teas, and chocolates—it's literally the queen's grocery store.

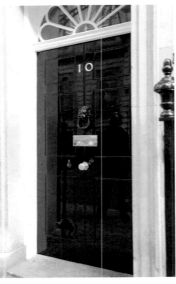

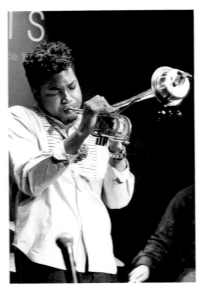

10 Downing St., home of the prime minister (p. 256).

Since the 1960s, stylish Ronnie Scott's (p. 241) has been London's premier club for such head-liners as American trumpeter Christian Scott.

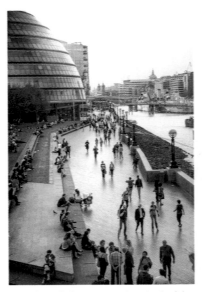

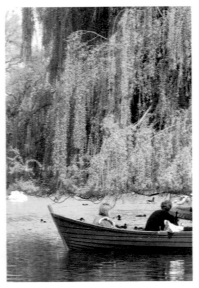

Once disused, the entire southern bank of the Thames is now alive with walkers day and night.

Locals from North London relax in Regent's Park (p. 191), where you'll find the London Zoo, an open-air theater, and vistas from Prim-rose Hill.

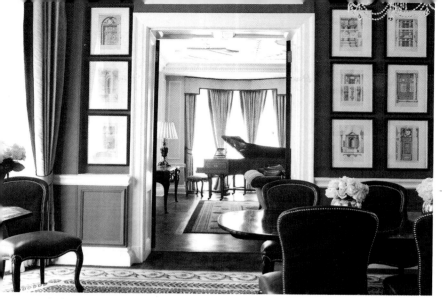

The hospitality at Claridge's (p. 52), which has catered to travelers since the 1800s, is considered a benchmark for luxury hotels around the world.

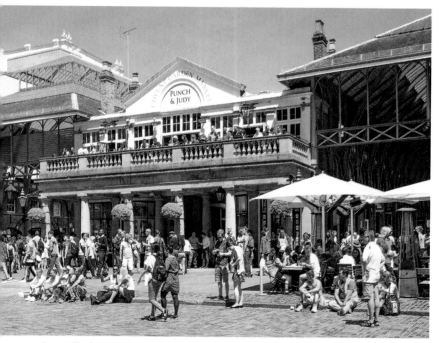

Covent Garden, once a common man's market, is now a central district for boutique shopping, dining, street performances, theater, and pubs.

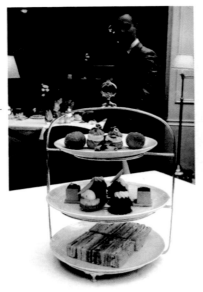

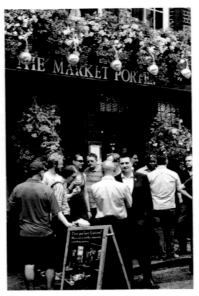

If you must indulge in the ritual of afternoon tea (and why not?), the Lanesborough Hotel's version is possibly London's classiest (p. 53).

The Market Porter (p. 104) pub appeared in the Harry Potter films.

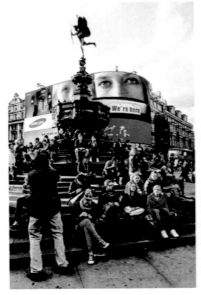

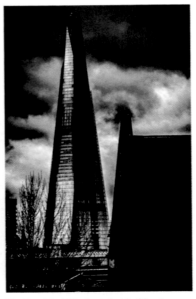

The "Eros" fountain in Picadilly Circus is a London fixture—but does it really depict Eros? See p. 127.

The Shard (p. 157), the tallest building in Europe, is visible from every quarter of town.

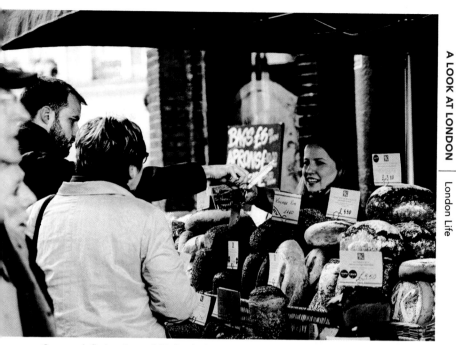

Gourmands flock to Borough Market for local delicacies, fine street food, and elbow-to-elbow grazing. See p. 95.

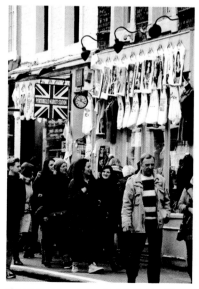

The weekend market at Portobello Road is touristy but fun (p. 222).

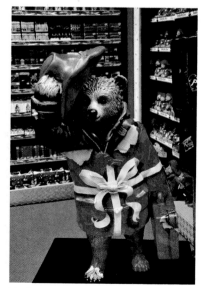

Hamleys toy store (p. 219) is a classic stop for families.

DAY TRIPS FROM LONDON

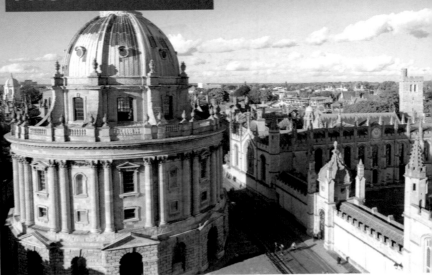

The neoclassical Radcliffe Camera library rises above Oxford University in what poet Matthew Arnold called "the City of Dreaming Spires."

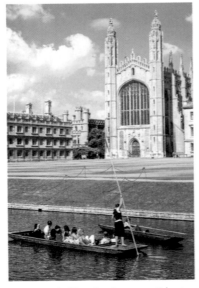

Punting on the River Cam is an essential outing for students at the University of Cambridge (p. 296).

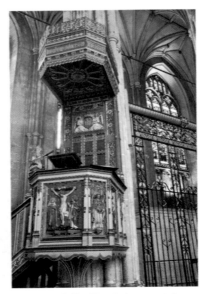

Ornate details like this polychrome pulpit enliven the austere beauty of Canterbury Cathedral (p. 304), one of the world's most historic churches.

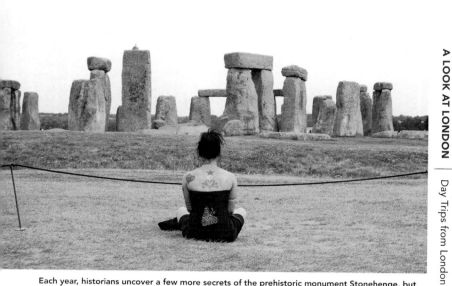

Each year, historians uncover a few more secrets of the prehistoric monument Stonehenge, but we may never unravel all of its mysteries. See p. 302.

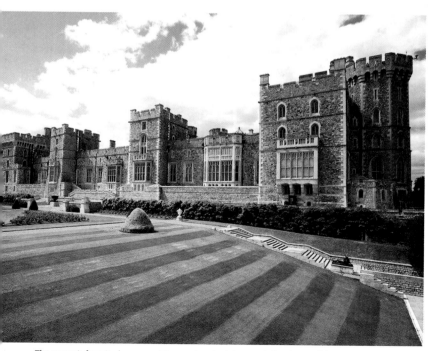

The queen's favorite home, and the modern burial grounds for the royal family, Windsor Castle is easily reached from London by train. See p. 286.

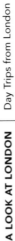

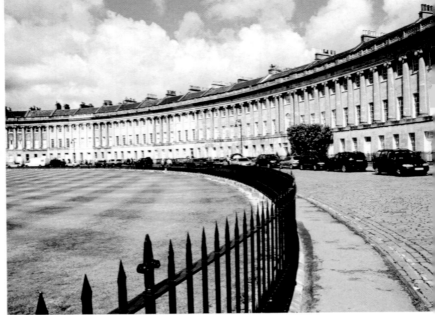

The elegant sweep of the Royal Crescent, a masterpiece of Georgian neoclassical architecture, dates to the 1760s, when Bath (p. 288) was England's most fashionable spa town.

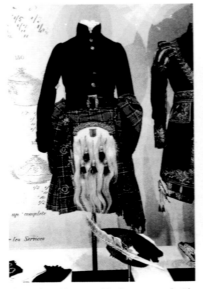

The Fashion Museum of Bath was started with the collection of Doris Langley Moore, a brilliant writer who also costumed Katharine Hepburn in *The African Queen*.

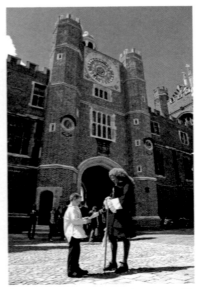

Curators at Hampton Court Palace (p. 179) fill the day with interactive performances by costumed historical characters.

THE BEST OF LONDON

Whether you realize it or not, London shaped your destiny. There's hardly a quarter of the globe that London, as the seat of England's government, hasn't changed. The United States was founded in reaction to London's edicts. Australia was peopled with London's criminals. Modern Canada, South Africa, and New Zealand were cultivated from London. India's course was irrevocably changed by the aspirations of London businessmen, as were the lives of millions of African slaves who were shipped around the world while Londoners lined their pockets with profits. That you bought this book, written in English somewhere other than in England, is evidence of London's reach across time and distance. And its dominion continues to this day: London is the world's most popular destination for foreign tourists.

London is inexhaustible—you could tour it for months and barely get to know it. Few cities support such a variety of people living in remarkable harmony. In 2016, this historically Christian country even elected a Muslim mayor. That diversity makes London like a cut diamond: Approach it from a different angle each day, and it presents an entirely fresh shape and color. From famous stories to high style, London is many things in every moment.

But at this moment, London holds its breath. Two monumental shifts—Britain's exit from its membership in the European Union (Brexit) and the passage of a beloved monarch after a record-breaking reign—will inevitably mold this place into something new, yet no one is confident about how these dual shocks will alter the color of the city and the mood of the nation. London is already an extremely difficult place to live. Foreigners have been overjoyed by the depression in the value of the British pound—it's cheaper to visit London right now than it has been in a generation. But locals aren't as excited. They pay the highest rate in the world for their public transit, and it's the fourth-most-expensive city for housing—the average monthly rent for a one-bedroom outside the center of the city is £1,600, but the average salary is only £300 more. Will industry trickle away? Are the high times coming to an end? For now, London waits.

LONDON'S best ATTRACTIONS

- **British Museum** (p. 113): Some of the most astounding treasures of the classical world are housed in one overwhelmingly glorious neoclassical building.
- **British Library** (p. 109): The finest and rarest books on the planet, plus the Magna Carta, are laid open for your eyes.
- **Churchill War Rooms** (p. 129): A time capsule of the tense days of World War II and the most advanced biographical museum in existence.
- **Museum of London** (p. 159): Beside a remnant of a Roman wall, the city's spectacular story is retold with the nonstop dazzle of precious finds.
- **National Gallery** (p. 122): Some 2,000 masterpieces, the cream of every genre, reside at what may be the best fine art collection in the world.
- **Natural History Museum** (p. 146): For kids, it's all about the dinosaurs, but this "cathedral of nature" has major chops as a research facility, too.
- **St Paul's Cathedral** (p. 161): Sir Christopher Wren's masterpiece is the icon of London and a shrine to historic events and people.

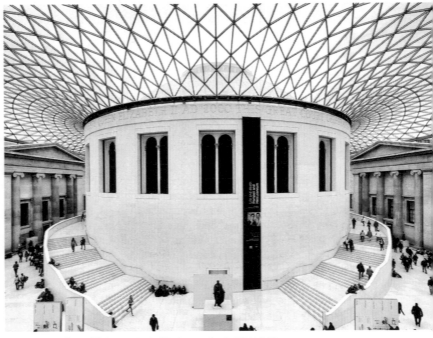

A stunning modern addition nestles inside the neoclassical British Museum.

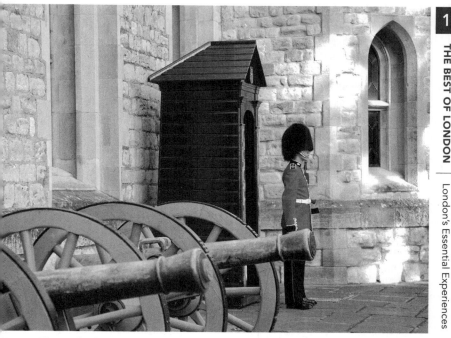

The guard and cannons at the Tower of London stand ready to impress.

- ✓ **Tate Modern** (p. 155): Bankside's hymn to the "shock of the new," a former power station, has just completed a milestone expansion.
- ✓ **Tower of London** (p. 164): Britain's gruesome underbelly and its glittering Crown Jewels coexist in one sprawling city castle of stone.
- **Victoria & Albert Museum** (p. 148): Always evolving and growing, this is probably the world's finest collection of decorative arts.
- ✓ **Westminster Abbey** (p. 134): Be awed by Britain's ancient spiritual heart, where nearly 1,000 years of monarchs have been crowned and many are buried.

LONDON'S essential EXPERIENCES

- **Promenading on South Bank:** In 1957, the Thames was declared "biologically dead." Today, it flows with life. Alongside it, as restaurants, bars, and creative developments continue to pop up, a walk along the South Bank from Westminster Bridge to Tower Bridge has become one of the world's great promenades. The ever-changing perspective from Parliament to the Tower is ceaselessly inspiring.

o **Following in Royal Footsteps:** London is where some of the most famous characters in history played their scenes. Nearly every British monarch since 1066 was crowned in **Westminster Abbey** (p. 134). Henry VIII strutted around **Hampton Court Palace** (p. 179), Charles I lost his head at the **Banqueting House** (p. 138), and Queen Elizabeth resides at **Buckingham Palace** (p. 128) and **Windsor Castle** (p. 286). And the story continues: The future King George VII and sister Princess Charlotte were diapered in **Kensington Palace** (p. 144).

o **Flying High on the London Eye:** Ride to the top of our generation's contribution to London's beloved landmarks for a far-reaching shot

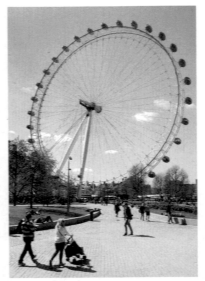

The London Eye on the South Bank is best visited in early evening for spectacular views.

of the cityscape. Time your trip for early evening as the sun starts to sink and the lights come on across the metropolis. See p. 154.

o **Climbing the Dome of St Paul's Cathedral:** Wren's baroque masterpiece stirs emotion in everyone who lays eyes on its lead-coated wooden dome. But it's the climb to the Golden Gallery for a 360° panorama that will stay with you forever. As for Wren, he was forced to add the balustrade for Queen Anne. "Ladies think nothing well without an edging," he complained. See p. 161.

o **Immersing Yourself in World War II:** More than 70 years later, the Blitz still isn't far from many Londoners' minds. Dig into the power of their resistance at the superlative time capsule of the **Churchill War Rooms** (p. 129), the immersive **Museum of London Docklands** (p. 172), the floating military museum **HMS** *Belfast* (p. 158), and the top-secret code breaking headquarters of **Bletchley Park** (p. 295).

o **Taking Afternoon Tea:** Look smart at **Brown's,** the **Goring, Fortnum & Mason,** or the **Langham** (p. 54), where the traditional tea ritual carries on as it did in Britain's colonial heyday.

o **Spending an Evening at a West End Theatre:** London is the theatrical capital of the world. The live stages of **Theatreland** around Covent Garden and Soho offer a combination of variety, accessibility, and economy—but the shows of the Fringe are where the future can be found. See p. 226.

LONDON'S best FOOD

○ **Tucking into Honest British Ingredients:** After many lost years of too much boiled cabbage and bread, the English have fallen back in love with farm-fresh ingredients. The gastropub movement, epitomized by its still-potent pioneer, the **Eagle** (p. 74), is just the beginning. Delectable English traditional cooking can be found from the oldest establishments (**Rules,** p. 86) to neighborhood holes in the wall (**Andrew Edmunds,** p. 80; **10 Greek Street,** p. 78).

○ **Sinking a Pint in a Traditional Pub:** From Tudor coaching inns to riverside taverns, London's pub culture spans the centuries. Raise a pint where Shakespeare did at the **George** (p. 103), immerse yourself in an ale at Dr. Samuel Johnson's local **Ye Olde Cheshire Cheese** (p. 107), and drink in a Victorian jewel box of etched glass at the **Princess Louise** (p. 106). Then repeat. See "20 Pubs You'll Love" on p. 101.

○ **Mining the Stalls at Borough Market:** The top weekend port of call for foodies is the market under the railway by London Bridge station—not least for the free samples dished out by vendors keen to market their wares. It's gourmet heaven. See p. 95.

○ **Enjoying the New English Comfort Food:** London's first Indian restaurant opened in 1810, and Asian food of every origin is now the capital's most popular genre of cuisine. The dozens of curry houses

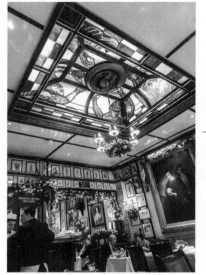

London's oldest restaurant, Rules, boasts a beautiful stained-glass ceiling.

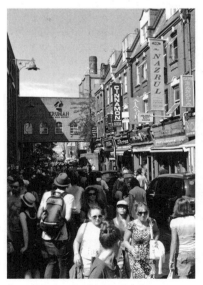

Curry houses on Brick Lane pitch for your business as you walk by.

on **Brick Lane** (p. 99) pitch for your business at the curb; or take in a traditional meal under the gold silk wallpaper at Covent Garden's **Punjab Restaurant** (p. 88), opened by an Indian wrestler back in 1947.

o **Chowing Down on Farmhouse Cheese:** England produces hundreds of artisan cheeses. Check out the West Country cheddars, red Leicester, and goat's cheeses at such cheesemongers as **Neal's Yard Dairy** (p. 95) or eat a gloppy, gooey plate of raclette at **Kappacasein** (p. 95). But get your fill while you're here: You can't get it back through Customs.

o **Tasting Britain's Fading Traditions:** As young English diners insist on flashier fare, the older ways of cooking become rarer. Whether it's jellied eels in the protected interior of **M. Manze** (p. 96), the deep-fried goodness at the linoleum-lined "chippie" **Fryer's Delight** (p. 76), or the traditional "caff" of the **Regency Café** (p. 93), mid-century Britain is still steaming along—affordably.

LONDON'S best HOTELS

By 2016, London will have 136,000 hotel rooms—some better than others.

o **Meet the Locals at a Family-Run B&B:** Mom-and-pop inns have taken a hit because of the dominance of corporate hotels. But you can still find some stellar homegrown hospitality where owners put you first, including the Valotis and Cabrals of the **Alhambra Hotel** in St Pancras (p. 38), the Beynons of Bloomsbury's **Jesmond Hotel** (p. 40), and the Callises of **22 York Street** in Marylebone (p. 56).

o **Lose Yourself in a Grande Dame:** The first all-service grand hotel in Europe, the **Langham** (p. 54) was built in 1865, and it's still extending top-flight hospitality to guests with taste—and cash. **Claridge's** (p. 52) and **Brown's** (p. 52) have attracted royalty and creative misadventures since the mid-1800s, while the world-famous **Savoy** (p. 43) still stands atop her field for Thames views. Best of all, you can tour their ground floors without being a guest.

o **Pay Less Than $50:** You may not think it's possible, but with advance planning, you can get a new, impeccably maintained private

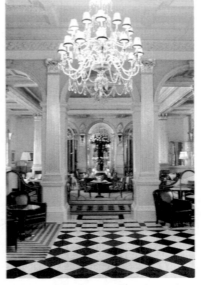

The lobby of Claridge's Hotel is truly grand.

room in the center of town for only £29 a night. Book way ahead with the British chains **Premier Inn, Travelodge,** or **easyHotel,** or with the imported budget brands **Ibis** and **CitizenM,** and London is yours, cheap. See p. 32.

o **Sleep Where History Happened:** Rather than tear it down, Londoners would rather revitalize it. Be party to the spy stories at **St. Ermin's Hotel** (p. 49), rest under the swoony spires of Gilbert Scott's neo-Gothic **St Pancras Renaissance Hotel** (p. 36), wake up where presses once printed the morning news at **One Aldwych** (p. 42), or relax in the onetime headquarters of the Ministry of Defense at the **Corinthia London** (p. 41).

o **Enjoy Style for Less:** "Boutique" hotels are encroaching deeper into budget territory than ever before. At the **Nadler** hotels (p. 45 and p. 51), **Z Hotels** (p. 35), and **hub by Premier Inn** (p. 34), you'll surrender some space, but not the chic. Buzzy Dutch boutique **CitizenM** (p. 32) has huge beds and a loopy personality, but a small price.

LONDON'S best FOR FAMILIES

o **Cruising London's Waterways:** In addition to the grand River Thames, London has a working canal system that once kept goods flowing to and from the city's docks. The best value trips are on the **Regent's Canal** (p. 191) and on the *Thames Clipper* passing under Tower Bridge (p. 318).

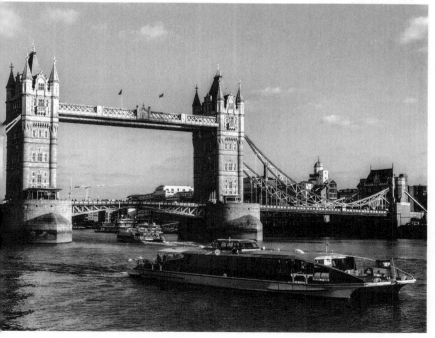

The *Thames Clipper* passing Tower Bridge offers a great value trip.

- o **Visiting Harry Potter:** Warner Bros.' deep dive into how it designed and made its seven blockbuster films, **The Making of Harry Potter** (p. 181), is one of the country's most popular family attractions, surpassing expectations. Potterheads could happily spend a whole day here.

- o **Losing Your Way in the World's Most Famous Hedge Maze:** The green labyrinth at **Hampton Court** twists and turns for almost half a mile. When you manage to extricate yourselves, stroll through centuries of architectural styles at this stunning palace, home of many an English monarch. Don't forget to pick up a kids' activity trail. See p. 179.

- o **Going Botanic in Royal Kew:** The **Royal Botanic Gardens,** Kew, house more than 50,000 plants from across the planet, including Arctic and tropical varieties. Youngsters will love the 200m (656-ft.) high Treetop Walkway, up in the Garden's deciduous canopy. See p. 180.

- o **Asking How, Where & Why:** Inside South Kensington's **Science Museum** (p. 147), interactive exhibits to keep inquisitive minds occupied. Or pilot a simulated ship at the kid-centric **National Maritime Museum** (p. 175), or learn how to drive a Tube train at the **London Transport Museum** (p. 120).

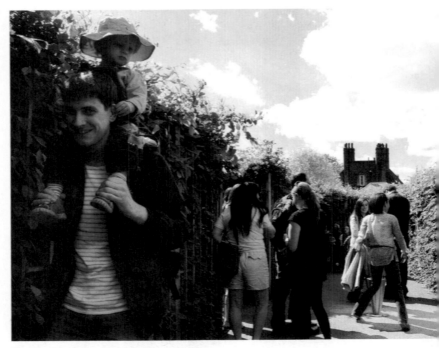

It's easy to get lost in the Hampton Court maze.

o **Learn the Panto Lingo:** From November to early January, join one of Britain's most delightful holiday experiences: pantomimes, which are slapstick musical romps through famous stories, usually starring D-list celebrities. Hiss at villains, shout instructions for heroes, and giggle at good-natured drag performers. Try the **Theatre Royal Stratford** (www.stratford east.com), the **New Wimbledon** (www.atgtickets.com), the **Hackney Empire** (p. 233), or the **Richmond Theatre** (www.richmondtheatre. net).

o **Seeing Peter Pan in Kensington Gardens:** You'll feel like a character from a Victorian novel as you see Sir George Frampton's beloved 1902 statue of the boy who played the panpipe. There's no bet-

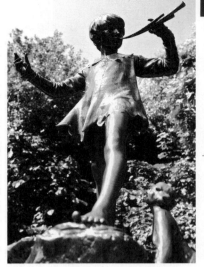

The Peter Pan statue in Kensington Gardens makes it easy to imagine this beloved character come to life.

ter way to admire and enjoy the "green lung"—the largest and most popular open space in a city that holds the record for the most green space for a city of its size. See p. 190.

LONDON'S best FREE & DIRT-CHEAP EXPERIENCES

o **Visiting the Great Museums:** London's state museums and galleries—including most of the big names—show off their permanent collections for free. They include the **British Museum, National Gallery, National Portrait Gallery, Tate Britain, Tate Modern, Natural History Museum, Science Museum, V&A,** the two **Museums of London,** and the **British Library.** See chapter 5.

o **Taking in Fresh Air & a City View:** North of the River Thames, **Hampstead Heath** (p. 189) offers miles of woodland trails, historic pubs, and sumptuous mansions. To the south, the flower beds of **Greenwich Park** (p. 189) enjoy a panoramic sweep over the Thames.

o **Dining on the Cheap:** Away from the Michelin-starred hotspots, London is surprisingly well equipped with affordable, tasty places to enjoy a full meal for under £10. Among the best is the West End's most venerable budget pit stop, **Café in the Crypt** at St. Martin-in-the-Fields church (p. 84).

- **The King of Libraries:** The **British Library** (p. 109) started as the monarch's private stash but now its doors yawn wide to the public with free exhibitions and priceless manuscripts that must be seen to be believed.
- **Catching a Free Event in the Center of the City:** From the **Lord Mayor's Show** to the **Notting Hill Carnival,** a large number of major public events cost nothing to attend. See "London's Calendar of Events" (p. 323).

THE best HISTORIC EXPERIENCES

- **Meeting the Heroes & Villains of History:** Get face-to-face with a rogue's gallery from the past at the **National Portrait Gallery,** where faces seem to watch you across time with a sparkle in their eye. The gang's all here, from a supercilious Henry VIII to a pugnacious Hogarth to a kind-eyed Princess Diana, already fading into a memory. See p. 124.
- **Taking a Tour of Royal London:** From palaces and parks to the royal art collections, history, geography, and culture have been shaped—or owned— by centuries of aristocratic rule. You can see the best of it in a day, including the queen's favorite grocer, **Fortnum & Mason** (p. 203), plus any one of 800 other Royal Warrant holders (p. 209). Roam the very rooms used in daily life by kings and queens at **Buckingham Palace** (p. 128), **Hampton Court Palace** (p. 179), **Kensington Palace** (p. 144), and **Windsor Castle** (p. 286).
- **Peering into a Time Capsule:** Some museums preserve scenes that were frozen in time. No reconstructions or fakery here: You'll gaze upon authentic World War II military operations at the **Churchill War Rooms** (p. 129); admire the graves of great artists and the location of epic rituals at **Westminster Abbey** (p. 134); see the home that made **Charles Darwin** want to stop traveling (p. 182); and marvel at the treasure-crammed townhouse of a 19th-century collector (**Sir John Soane's Museum,** p. 126).
- **Shopping in the Grandest Department Stores of Them All:** And, no, it's not Harrods. **Liberty of London** (p. 205), founded in 1875 and moved to its current half-timbered, mock-Tudor home in 1924, and **Selfridges** (p. 206), both designed and built by Americans, redefined sales methods and played crucial roles in world history.
- **Imagining Domestic Life Through the Ages:** At the **Geffrye Museum** (p. 170) period re-creations of interiors from the spartan 1630s to the flashy 1990s allow visitors to understand how home life has changed. But nothing immerses you in the past quite like the brain-bending role-playing of a night visit to **Dennis Severs' House** (p. 170).

SUGGESTED ITINERARIES & NEIGHBORHOODS

Few great modern cities are as multilayered, intricate, and, yes, *messy* as London, Western Europe's most populous city (8.7 million in 2017, and growing). Perhaps that's because history was knitted into its layout. London is mostly the haphazard product of blind evolution, which piled up over successive generations to produce a complicated metropolis. One could say that London simply happened.

As recently as the early 1800s, London—and by London, I mean what we now call The City, between St Paul's and the Tower—was a frenzied cluster where many lives, birth to death, were carried out within the same few blocks. The main streets ran south to the river (not east or west, as they do now), the smoke of industry was banished downwind to the east, and kings lived near the Thames for easy transportation. All around The City were dozens of villages, many of which retain their names as modern neighborhoods—and, if you're lucky, a whiff of their original personalities, but not of their original pestilence.

Quickly, London swelled to swallow its current territory. Yet because of ancient echoes, neighborhoods remain surprisingly small—many are just minutes across by foot, and even crucial streets can change names several times. It's still possible to stroll along and sense sudden shifts in energy and character. In many ways, London is still a complex system of hamlets. It's one of the many delights that makes it so surprising. It also means it can take a lifetime to scratch its surface.

Addresses sometimes reflect this improvisation; a building numbered 75 may sit across the street from one numbered 32. Despite this, it's immensely difficult to get lost. The City maintains some 1,200 Legible London map **"Finger Posts"** throughout town. Wherever you are, a map is near.

If you want a map, forgo the oversimplified one your hotel might offer and don't tax your data plan. The most cherished paper map

London's Neighborhoods

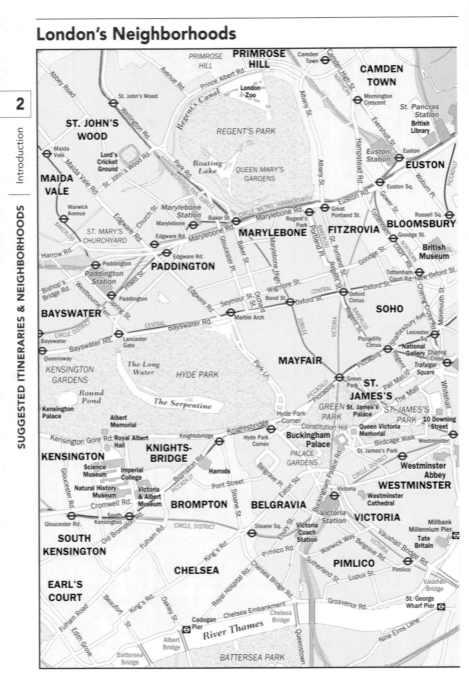

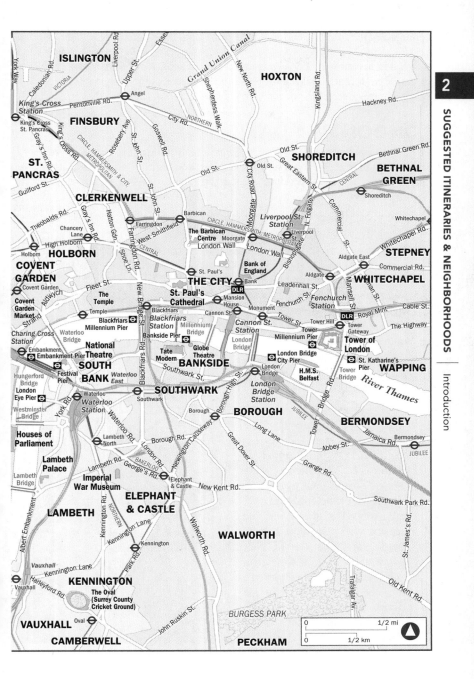

is the **London A–Z** (www.az.co.uk), first compiled by the indefatigable Phyllis Pearsall, who walked every mile of The City for the 1936 debut edition and commanded the resulting cartography empire until her death 60 years later. Its *London Mini A–Z Street Atlas* (£6) fits into a pocket. (Don't buy the app, which drains your smartphone's battery.) Just be sure to call it the "A to Zed" or you'll get a funny look; in England, the last letter the alphabet is, quite sensibly, pronounced so it doesn't rhyme with eight other letters.

LONDON IN 1 DAY

First of all, what were you thinking? If you're in town on a layover, didn't you know that many airlines will allow you to stick around for a few days at no charge? Never mind. What's done is done. Eat a huge breakfast and make your way to Tower Hill.

1 The Tower of London ★★★

Start here (p. 164) because it usually opens an hour earlier (9am) than most attractions. Spend about 2 hours making stops at the **Crown Jewels** and the **White Tower,** and snap that requisite photo of the **Tower Bridge** (p. 164) from the quay. Grab a triangle sandwich (the quintessential London lunch).

Tube it west on the Circle or District lines to Westminster.

2 Westminster Abbey ★★★

Allot a rushed 2 hours to see the effigies of kings and queens (p. 134). Of the **Chapel of Henry VII,** Washington Irving wrote: "Stone seems, by the cunning labor of the chisel, to have been robbed of its weight and density, suspended aloft as if by magic, and the fretted roof achieved with the wonderful minuteness and airy security of a cobweb." Outside, take in the **Houses of Parliament** (p. 130) and **Big Ben's Elizabeth Tower** from across the street.

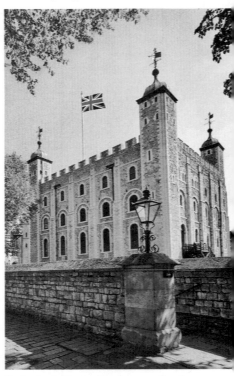

Don't miss the Tower of London, even if you're just in The City for a day.

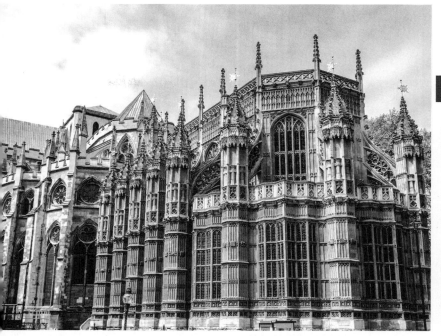

The Chapel of Henry VII at Westminster Abbey is an essential stop in London.

Walk up Whitehall, passing No. 10 Downing St. (the Walking Tour on p. 249 will guide you).

3 The National Gallery ★★★

At **Trafalgar Square,** a symbolic heart of the city, you can finally see some of the world's most famous paintings in person (p. 122). Park guards also turn a blind eye to tourists climbing alongside those famous bronze couchant lions, each of them 20 feet long. But don't mount them—they're cracking.

From the Strand, head to the back of Charing Cross station and cross the Thames.

4 London Eye ★★

There's time for a revolution on London's favorite contemporary icon and the new focal point of national celebrations (p. 154). In the colder months, you'll be there to watch the sun go down slowly as **Big Ben** gongs.

Finish just north of the Gallery, around Leicester Square.

5 West End Show ★★★

Curtains go up around 7:30pm (p. 226). Enjoy an ice cream during interval (intermission)—it's a custom. Afterward, hurry to a **pub** and raise a pint to a city where you've barely scratched the surface (see p. 101 for ideas).

LONDON ON A 2ND DAY

You're going to have to move fast, but you'll be able to see some highlights. Take the Tube to Mansion House, Blackfriars, or St Paul's.

1 St Paul's Cathedral ★★★

As you appreciate the underside of her dome, also appreciate the grave fact that before the 1940s, her flanks were crowded with buildings. Bombings devastated the structures that once hemmed her in.

Cross the Thames on the Millennium Bridge (the Walking Tour on p. 262 will help).

2 Tate Modern ★★★

Here's a museum (p. 155) in a colossal structure with river views that can be more memorable than what's on display inside it—although Rothko's paintings for the Four Seasons restaurant can't fail to put you in a restive mood. If it's summer, catch a matinee at **Shakespeare's Globe** (p. 231), just a few yards east; an afternoon pint across the bridge at the Art Nouveau the **Black Friar** (p. 102) will recharge you.

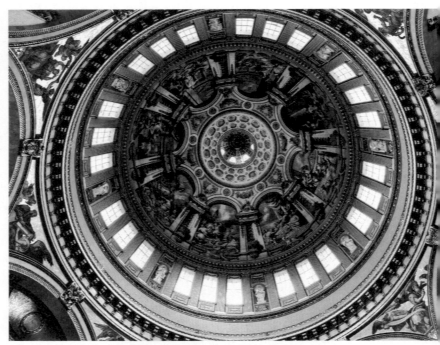

The ornately detailed underside of the dome of St Paul's Cathedral.

Take the Jubilee line from Southwark to Green Park.

3 Green Park ★★

Walk south through Green Park (p. 188) to behold the front of **Buckingham Palace** (p. 128); if you're here in March, you may be lucky enough to see fields of daffodils in bloom. Return to Piccadilly to browse the classy shops lining it, including **Fortnum & Mason** (p. 203).

Take the Tube's Piccadilly line (notice the century-old tilework) to Russell Square.

4 The British Museum ★★★

You'll spend the afternoon roaming its vast halls (p. 113), but you'll scarcely be able to wrap your brain around the age, rarity, and craftsmanship of what you see. Such aesthetic exertions may induce cravings for cream tea at its Great Court Restaurant or another pint at a Victorian valentine of a pub, the **Princess Louise** (p. 106).

Catch Bus 55 toward Oxford Circus. Sit on the top level for the views!

5 Oxford Circus ★★

Wind up the afternoon with a dive into the bustling fitting rooms of the shops on **Oxford Street, Regent Street,** and **Carnaby Street** (p. 274), where you'll find a huge selection of cool clothes at what Londoners call "High Street" prices— meaning they're sane. Walk southeast for a few minutes to Frith Street in Soho and have dinner at **Andrew Edmunds** (p. 80), a neighborhood gem with a changing menu that charges prices far below its rank,

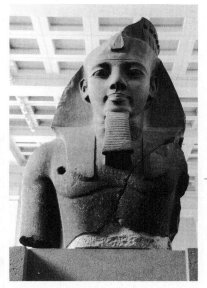

Ancient treasures, such as this statue of Ramses II, fill the British Museum.

and afterward, stroll past the lights of **Piccadilly Circus.** If you still have juice left, walk down Haymarket, turn left on Cockspur, and follow it down the Strand to Aldwych.

6 South Bank ★★★

Cross the Waterloo bridge and wander east along the popular promenade of **South Bank.** During the evening, couples stroll, theatres light, cafés buzz, and the water of the Thames glitters in the light reflected from the ancient grey dome of St Paul's. It makes for an unforgettable evening.

LONDON ON A 3RD DAY

Follow the itinerary for 2 days in London, but add in one of The City's South Kensington museums, preferably the **Victoria & Albert** (p. 148), and follow that with a walk through **Hyde Park** (p. 190), possibly to see the **Diana Memorial Fountain** (p. 144), and to tour the public areas of her son's and grandchildren's London home, **Kensington Palace** (p. 144), in adjoining **Kensington Gardens.** Take the Tube or a bus to Westminster and dive into the time capsule of the **Churchill War Rooms** (p. 129). Follow that with a stroll along the South Bank from Westminster to London Bridge, taking your pick among the pubs and restaurants you find along the path.

AN ITINERARY FOR FAMILIES

There's no bad neighborhood to stay in if you've got kids, because London is low-rise and manageable. But make sure they're ready to climb stairs if you're taking the Tube. On paper, some of London's museums sound as if they'd be too dry, but in reality, they bend over backward to cater to children—maybe

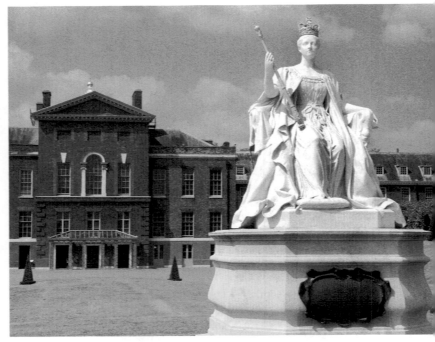

A statue of Queen Victoria rules from in front of Kensington Palace.

too much, as it's often at the expense of adult minds. Every major museum, no exceptions, has an on-site cafe for lunch.

Day 1: Double-Deckers & *Thames Clippers*

Forget expensive open-top tours: Start your day seeing Piccadilly Circus, Trafalgar Square, St Paul's Cathedral, the Tower of London, and much more for the price of bus fare on an antique, double-decker **Routemaster bus** with an old-style staircase on the end. Take route 15, every 15 minutes. After visiting the **Tower of London** (p. 164), head to the ferry dock and see The City from the river on a *Thames Clipper* (p. 318). Disembark at **Tate Modern** (p. 155), which comes fully loaded for young exploration with family trails, a learning zone on Level 5, and some very cool video tablets for interpreting the art. Take the Tube to Leicester Square for a **West End musical** (p. 226).

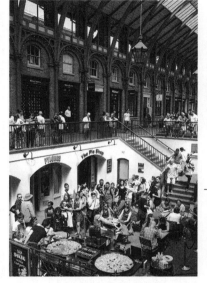

Day 2: Covent Garden & Coram's Fields

Make your way to Covent Garden's **London Transport Museum** (p. 120), where kids can pretend to drive a bus and explore other eye-level exhibits. Then bring your brood on a 15-minute walk north to the **British Museum** (p. 113) and hook them up with crayons and pads, exploration backpacks, and the special object collections tour geared to young minds. If

Covent Garden offers several family-friendly bars and restaurants.

they're the daring types, the mummies never fail to impress. Just east you'll find a city park just for children: The 7-acre **Coram's Fields** (www.coramsfields.org), which was set aside in 1739 for an orphanage at a time when 75% of London kids died before the age of 5. Its southern gate is where mothers once abandoned their babies in desperation. Today, no adult may enter without a child, and this once sad spot is now the scene of daily family joy; there's a petting zoo, two playgrounds for all ages, sand pits, and a paddling pool.

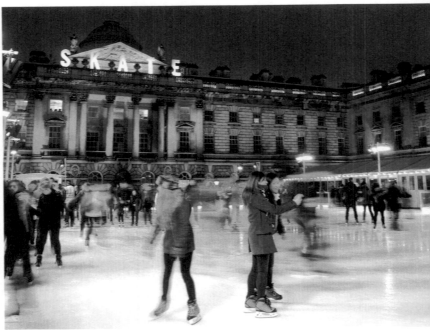

Ice skating at Somerset House is available in winter, when the water jets are transformed into a skating rink.

Day 3: The Brompton Road Museums

Today is devoted to exploration of the Brompton Road museums, a trio of world's-bests for kids: Take the Piccadilly line to South Kensington, where the **V&A** (p. 148) has hundreds of hands-on exhibits for kids (look for the hand symbol on the maps), such as trying on Victorian costumes or donning armor gauntlets. Next door, the plain-speaking signs and robotic dinosaurs of the **Natural History Museum** (p. 146) impress kids as much as the airplanes and space capsules over their heads at the **Science Museum** (p. 147)—both institutions furnish even more kids' trails and activities for free. Go east on the Circle or District Tube lines to Temple, and you're at the dancing water jets (transformed in winter to a skating rink) of the **Somerset House** courtyard (home of the Courtauld Gallery, p. 119). If the weather doesn't suit that, the **London Eye**'s capsules are safe, climate-controlled, and move imperceptibly—the view will stimulate and inspire kids.

A DISCOVERY WEEKEND

The *Frommer's EasyGuides* are designed to give you a firm introduction to the sights, hotels, and restaurants that speak most to a visitor about what's going on in each destination. But authentic London doesn't begin and end with these pages, and if you dip into neighborhoods where more locals live, your visit will be immeasurably richer.

Day 1: Brixton & Bollywood

When Victoria was queen, families flocked to live near the incandescent lights of Brixton's Electric Avenue, which in 1888 became one of London's first shopping streets lit by electricity. Today, it's a boisterous immigrant community. By day, explore the glazed awnings of its markets, where to inhale the aroma of meat and exotic spices is to walk through a portal to Jamaica, India, or China—and to be reminded that London, like few others, is a truly worldly city. In the evening, experience London's huge South Asian population—Indians are nearly 2% of the population, and one of Britain's richest men, Lakshmi Mittal, is

Use the Code

London is chopped into geographic parcels, and you'll see those postcodes on street signs. The heart of The City, in postcode terms, is near the Chancery Lane Tube stop. From there, areas are given a compass direction (N for north, SW for southwest, and so on) and a number (but ignore that, since a number greater than 1 doesn't mean the area is in the boonies). In the very heart of town, addresses get an extra C for "centre," as in WC1, which is where Covent Garden is located. Every address in this book includes its postcode, which corresponds to the neighborhood in which you'll find it. Don't worry—you won't need to memorize these because each listing also includes the nearest Tube stop to help you quickly place locations on a map. Here are some of the most common postcodes:

WC1 Bloomsbury
WC2 Covent Garden, Holborn, Strand
W1 Fitzrovia, Marylebone, Mayfair, Soho
W2 Bayswater
W6 Hammersmith
W8 Kensington
W11 Notting Hill
SW1 Belgravia, St James's, Westminster
SW3 Chelsea
SW5 Earl's Court
SW7 Knightsbridge, South Kensington
SE1 Southwark
SE10 Greenwich
EC1 Clerkenwell
EC2 Bank, Barbican, Liverpool Street
EC3 Tower Hill
EC4 Fleet Street, St Paul's
E1 Spitalfields, Whitechapel
E2 Bethnal Green
E14 Canary Wharf/Isle of Dogs
N1 Islington
NW1 Camden Town
NW3 Hampstead

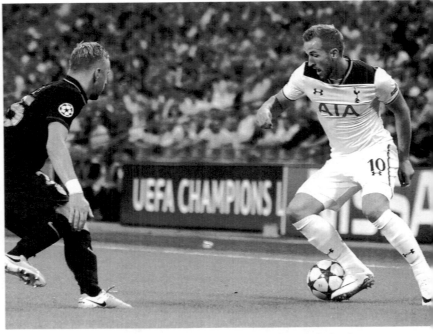

Tottenham Hotspurs are one of five Premier League football teams playing in the London area.

Indian-born—by attending a Bollywood film at the Boleyn Cinema (www.boleyncinemas.com; Upton Park tube), a historic 1938 Art Deco building and the second-largest Bollywood screen in a country that loves the genre.

Day 2: Go Football Mad or Cricket Crazy

London hosts 13 professional football (soccer) teams, more than any other city on Earth. From mid-August to mid-May, catch matches at some of the best Premier League teams: **Chelsea** (www.chealseafc.com), **Arsenal** (London's first club; www.arsenal.com), **Tottenham Hotspur** (www.tottenhamhotspur.com), **Fulham** (www.fulhamfc.com), or **West Ham United** (www.whufc.com), which took up residence in the former Olympic Stadium at Stratford. Filling the gap from April to September, and less likely to pelt you in the skull with a beer bottle, is cricket. Attend "test matches" at Marylebone's **MCC Lord's Cricket Ground** (www.lords.org) or Oval's **Surrey County Cricket Club** (www.surreycricket.com). If you figure out how the game works, fill me in, won't you? It's a little like baseball—and a lot like watching grass grow.

Day 3: Ale, Yorkshire Pudding & Tough Questions

On Sunday afternoons, find a pub with an inviting garden for a traditional
Sunday Roast, a spread of roasted meats with all the trimmings such as
Yorkshire pudding (a popover-like pastry) and gravy, washed down with
copious amounts of beer. It's the more leisurely equivalent of brunch:
After a long week of working to keep their exorbitantly priced shared
flats, Londoners hang out until Monday. Some pubs also hold **pub quiz-
zes,** another staple of British life. Form teams and answer trivia for lame
prizes, but be warned: Foreigners always fold on the sports and politics
questions.

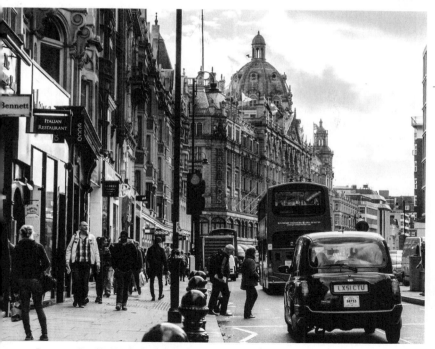

Brompton Road in Knightsbridge, in the SW7 postcode.

Neighborhoods in Brief

London's neighborhoods were laid out during a period of wagon and foot traffic, when districts were defined in narrower terms than we define them today; indeed, for centuries people often lived complete lives without seeing the other side of town. Ironically, in our times, the Tube has done much to divide these districts from each other. Visitors are likely to hop a train between them and don't often realize how remarkably close together they really are.

Are these the only areas of interest? Not even close. Literally hundreds of fascinating village clusters abound, many with names as cherishable as Ponders End, Tooting, and The Wrythe. And considering that a third of Londoners now belong to an ethnic minority and more than 200 languages are spoken, the flavor of your experience shifts as you go. But visitors are likely to spend time here:

BLOOMSBURY & FITZROVIA

Best for: *Museums, affordable inns, residential streets, universities, and homewares and electronics shops on Tottenham Court Road*
What you won't find: *Evening entertainment, nightclubs*

Bloomsbury's dark-brick, white-sashed residential buildings and leafy squares date mostly from the Georgian period, when the district became the first in a chaotic city to be planned—it was an early version of the modern suburban development. The refined air attracted the intelligentsia nearly from the start, and its two universities are both 19th-century institutions. The British Museum settled here, too. Bloomsbury became a place of remembrance on July 7, 2005; of the 52 who died that day, 26 perished underground on a bombed Piccadilly line train between King's Cross and Russell Square stations, and 13 were killed on a double-decker bus passing above through Tavistock Square. Bloomsbury's cozier sister Fitzrovia, similar in character but devoid of major attractions, lies on the western side of Tottenham Court Road. Famous residents include George Bernard Shaw and Virginia Woolf, who both lived (at different times) at 29 Fitzroy Square.

KING'S CROSS

Best for: *Budget hotels, trains heading north (and south to Paris), alternative/down-and-dirty nightlife, student housing, takeaway counters*
What you won't find: *A large restaurant selection, shopping*

A decade ago, the area around King's Cross station was an unsavory tenderloin of porn stores and warehouses. Behind the station, millions of pounds have just transformed once-derelict industrial infrastructure into Granary Square, a canalside center for arts hotspots, restaurants, colleges, and tech HQs. Legend (surely apocryphal) says the Celtic queen Boudicca rests somewhere near Platform 8 of King's Cross. Fans of Harry Potter know that the young wizard boards the Hogwarts Express at the (fictitious) Platform 9¾; the movie versions have shot at Platforms 4 and 5 but used prettier St Pancras station, next door, as a stand-in facade. Change came, as it often has in English history, from France: The Channel Tunnel Rail Link is the starting point for Eurostar train trips to France and beyond.

MARYLEBONE & MAYFAIR

Best for: *Luxe shopping, hotels, restaurants, small museums, strolling, embassies*
What you won't find: *Historic sights, savings*

The middle-class hubbub of Oxford Street west of Regent Street divides high-hat Marylebone from its snobbish southern neighbor, Mayfair. Both play host to upscale shopping and several fascinating, if overlooked, museums, but there the similarities end. World-famous Mayfair, typified by hyperluxe bauble shops and blue-blood heritage (the present queen was born at 17 Bruton St. in a building that is no longer there), has a high opinion of itself as a starchy enclave of wealth, much of it from other countries. Yet Mayfair has less to offer the casual tourist, although it is the city's hot zone for cushy hotels. (The title of the musical *My Fair Lady* is witty wordplay on how its

Cockney heroine, Eliza, would have pronounced "Mayfair lady.") Marylebone (Mar-le-bun), on the other hand, benefits from convenient Tube and bus connections and lively sidewalks crowded with evening celebrants, particularly around James Street. Also, thanks to a territorial local authority, its main shopping drag (Marylebone High St.) remains one of the last important streets in London that isn't awash with the ubiquitous corporate chain stores. Oxford Street is The City's premier shopping corridor; the western half between Oxford Circus and Marble Arch is the classier end, with marquee department stores such as Selfridges and Marks & Spencer.

SOHO, COVENT GARDEN & CENTRAL WEST END

Best for: Shopping, restaurants, theater, cinema, nightlife, opera, free art (National Gallery and National Portrait Gallery), star sightings

What you won't find: Elbow room, silence

London's undisputed center of nightlife, restaurants, and theater, the West End seethes with tourists and merry-makers. After work, Old Compton Street and Covent Garden overflow with people catching up with friends; by 7:30pm, the theaters and opera houses are pulsing; by midnight, the action has moved into the nightclubs of Leicester Square and lounges of Soho; and in the wee hours, you might find groups of partiers trawling Gerrard Street, in a teeny Cantonese Chinatown, hunting for snacks. Prim Trafalgar Square, dominated by the peerless National Gallery, has often been called London's focal point. On a sunny day, you'll find few places that exude such well-being.

WESTMINSTER, INCLUDING ST JAMES'S

Best for: Historic and government sights, river strolls, St James's Park

What you won't find: Affordable hotels, a wide choice of restaurants

Though it's near the West End, this area's energy is more staid. It's a district tourists mostly see by day. South of Trafalgar Square,

you'll find regiments of robust government buildings but little in the way of hotels or food. Whitehall's severity doesn't spread far: Just a block east, its impenetrable character gives way to the proud riverside promenade of Victoria Embankment overlooking the London Eye, and just a block west, to the greenery of St James's Park, which is, in effect, the queen's front yard, since Buckingham Palace is at the western boundary of this area. North of the park, the tidy streets of St James's are even more exclusive than Mayfair's, if that's possible.

THE CITY

Best for: Old streets, the Tower of London, St Paul's, financial concerns

What you won't find: Nightlife or weekend life, affordable hotels

Technically, this is the only part of London that's London. Other bits, including the West End, are under the jurisdiction of different local governments, such as Westminster or Camden. The City, as it's called, is where most of London's history happened. It's where Romans cheered gladiators. It's where London Bridge—at least 12 versions—touched shore. It's where the Great Fire raged. And, more recently, it's where the Deutsche Luftwaffe focused many of its nocturnal bombing raids, which is why you'll find so little evidence of the aforementioned events. Outside of working hours, the main thing you'll see in The City is your own reflection in the facade of corporate fortresses; west of Liverpool Street station, even most of the pubs close on weekends. Although it encompasses such priceless relics as the Tower of London, St Paul's Cathedral, the Tower Bridge, the Bank of England, and the Monument, many of the area's remnants are underfoot—the spider web of lanes and streets dates to the Roman period, with names that hint at their former lives (Walbrook is where the river Walbrook, now hidden underground, flowed down to the Thames; Honey Lane, Bread St., Milk St., and Poultry all once hosted food markets.) Buildings have come and gone, but the veins of The City have pumped in-situ for thousands of years.

THE SOUTH BANK, SOUTHWARK & BOROUGH

Best for: Museums, memorable pubs, strolls, gourmet foods and wines
What you won't find: Shopping, parks

During the recent rehabilitation of Southwark (Suth-urk) from a crumbling industrial district, its blighted power station became one of the world's greatest museums (the Tate Modern), a master playwright's theater was re-created (the Globe), and a sublime riverfront path replaced the coal lightermen's rotting piers. Now it's where London goes to fall in love with The City. It's a 1-mile riverside stroll between the London Eye and the Tate Modern, and every step is a pleasure. Once-dank railway viaducts are filled with cafes and reasonable restaurants; Western Europe's tallest skyscraper, The Shard, lords over from above; and the nation's dramatic showpiece (the National Theatre) anchors them at South Bank. But it's gratifying to see that some things never change: Borough Market, which attracts gourmet foodies from around the world, is the descendant of a market that fed the denizens of that medieval skyscraper over the water, London Bridge.

VICTORIA & CHELSEA

Best for: Boutiques, low-cost lodging, town homes, wealthy neighbors
What you won't find: Transit options, street life, museums

Victoria doesn't technically apply to the neighborhood around the eponymous train station—Belgravia (to the west) and Pimlico (south and east) take those honors—but the shorthand stuck. Most of the area, which is residential or uninterestingly workaday, was developed starting in the 1820s in consistent patterns of white stucco-terraced homes. The area around the station, which is being redeveloped in a massive works project, contains two outlier West End theatres, but little else. Just north, you'll face the brick walls of Buckingham Palace Gardens. Chelsea, to its south, has a history of well-heeled bohemianism—Oscar Wilde, James McNeill Whistler, and the Beatles all lived here—although it's known more as one of The City's most exclusive (and some would say

insular) communities. A stroll past boutiques and pocket-squared residents on the King's Road, turning ever-more corporate and indistinct, is not the adventure it once was.

KENSINGTON, KNIGHTSBRIDGE

Best for: Museums, shopping, ultra-luxe boutiques, also-ran hotels
What you won't find: Historic sights

Here, one expensive neighborhood genuflects to another, and barely anyone you meet was born in England. South Kensington and Brompton draw the most visitors to their grand museums; and Knightsbridge is where moneyed foreigners spend and show off—London now has the most billionaires in the world, nearly twice as many as New York or Moscow. They can't legally change most of the facades, so to satisfy their hunger for more space, the big trend among the rich is to burrow downward to build underground rooms—the "pleasure caves" of Kensington. Privilege has long had an address in Kensington—that's a reason those edifying institutions were located here to begin with, away from the grubby paws of the peasants—but it also is home to a core of French expats; you'll find the cafes catering to them on Bute Street. Kensington Palace, at the Gardens' western end, is where Prince William and Kate live when they're in town. When you travel west to Earl's Court, you experience a considerable drop in voltage. It's a frumpy zone deprived of a contingency to the park with undistinguished eats and sleeps; the rise of King's Cross and Shoreditch for younger travelers has reduced it to near-negligible stature. Your parents may have stayed here once, but you shouldn't.

SHOREDITCH, SPITALFIELDS & HOXTON

Best for: Nightclubs, music, food of all types, galleries, clothing
What you won't find: Museums, parks

If Mayfair is London's champagne, the East End hoods have been its hangover. For centuries it was an impoverished, squalid slum for poor immigrants and shifty souls. Jack the Ripper slashing and the Elephant Man suffering jibes—it happened here. That's in the history books now. Spitalfields (Spit-all-fields), named for its excellent covered market (p. 223) and increasingly threatened by an unstoppable cancer of soulless, open-plan office buildings from The City, blends into Shoreditch, big on name-dropping up-and-coming designers and party promoters as if you knew who they were. Shopping, restaurants, bars, hipsters—it's all here now. Dalston, young and bohemian, is north of these. East of Spitalfields, in ancient homes that have long housed waves of immigrants (French, then Jewish, now South Asian), you'll find the famed restaurants of Brick Lane (p. 99), the cafes and dance clubs of the converted Old Truman Brewery, and the art-savvy neighborhood of Whitechapel. Prostitutes are out, £4.50 coffee is in—which may not be an improvement.

GREENWICH

Best for: *Museums, antique and food markets, river views, strolls, boats*

What you won't find: *Hotels, bustle*

Greenwich, on the south bank across from the Canary Wharf developments, retains the tranquility of an untouched village. Such lovely insularity exists because the Tube (well, the DLR) didn't connect it to the greater city until 1999—all the more remarkable when you consider the town's illustrious pedigree as a royal getaway (it's got the oldest royal park in London), as a scientific capital, and as one of the world's most crucial command centers. If it all sounds like a living museum, it is: On top of being a UNESCO World Heritage Site (Maritime Greenwich), the village is literally the center of time and space, since it inhabits the exact location of Greenwich Mean Time, and of longitude 0° 0' 0". Set away from Greenwich town there's the colossal O₂ dome, The City's iconic concert venue.

Other Popular London Neighborhoods

Mostly because of iffy transit connections (for example, service by a single Tube line that, should it go on the blink, would derail your vacation), this book doesn't focus on these neighborhoods as prime places to stay, but they're still vital parts of town.

BAYSWATER & PADDINGTON

Best for: *Sub-par inns, ethnic food, well-preserved Victorian thoroughfares*
What you won't find: *Attractions, non-chain stores, street life, adorable bears*

Its whitewashed, terraced houses were briefly the most fashionable in The City (Churchill and Dickens were residents), yet today, the sizable transient population of this area deprives it of sustained energy, and its hotels tend to be for immigrant tradesmen. Crowning the muddle is Queensway, a popular shopping street containing Whiteleys, a 1911 department store edifice converted into a mall with fairly unexciting tenants. Although Paddington station is one of London's most beautiful train hubs (it was built by the legendary architect Isambard Kingdom Brunel in 1838), it's also the most inconvenient—although Heathrow and Windsor trains go from it.

DOCKLANDS

Best for: *Development, ancient warehouses, super-cheap chain hotels*
What you won't find: *Street life, nightlife*

Most of far east London along the north side of the Thames is ignobly called by a single, sweeping name: Docklands. The past is rich here: Captain Cook set off on his explorations from here, and its hand-dug basins once teemed with ships bearing goods from around the planet. Docklands made colonial Britain successful—and thus America, Canada, Australia, and South Africa, too. After a fallow generation, East London's hand-dug pools are under constant redevelopment by corporations in stacks of fluorescent-lit office cubes, and the Olympics settled here in 2012 near the Stratford Tube stop. Away from the river, in salt-of-the-earth neighborhoods like Bethnal Green, Stratford, and West Ham, The City's Pakistani and Indian populations flourish, with marvelous but unglamorous food and shops.

ISLINGTON

Best for: *Antiques, gastropubs, theater, street markets, cafes, strolls*
What you won't find: *Museums, hotels*

Few neighborhoods retain such a healthy balance between feisty bohemianism and groomed prosperity, and almost none retain streetscapes as defiantly mid-century as Chapel Market. Islington's leafy byways are dotted with antiques dealers, hoary pubs with backroom theater spaces, beer gardens, and most pleasingly on a sunny day, pedestrian towpaths overlooking Regent's Canal. Why more tourists don't flood Islington is a mystery—and a blessing—but that hasn't stopped its ascendancy as a choice neighborhood for those with money.

CAMDEN

Best for: *Alternative music, massive clothing markets, junk souvenirs, pubs*
What you won't find: *Elbow room, hotels, upscale restaurants*

Name a British tune that got under your skin, and chances are it received its first airing in the beer-soaked concert halls of Camden Town. London's analogue to San Francisco's Haight-Ashbury District, it was big in the countercultured '60s and '70s and is still grotty enough for Amy Winehouse to have expired in. The area's shoulder-to-shoulder markets, which hawk touristy hokum, cheap sunglasses, and £5 falafel in the former warehouses and stables serving Regent's Canal, can be pretty awful, and the sort of places where you feel compelled to carry your wallet in your front pocket. Tourists come more out of duty than for any true mission for commerce and they cram the inadequate Tube stop on weekends.

NOTTING HILL

Best for: *Markets, village vibes, restaurants, pubs, tourists, antiques*
What you won't find: *Well-priced shopping, museums, Hugh Grant*

Thanks partly to Hollywood, this westerly nook known to locals for race riots and, in 2017, the horrible Grenfell Tower fire, appears high on many visitors' checklists. Its Saturday Portobello Road market, the principal draw, is fiendishly crowded but short on truly wonderful wares. In fact, it's touristy. Like Camden, people go because they think they should. But if you feel compelled, Hugh Grant's blue door from *Notting Hill* (1999) is at 280 Westbourne Park Rd.

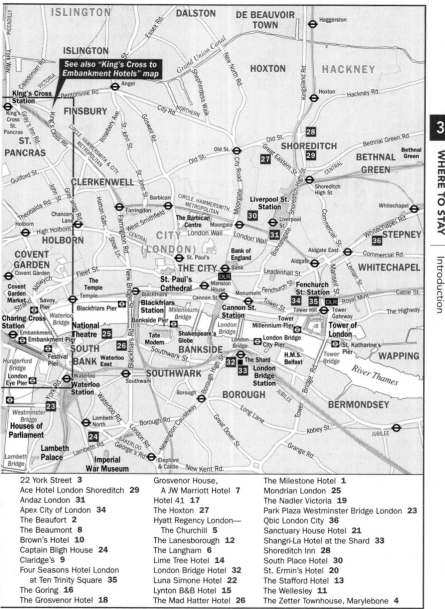

22 York Street **3**	Grosvenor House,	The Milestone Hotel **1**
Ace Hotel London Shoreditch **29**	A JW Marriott Hotel **7**	Mondrian London **25**
Andaz London **31**	Hotel 41 **17**	The Nadler Victoria **19**
Apex City of London **34**	The Hoxton **27**	Park Plaza Westminster Bridge London **23**
The Beaufort **2**	Hyatt Regency London—	Qbic London City **36**
The Beaumont **8**	The Churchill **5**	Sanctuary House Hotel **21**
Brown's Hotel **10**	The Lanesborough **12**	Shangri-La Hotel at the Shard **33**
Captain Bligh House **24**	The Langham **6**	Shoreditch Inn **28**
Claridge's **9**	Lime Tree Hotel **14**	South Place Hotel **30**
Four Seasons Hotel London	London Bridge Hotel **32**	St. Ermin's Hotel **20**
at Ten Trinity Square **35**	Luna Simone Hotel **22**	The Stafford Hotel **13**
The Goring **16**	Lynton B&B Hotel **15**	The Wellesley **11**
The Grosvenor Hotel **18**	The Mad Hatter Hotel **26**	The Zetter Townhouse, Marylebone **4**

nights like zombies. The hotels in this chapter strive to keep you out of dead tourist-hotel zones and keep you in the middle of the action.

Accommodations are subject to a Value Added Tax (VAT) of 20%. Happily, almost all small B&Bs include taxes in their rates, although you may be charged 3% to 5% to use a credit card. More expensive hotels (those around £150 or more) tend to leave taxes off their tariffs, which can result in a nasty surprise at checkout, so it never hurts to ask if the rate "excludes VAT."

THE BUDGET HOTEL CHAINS

We put this section first because it includes a huge number of the best-priced rooms in the best neighborhoods. Expect reliable standards, decently sized rooms with private bath, and unbeatable lead-in rates for people who pay months ahead of time. Also, so many people habitually turn to these brands that prices frequently rise far past the point of value, particularly close to the dates of stay. In addition to these names, look into **Motel One** (24–26 Minories, EC3; www.motel-one.com; ✆ **020/7481-6420;** doubles from £98), a stylish and ultra-cheap but cramped German newcomer with a single location in the somewhat inconvenient neighborhood of Tower Hill. For specific locations, look on the chain's websites, listed below.

CitizenM ★★★ My favorite affordable London chain is actually Dutch. Their glassy open-plan lobbies lined with shelves of orange-and-white Penguin classic paperbacks (which every self-conscious interior designer in London displays to denote postmodern intellectualism), churn day and night with people sipping fine coffee and telecommuting. Check-in is self-guided by kiosk, and rooms are compact—almost podlike—but arranged with genius. Expect massive platform beds piled with body pillows, curvy unit bathrooms slotted into the space with calculated aplomb, and a bedside tablet that lets you control everything from motorized blinds to the color of the room's mood lighting. There's even a hefty library of free movies (including porn—like I said, it's Dutch). My favorite locations are Bankside (near the Tate Modern) and Tower of London, with rooms and a fab rooftop bar overlooking said eternal fortress.

www.citizenm.com. 3 locations around London. From £125 double. **Amenities:** Free movies; free Wi-Fi.

easyHotel ★ This is how you do London super-cheaply while avoiding hostels. Reservations typically cost £25 for double rooms if you book 6 months ahead, and £35 to £90 if you procrastinate. Prefabricated room units

King's Cross to Embankment Hotels

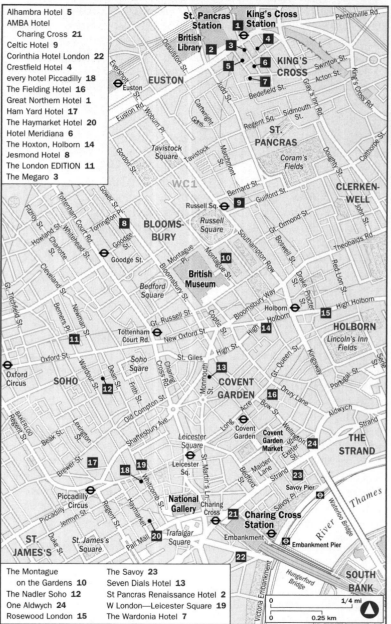

Alhambra Hotel **5**
AMBA Hotel
  Charing Cross **21**
Celtic Hotel **9**
Corinthia Hotel London **22**
Crestfield Hotel **4**
every hotel Piccadilly **18**
The Fielding Hotel **16**
Great Northern Hotel **1**
Ham Yard Hotel **17**
The Haymarket Hotel **20**
Hotel Meridiana **6**
The Hoxton, Holborn **14**
Jesmond Hotel **8**
The London EDITION **11**
The Megaro **3**

The Montague
  on the Gardens **10**
The Nadler Soho **12**
One Aldwych **24**
Rosewood London **15**

The Savoy **23**
Seven Dials Hotel **13**
St Pancras Renaissance Hotel **2**
W London—Leicester Square **19**
The Wardonia Hotel **7**

differ only in how little space you're given (the smallest are 6 sq. m/65 sq. ft., space only for a bed and a breath), with rarely an inch of space between mattress and wall. No phone, no hair dryer, no frills at all. Bathrooms are just plastic cubicles combining a shower, toilet, and sink in one water-splashed closet. The cheapest rooms don't even have windows, and you cannot change the thermostat. Want to watch TV? You'll pay £5 for 24 hours. Want housekeeping? £10. Wi-Fi is pay-as-you-use. This no-nonsense concept humiliates some and delights others by being so incredibly affordable.

www.easyhotel.com. No phone reservations. 5 locations in Central London. Rooms £25–£90. **Amenities:** Wi-Fi £10/day.

hub by Premier Inn ★★   Sleek, cannily designed rooms (just 11.4 sq. m/123 sq. ft.) are tight as airlocks, packing in a platform bed for two with storage underneath, a bright and clean-lined shower/toilet module, well-located power outlets and USB charging ports, a fold-down desk, a lime green chair. The staff won't do much for you, but using an app, you can dim or extinguish the lights, watch TV (all movies are free—the Wi-Fi is mercury-fast, too), or turn on the "do not disturb" light. Downsides: You may not get a mobile phone signal and you won't be able to look out a window, but the location is unmatched and there's a cafe for breakfast (under £10). Deservedly, the best rates sell out months in advance—book online only. My favorite location: Covent Garden.

www.hubhotels.co.uk. 6 locations around London. £69–£161 double. **Amenities:** Breakfast (fee); free movies; free Wi-Fi.

Ibis Hotels ★★   This 600-strong French chain by the Accor hotel giant is distinguished by simple but cheerful decor. You'll get a double bed, bathroom with shower, climate control, a 24-hour kitchen, TV, phone, free Wi-Fi, at least one outlet, and a built-in desk. The breakfast charge varies per property (£8 is typical), but food is usually served from 4am, making this a smart choice if you need to catch an early flight or train. The fresh-baked breakfast baguettes are delicious—hey, it's French. There's also **Ibis Styles,** the "all-inclusive" brand that is slightly more upscale and includes breakfast and Wi-Fi, and **Ibis Budget,** a bare-bones, shower-only crash pad once known as Etap or Formule 1; rooms there are ultra-simple (though with style), sleep up to three people, and have free Wi-Fi and TV, but practically nothing else.

www.ibishotel.com. No English-reservations hotline. 6 locations around London. Rooms £101–£218, varying by season and location. **Amenities:** Free Wi-Fi.

Point A Hotels ★   This modern-design import, once Tune Hotels, provides everything you need but nothing else: en-suite power shower, round-the-clock reception, air conditioning, but not even a closet—you get hangers. Even windows come at a price. The a la carte model keeps costs down but isn't a path to luxury, yet the facilities are clean and designed with minimalist zip. Don't write off a windowless room's power to mediate jet lag. Too often, however, rates are around £175, which is too much for this simplicity—around £110 would be more reasonable.

www.pointahotels.com. No phone. 5 locations in the city. Rooms £35–£125. **Amenities:** Wi-Fi £4 per device per day.

Premier Inn ★★ The largest hotel chain in the country, Premier offers rooms (maximum of two adults) with a king-size bed, bathtub and shower with all-purpose shower gel, tea- and coffee-making facilities, TV, phone, iron, air conditioning (sometimes), at least three outlets, and a desk. Increasingly, it requires you to check in at a kiosk, eliminating human interaction, but that tells you about the tourist churn that this company is going for. Many locations include a mass-appeal bar/cafe, Thyme. Like airline tickets, prices rise as availability dwindles. Its prices start at £19 nearly a year ahead, but final prices can be poor value, so the key is early booking. Clip £10 off prices by booking ahead with a nonrefundable reservation. *Note:* Reservation search engines may return results that are deep in distant suburbs, so consult a map before taking the bait of a low price. My favorite locations: Southwark and County Hall.

www.premierinn.com. ⓒ **0845/099-0095.** More than 12 locations around the city. Rooms £80–£126, depending on season and location. **Amenities:** Bar/cafe; 30 mins. free Wi-Fi daily, then £3 per 24 hr.

Travelodge ★ Rates start around £88 for a non-flexible reservation if you book 11 months ahead. That more than makes up for the thin amenities of this economy brand, which has some two dozen properties in Greater London. It's nicer than the American Travelodge brand, which isn't related to it. Expect king-size beds, bathtub and shower, TV (but no phone, hair dryer, or toiletries), paid in-room movies, a wardrobe, at least one power point, and a desk. Breakfast, if your property offers it, is about £8 more. "Family rooms" have a pullout couch for two kids but cost the same as a double. Prices go down to £25 if you're first to book but they skyrocket in peak periods.

www.travelodge.co.uk. ⓒ **08719/848484.** More than 20 locations around the city. Rooms £65–£116, depending on season and location. **Amenities:** Bar/café (often); Wi-Fi £3 a day.

Z Hotels ★★★ Please say it "Zed," which rhymes with "bed." Now that you've got that down, here's the formula: extremely compact rooms, but lots of room under the duvets; glassy sleek style; and a lobby that's always abuzz with breakfast, coffee, or free daily wine. The formula works because there are design smarts where they count: Shower nozzles swivel the way you need them to, towels are plump and copious, you can control your thermostat. They poured cash into the bedding and the 40-inch TVs but did without closets and drawers. Very cheap rooms may not have windows. Note that if you share a room with a platonic friend, bathrooms are enclosed only by panels of fogged glass. My favorite locations: Soho and Piccadilly.

www.thezhotels.com. 8 locations around the city. Rooms £80–£130. **Amenities:** Cafe/bar; air conditioning; free evening wine and cheese; free Wi-Fi.

KING'S CROSS & BLOOMSBURY

King's Cross hotels offer small rooms in old buildings, but they are close to six important Tube lines. Bloomsbury's chocolate-colored Georgian brick town houses lie within a 20-minute walk of Soho and Covent Garden, and they're near the Piccadilly Line to Heathrow. To be honest—and let's spill a dirty secret here—these places are better located than some of London's most expensive hotels.

Expensive

Great Northern Hotel ★★   Of all of London's railway terminal hotels, from the outside the Great Northern seems the plainest—and the smallest. Its crescent-shaped building went up quite early, in 1854, and as a consequence it isn't as bombastic as its brethren. Rooms aren't huge, but they have a smart modern edge that includes—daringly for a hotel—cream-colored carpeting. The smallest rooms are called "couchette" because the sled-style queen beds, attached at head and foot to the walls, are said to have been inspired by railway sleepers. (Don't worry—they have much more space for your luggage, although the result is something less than ideal for families.) Etched glass and cute little curved banquettes complete the allusions to trains. High-standard perks pack the other spaces—a good British restaurant, Plum & Spilt Milk (named after a color scheme), is one. *Note:* If you're quoted a rate over £300, you can do better elsewhere.

Kings Cross St Pancras Station, Pancras Rd., N1. www.gnhlondon.com. ℂ **020/3388-0800.** 91 units. Doubles from about £195. Tube: King's Cross St Pancras. **Amenities:** Restaurant; bar; snack bar; free Wi-Fi.

The Montague on the Gardens ★★   It's not easy these days finding typically British midpriced hotels that aren't mired in gloomy tour-group dinginess, but the conjoined town houses of the Montague deliver Englishness in demonstration as much as in word. Downstairs, a large staff pays close attention to guest needs, and rooms, always tasteful and richly comfortable, are a mishmash of styles as if in a moneyed home. They're also a mix of sizes, given the age of the buildings, but they're silent, plush, and otherwise appointed with more than you'll need. It's comfortable, dignified, and a homey bolthole for Central London explorations, with the British Museum literally across the road. It's family-friendly as well.

15 Montague St., WC1. www.montaguehotel.com. ℂ **020/7858-7731.** 100 units. Rooms £194–£356. Tube: Russell Square. **Amenities:** Restaurant; bar; air conditioning; free bottled water; free Wi-Fi.

St Pancras Renaissance Hotel ★★   This Gothic red-brick palace, built in the 1870s as a terminal hotel for a railway line, is one of London's most distinctive buildings; its meticulous 2011 restoration not only rescued a Victorian icon from neglect but also created a distinctive property. Premium rooms have an unforgettable view down the ribbed, cast-iron cavern of the train shed, where Eurostar arrives and departs for Paris. There, the epic

WHAT TO EXPECT AT town house hotels

Unfortunately, the once-famous English B&B is an endangered species, at least in central London. Neighborhoods that were recently dependable for cut-price lodging (Gloucester Place in Marylebone, Ebury St. in Victoria, Gower St. in Bloomsbury) are being sold to the ultra-rich, and B&Bs are converting to luxury apartments or selling out. Most desk staff now know London little better than you do.

The ones that survive usually occupy "listed" buildings. What does that mean? It means that it has historical or architectural importance—for example, it's an example of a fine Georgian town house or an original stately Victorian terrace home. To keep developers from knocking down a gem, "listed" buildings are protected. Changing anything requires permission, down to the color of the paint. American tourists who are unused to London's listed buildings often post huffy online reviews about the very things that define town house hotels, penalizing London inns for being London inns. That hotel is not a dump! It's historic.

Rooms are small by American standards. Interior walls were added to subdivide the original rooms, but don't blame the current owners. Most subdivision was done after World War II, to fill a housing gap after many of the city's big hotels were destroyed, and now even removing those slapped-up walls requires civic approval, which is nigh impossible. You are unlikely to have a closet, and in some rooms suitcases can be hard to open without using the bed. The largest rooms in such B&Bs usually face the front.

Bathrooms are even smaller. In the old days, guests shared bathrooms. To suit changing tastes, landlords wedged booths containing the staples (toilet, shower, sink) into rooms that weren't designed to have them.

Don't expect an elevator, or "lift." It takes years of begging and a small fortune to convince the council to permit the installation of an elevator. Assume you'll have to use the stairs. They may be narrower than you're used to. Rooms on higher floors require climbing, but they also receive more light, less noise, and often cost less.

Ceilings get lower as you go higher. Until the 20th century, the floors of fashionable town houses served distinct functions. The cellar was for kitchens and coal storage. The ground floor was usually used for living rooms. The first and second floors were reserved for bedrooms, and the top floor was for servants and for the children's nursery, which accounts for the slightly lower ceilings there.

Not all windows are double glazed. You think you hear traffic now? Imagine when horses and carriages clattered up the cobbles at all hours. If you're a light sleeper, simply ask for a room at the back. Rooms on back stairway landings often don't adjoin other rooms, either, which takes care of more ambient noise.

Chambers rooms have 5.5m (18-ft.) ceilings and details such as (now-decorative) fireplaces, arched windows, and substantial wooden doors. Rooms in the new Barlow wing lack those long views and suit corporate hotel tastes—the real show is in the original building. Echoing public spaces are a gilt-and-tile parade of self-important Victorian excess, from the winged Grand Staircase to the lushly carved The Gilbert Scott brasserie (named for the architect; local star Marcus Wareing oversees it) and the old wooden Booking Hall, now a bistro where old English punch cocktails are revived. The building was "too good for its purpose," lamented Scott, whose own son went mad and died in one of the rooms. It's worth a wander even if you're not staying here—management knows it's a jewel, and it welcomes visitors.

Euston Rd., London, NW1. www.stpancrasrenaissance.co.uk. © **020/7841-3540.** 245 units. Doubles £250–£450. Tube: King's Cross St Pancras. **Amenities:** Restaurant; 2 bars; indoor pool; gym; spa; free Wi-Fi in Chambers rooms, otherwise £15/day.

Moderate

The Megaro ★ This old office building has been tarted up with brassy colors and a cluttered exterior mural, which the neighbors must hate, but inside, the theme is spacious and virtually Scandinavian, with open wood floors, unadorned paneling, smart slide-out make-up desks and workspaces, and fresh tea leaves for your cuppa. Rooms on the main road have killer views of St Pancras and the plaza in front of King's Cross (no. 504, a corner, is the best for that), but if traffic noise irritates you, go for one facing the other way (no. 508, with a small balcony, picturesquely peeks over the pipe chimneys of nearby town houses). The tariff comes with a free newspaper you can download to your iPad. If you're traveling with a platonic companion, ask for a room in which your bathroom isn't encased in glass walls; some are, some aren't. Next door, its sister the **California** (www.thecalifornialondon.com; © **020/7837-7629**), a converted town house, is much tighter and lift-free, but 40% cheaper.

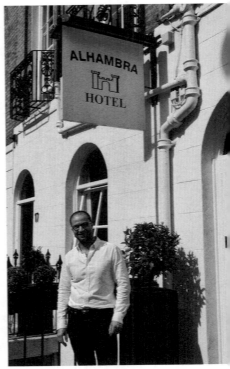

Belgrove St., WC1. www.hotelmegaro.co.uk. © **020/7843-2222.** 49 units. Average price £165 single, £185 double, save £15 on website. Rates include breakfast. Tube: King's Cross St Pancras. **Amenities:** Restaurant; bar; free Wi-Fi.

Inexpensive

Alhambra Hotel ★★★ My favorite budget family-run B&B in London, the comforting Alhambra is an inn with heart, and a top value in Frommer's ever since *Europe on $5 a Day.* They care. Its proprietors, whose lineage has owned the land for decades and aren't at risk of being elbowed out like so many others, take pride in the business and they keep prices low. Picture simple, small, but dignified rooms squeezed into old spaces, but always spotless and

The family-run Alhambra Hotel keeps prices low and amenities high.

freshened up with bright bedspreads, inviting royal-blue carpeting, built-in desks with chairs, and flat-screen TVs (but no phones). Bruno Cabral handles the hotel's modern service, such as the addition of free fiber-optic Wi-Fi and in-room safes, rarities for this price point. If you share a bathroom, there are plenty to go around. Guests can use the lobby computer. The same family runs an annex across the street that has the same high standards. In winter, it's easy to negotiate rates down by as much as 30%.

17–19 Argyle St., WC1. www.alhambrahotel.com. ℗ **020/7837-9575.** 52 units. £85–£110 single, £95–£135 double. Rates include full breakfast. Tube: King's Cross St Pancras. **Amenities:** Lobby computer; free Wi-Fi.

Celtic Hotel ★★   The eccentric but dedicated Marazzi family, beloved in London's affordable-travel world, transformed a guesthouse near the British Museum (and the Tube to Heathrow) into this memorable budget citadel. Few other hoteliers put as much heart into making sure guests are acclimated to London by answering questions, obliging special dietary requests, and filling bellies with a cooked breakfast that's so enormous (try the banana yogurt) that lunch might become optional. To keep attracting longtime regulars—there are many, going back a half a century, because the Marazzis owned the departed St Margaret's Hotel for 56 years—the Celtic retains quirky features: Rooms don't have TVs or phones, furniture is endearingly mismatched, and the lounge is a hub for socializing with fellow guests. Add £6–£21 if you don't want to share a shower or toilet. You must book directly.

61–63 Guilford St., WC1. www.celtichotel.com. ℗ **020/7837-6737.** 30 units. Singles from £63, doubles from £85. Rates include cooked breakfast. Tube: Russell Square. **Amenities:** 2 lounges; free Wi-Fi.

Crestfield Hotel ★   Every city needs a few basic, secure choices that aren't grim. It will never be your favorite hotel, but the price could make London do-able for you: Rooms are tiny, painted in grey-blue, with wee TVs but no phones. Their bathrooms are essentially tiled cubicles with drains, but the £100 family room for four is a true steal. Room no. 9, a double, is located on a landing facing the back, so it's even quieter than most. There's no lift. This building has been a guest house for more than a century. Seriously, what more do you require?

2–4 Crestfield St., WC1. www.crestfieldhotel.com. ℗ **020/7837-0500.** 58 units. Singles from £50, doubles from £65. Rates include continental breakfast. Tube: King's Cross St Pancras. **Amenities:** Bar, free Wi-Fi.

Hotel Meridiana ★   This is what a value hotel should be: not lavish, but you happily get what you pay for. Walls can be thin, rooms truly teeny, and many share bathrooms, but everything is spotless, and breakfast (served in a room so small that sometimes you have to wait your turn) is a proper cooked one. Heating and hot water are reliable, too, which isn't always the case in buildings of this age, and some rooms have drawers, another relative curiosity. If you just want a dead-cheap place to sleep where you'll have no regrets about hygiene, this no-frills B&B is a decent choice. You're unlikely to get as much value for the price elsewhere.

43–44 Argyle Sq., WC1. www.hotelmeridiana.co.uk. © **020/7713-0144.** 27 units. Singles from £65, doubles from £85. Rates include full breakfast. Tube: King's Cross St Pancras. **Amenities:** Free Wi-Fi.

Jesmond Hotel ★★★ I have a soft spot for this place near the British Library. I stayed here often when I was just out of college (in room no. 3, a cozy single on the rear landing—still there, still snug). Back then, the Beynon family had a young son, Glyn. Today, Glyn is a grown family man, and he's in charge—and he's doing a proud job of updating the family B&B in a 1780s town house (ask him about its history) far beyond the expectations of its tariff range. He installed new bathrooms with all-new piping, accounting for the larger-than-average showers; he soundproofed the front windows to keep out the roar of Gower Street's traffic. He also converted the former parlor, with its antique (nonworking) fireplace, into room no. 2, a spacious double. It's classic (not all units have bathrooms), and in fact, has been a Frommer's selection ever since *Europe on $5 a Day* (when it cost $3.20). It's still one of London's last "they're charging *how* much?" values. Pay for 6 nights from November to February, and you can stay for 7. Don't confuse this place with the Jesmond Dene, a B&B on Argyle Square—it's very good, too, but not as central.

63 Gower St., WC1. www.jesmondhotel.org.uk. © **020/7636-3199.** 15 units. £75–£85 single, £95–£125 double, £150 quad, often a 3-night minimum. Rates include full breakfast. Tube: Goodge St. **Amenities:** Free Wi-Fi.

The Wardonia Hotel ★ For almost half a century in the pages of Frommer's, the Wardonia has been suggested for those times when you need a place to be super cheap, no matter the sacrifice: Rooms are wee—like *sooooo* tiny, as if the walls and the bed are in a death match for dominance, recalling the compactor scene in *Star Wars*. Thus warned, you will now be prepared for the impossible value. Very simple in plain brown wainscoting, crash-pad rooms have bathroom cubbies with showers but not tubs, and you don't get breakfast—all reflected in the crazy low rates, which are a third of what other budget places charge and have barely budged in a decade. The Wardonia is plainly a value champion. Prices dip about £10 lower in winter.

46–54 Argyle St., WC1. www.wardoniahotel.co.uk. © **020/7837-3944.** 65 units. £50 single, £60 double/twin, £70 triple. Tube: King's Cross St Pancras. **Amenities:** Free Wi-Fi.

SOHO, COVENT GARDEN & WEST END

This is the middle of London. The part of town that offers everything you need outside your door. The area that also offers streets crawling with inebriated 20-year-olds singing drinking shanties in full voice after midnight. You may not care, because staying centrally can save on Tube fare more than it costs in shoe leather. Sunday through Thursday are the cheapest nights here.

Expensive

Corinthia Hotel London ★★ In 1885, this proud wedge-shaped block between Trafalgar Square and the Thames opened as the Hôtel Métropole, one of London's finest. Then, for 70 years, the Ministry of Defence commandeered it and drabbed it into its desultory HQ, leading the war effort from here. It's now again one of London's finest hotels, leading the fight against frugality with an epic breakfast buffet (extra fee), two gourmet restaurants (one modern English, one Italian), a moody jazz cocktail bar where celebrities are spotted but not disturbed, and a four-level subterranean ESPA Life spa—in some ways the Corinthia's heart—a smooth-edged windowless realm of white and water, like being swaddled in a fragrant egg. Rooms lapse slightly (outlets are inconvenient, and only the most expensive categories glimpse the river), but overall, a splendid splurge, even if it's one that charges above its grade.

Whitehall Place, SW1. www.corinthia.com/london. ℘ **020/7930-8181.** 127 units. Rooms £200–£570. Tube: Charing Cross. **Amenities:** 2 restaurants; bar; spa; fitness center; free Wi-Fi.

Ham Yard Hotel ★ Firmdale Hotels is a revered name in London's vanity circles, and the design penchant of its co-owner, Kit Kemp, has made her a style celebrity. Tucked into a mews north of Piccadilly Circus, it's preferred by social butterflies—the huge ground floor bar and four-lane basement bowling alley/cinema complex swarm during the weekend, and not with fellow guests. The hive of activity can put a frenetic spin on breakfast or a sundowner, but rooms (no two identical, each one seemingly ripped from a design magazine) are buffered from the buzz with soundproofing, plump queen beds, floor-to-ceiling windows, and generous bathrooms of granite and oak with walk-in showers. You're paying for coolness.

1 Ham Yard, W1. www.firmdalehotels.com. ℘ **020/3642-2000.** 91 units. Rooms from £400. Tube: Piccadilly Circus. **Amenities:** Bar/restaurant; fitness center; cinema; bowling alley; rooftop bar; free Wi-Fi.

The Haymarket Hotel ★★ Bubbly colored textures, mismatched but impeccably selected furniture—this Firmdale property is like staying at the country house of a fabulous friend who has made a fortune in coffee table books. This elegant (but never stuffy) choice takes its cues from nearby St James's, regally situated in a cluster of rehabbed buildings beside the Theatre Royal Haymarket, and it backs up its bright Modern English visuals with five-star features such as a sharp staff, indulgent showers, and an indoor swimming pool. There are no high-end choices closer to the West End action yet serenely removed from its tumult—it's the one property in the Firmdale group not to be routinely mobbed with cocktail-swilling fashion chasers, which makes it a delicious place to land and recharge after a tiring day.

1 Suffolk Pl., SW1. www.firmdalehotels.com. ℘ **020/7470-4000.** 50 units. Rooms from £400. Tube: Piccadilly Circus. **Amenities:** Bar/restaurant; fitness center; basement pool; free Wi-Fi.

The London EDITION ★ Hotel superstar Ian Schrager launched this impudent lifestyle brand, which now has seven worldwide locations. It's a calculated mix of classy and irreverent—look closely and you'll see those photographic homages to Rembrandt depict a girl wearing toilet paper rolls around her ears. Rooms slouch just enough to please wealthy people who can't relinquish their hipness—faux fur sculpturally strewn on your bed, pre-fab wood panel decor slumming it like a 1970s basement rumpus room. It's also—this must be said—the place to stay if you love a hot hotel staff, since the porters and desk staff seem to have been hired as much for the cornflower blue of their eyes as for their service credentials. The adjoining lobby bar and Berners Tavern restaurant are scenes for one and all.

10 Berners St., W1. www.editionhotels.com. ℂ **020/7781-0000.** 173 units. £319–£505 double. Tube: Tottenham Court Rd. **Amenities:** Restaurant; bar; room service; 24-hr. fitness center; free bottled water; loaner laptops; free Wi-Fi.

One Aldwych ★★★ The domed one-time headquarters of the *Morning Post*, built in 1907, is now home to this consistently high-quality boutique hotel with two restaurants (one of which serves Basque gourmet); a double-tall, sculpture-filled lobby cocktail lounge; and a theatrically lit underground swimming pool where the printing presses were once housed. Rooms are mildly contemporary; some sneak a view of the Thames and others admire the Lyceum Theatre. The staff is five-star, usually meeting guests' needs without being asked, and the location feels impossibly considerate, too: steps from Covent Garden and Trafalgar Square, a walk down Strand to St Paul's, and a brief stroll over the Waterloo Bridge to the glories of Southbank. This well-kept secret is a favorite of those in the know.

1 Aldwych, WC2. www.onealdwych.com. ℂ **020/7300-1000.** 105 units. £264–£471 double. Tube: Covent Garden or Temple. **Amenities:** 2 restaurants, cocktail bar, indoor pool, gym, spa treatments, free Wi-Fi.

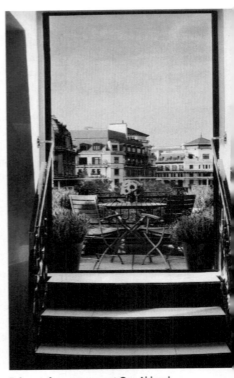

Balcony of a guest room at One Aldwych, which used to be the home of the Morning Post.

Rosewood London ★★★   The city's lushest modern hotel is entered through a stone courtyard arch of a gloriously elaborate edifice (constructed with pomp in 1914 as the Pearl Assurance insurance citadel). The foyer is amazingly sheathed in brass, and rooms are so quiet you could hear your champagne bubbles pop. They're also exquisite: Giant 46-inch flatscreen TVs are standard, as is Italian bedding you sink into like a swimming pool. Push a button to bring down your window blinds and sip homemade sloe gin from the minibar (there's also a gin bar in the restaurant downstairs, plus a gimmicky bar themed to Scarfe, a cartoonist who is London's modern-day version of Broadway's Al Hirschfeld). If it weren't for the hard reality of the tariff, it'd be enough to sour you to the rest of the planet. The neighborhood seems at first to be too dry, but the pleasures of the British Museum and Covent Garden are both 5 minutes away.

252 High Holborn, WC1. www.rosewoodhotels.com/london. © **020/7781-8888.** 262 units. Rooms £320–£510. Tube: Holborn. **Amenities:** Restaurant; bar; lounge; fitness center; spa; free Wi-Fi.

The Savoy ★   Few cities can claim hotels as iconic as the Savoy, which merits a visit even if you, like most people, cannot afford to stay there. From the polished gleam of its iconic drive-in porte cochere to the palatial receiving rooms off the lobby, The Savoy has vibrated with high history, half Edwardian

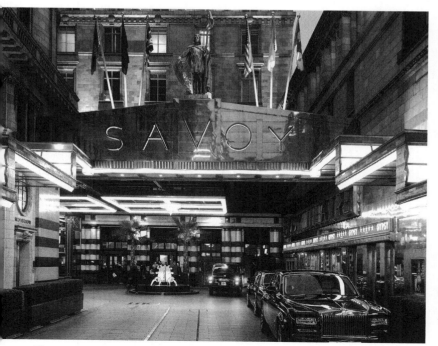

The entrance to the iconic Savoy is sure to impress.

and half Jazz Age, since 1889. The American Bar has been a hushed labora-tory for upscale cocktails for a century. A small museum about the Savoy's pedigree, open to anyone, reminds you how much happened here: Churchill puffing, Chaplin mugging, Wilde and Bosie dallying, Gilbert and Sullivan pattering in its theater, Monet and Whistler painting the Thames from their windows—but to be fair, as it gets more touristy, the Savoy, now run by Fair-mont, is more likely to revel in that past than create such yarns for the future. Still, your every need, from floral to gourmet, will be addressed with abject elegance and for a dear price. A fine honeymooners' selection.

Strand, WC2. www.fairmont.com/savoy-london. © **800/257-7544** (U.S.) or 020/7836-4343 (London). 268 units. Rooms from £445. Tube: Embankment or Temple. **Amenities:** 3 restaurants; 2 bars; indoor pool; gym; spa; business center; Wi-Fi £10/day.

W London—Leicester Square ★   London's only outpost of Starwood's self-consciously cool brand looks like a glass hippopotamus wallowing beside Leicester Square, and it effortfully preens (crowd-control ropes appear at the entrance at night whether they're needed or not). Standard ("Wonderful") rooms are funky. Maybe *too* funky: A central bar contains both bathroom sink and desk (not a great pairing), walls are hung with silvery curtains instead of art, the shower and WC are concealed behind mirrored doors (*lots* of mirrors in this hotel, including hundreds of disco balls). Frustratingly, your exterior view is obscured by a dotted glass curtain so outsiders can't see in. You either dig W's shtick or roll your eyes to its beat. Or you were just cashing in Star-wood points.

10 Wardour St., WC2. www.wlondon.co.uk. © **020/7758-1000.** 192 units. Rooms from £299. Tube: Leicester Square or Piccadilly Circus. **Amenities:** Restaurant, bar, spa, gym, free Wi-Fi.

Moderate

AMBA Hotel Charing Cross ★★★   The railway terminal hotel above Charing Cross Station opened a month after Lincoln's assassination and underwent many lives (and Blitz damage). Now the Charing Cross is an upper-moderate hotel that dips its toes into luxury trimmings (heated bath-room floors, walk-in showers, Nespresso coffee, free minibars that even include beer, and so forth) without going over-the-top on price. The location is spectacular and could command much higher rates: With Trafalgar Square steps in one direction and morning strolls on the Thames a block away in the other, you're truly spoiled. Breakfast (crowded; the staff isn't always on top of things) is taken with a view toward St Martin-in-the-Fields, and at night, some 350 LED candles flicker throughout the hallways and up the sweeping central grand staircase. Such echoes of a more genteel age treat you to the grandeur of old London at a good price.

The Strand, WC2. www.amba-hotel.com/charing-cross. © **0800/330-8397.** 239 units. Rooms £171–318. Tube: Charing Cross or Embankment. **Amenities:** Restaurant, bar, business center, free Wi-Fi.

every hotel Piccadilly ★   Steps from Leicester Square, this hotel shares a concept with other trendy budget brands: Give them comfortable beds and free Wi-Fi, let them check in by kiosk, and then leave them alone. You get a Nespresso coffee machine, a Smart TV, an upper-grade bed, and access to a printer for boarding passes. The stripped-down staff has its drawbacks (if you need someone, you may have to wait), but for what you're saving and the prime spot you're scoring, big deal. Prices are £20 to £30 lower if you book many months ahead.

Coventry St., W1. www.every-hotels.com/Piccadilly. ⓒ **0800/330-8395.** 127 units. Rooms from £177. Tube: Leicester Square. **Amenities:** Restaurant; fitness center; free Wi-Fi.

The Fielding Hotel ★   It's nearly impossible to beat the location, just steps from Covent Garden's food and shopping, which is why you overlook the cramped, lift-less quarters at this family-owned hotel. In this early-19th-century warren of tight staircases and fire doors, the sometimes slightly airless rooms snuggle you with a certain throwaway charisma. It's not top of the line, but it feels like home. Room no. 10 is a double with a sitting area that catches lots of afternoon light, thanks to its corner position and copious windows. Everything's en suite (but mostly shower only) and there are no common areas to speak of. Trivia: Oscar Wilde was convicted of gross indecency in the Bow Street Magistrates' Court next door.

4 Broad Ct., Bow St., WC2. www.thefieldinghotel.co.uk. ⓒ **020/7836-8305.** 24 units. £90–£100 single, £140–£180 double. Tube: Covent Garden or Holborn. **Amenities:** Pass to nearby fitness center; free Wi-Fi.

The Hoxton, Holborn ★   It's called Hoxton because that's where this boutique hipster hotel brand began (the original is listed on p. 63). This one is newer (2014), busier, and delightfully it's also a few minutes' walk south of the British Museum, in the middle of it all. There's a restaurant, a bar, and a too-cool-for-school beauty salon. It may be off-puttingly millennial: The lobby is always packed with Wi-Fi spongers (good luck finding a seat as a paying guest). You get a smallish, winkingly antique-styled room with a double bed, fun throwback touches like wooden desks, vintage-looking music players, a chubby duvet, and an hour's worth of free calls every day. The bathroom is less smart; tiled showers are faux-Victorian but don't have doors. Continental breakfast is delivered in a bag. Every room is a good value—that's the point—but they all have the same amenities no matter the size, so why not go for the cheapest, the 129-square-foot "Shoebox"?

199–206 High Holborn, WC1. www.hoxtonhotels.com. ⓒ **020/7661-3000.** 174 units. Rooms £159–£255. Rates include continental breakfast. Tube: Holborn. **Amenities:** 2 restaurants; bar; coffee house; salon; 1 hr. free calls daily; free water and milk; free Wi-Fi.

The Nadler Soho ★★★   The Nadler gets moderate lodging exactly right by providing style without pretension or henpecking guests with fees. Quiet, high-design rooms are compact but nonetheless kitted out with twists such as

ALL IN THE timing

To save money on guesthouses and inns, remember five simple rules:

1. **Off-season is cheaper.** Many big hotels have two seasons: April through September vs. October through March (excluding holidays). Prices will be 10% to 25% cheaper in winter. Interestingly, very few family-owned B&Bs and inns bother with this system, pricing uniformly.

2. **To save, stay longer.** I haven't found a family-run hotel that wasn't willing to lower prices for anyone staying more than 5 or 6 nights.

3. **Mind the crowds.** Soho, a party zone, is cheaper on weekdays; The City, a business enclave, is cheaper on weekends.

4. **Go mom-and-pop.** Their rates usually include taxes, but big hotels' rates don't.

5. **Last-minute deals are rare but do exist.** Routes for looking into deals are Hotwire.com, Priceline.com, and the same-day booking app Hotel Tonight.

wide beds, mini-kitchens with a third tap for filtered water, a microwave, big glassy bathrooms with rain showers, plenty of power points plus a loaner plug adapter, a half-hour of free national calls a day, and flat-screen TVs that double as music players. Deluxe rooms, at the top of the middle-rate scale, sleep up to four. There's no restaurant (breakfast can be delivered at prices that aren't marked up), but all of Soho is teeming right outside your door—reason alone to book here. A very strong budget choice in the central West End.

10 Carlisle St., W1. www.thenadler.com. ✆ **020/3697-3697.** 78 units. Rooms £140–£275. Tube: Tottenham Court Rd. or Piccadilly Circus. **Amenities:** Free Wi-Fi.

Inexpensive

Seven Dials Hotel ★   There are almost no budget hotels near Covent Garden, so hoteliers get away with merely functional facilities. Here, everything is little: the stairway, the rooms, the charm. And correspondingly, the rates. There's usually barely enough storage space, a TV mounted on an armature, a basic writing desk, teeny clean bathrooms, and firm beds, albeit ones covered with dowdy bedspreads. Forget the lack of a lift and all the ways it's average and slipping year by year. Its footing on Monmouth Street, steps from a rainbow of pubs, shops, and bars clustering around Covent Garden, is without comparison. Dump your bags and go play, because the price is right.

7 Monmouth St., WC2. www.sevendialshotel.com. ✆ **020/7681-0791.** 18 units. £90–£100 single, £85–£120 double. Rates include full breakfast. Tube: Covent Garden. **Amenities:** Free Wi-Fi.

KENSINGTON, VICTORIA & KNIGHTSBRIDGE

As affordable prospects develop in King's Cross and South Bank, it makes less sense to put up with the Tube ride required to stay here, so for budget tourists, South Ken and Victoria have slipped many notches in desirability, although people with higher budgets who don't require nightlife or cheap transportation are still attracted. The stores and restaurants of Knightsbridge are now so skewed to free-spending Persians that it's not a prime tourist hotel spot anymore, and the increasingly obsolete fleabag hotels in Earl's Court, just west, are now pretty much off the radar.

Expensive

The Beaufort ★   Quiet as a dropped pin, this tidy upscale hotel down a dead-end residential street just west of Harrods (your neighbors: the 1%) distinguishes itself by offering more services than the standard: free afternoon tea with homemade scones, free cocktails by evening. Rooms—most of which are tucked away in a tortuous maze of corridors resulting from the combination of several town houses—are spacious for London, tastefully and conservatively decorated with delicate wallpaper and big cushy beds, and finely equipped. It's fairly good with options for families. The museums of South Kensington are a 5-minute walk away, as is Hyde Park.

33 Beaufort Gardens, SW3. www.thebeaufort.co.uk. © **020/7584-5252.** 29 units. Doubles from £255. Tube: Knightsbridge. **Amenities:** Free cocktails; free afternoon tea; free Wi-Fi.

The Goring ★   Only one five-star hotel has the Royal Warrant from the queen for Hospitality Services. Only one has been run by the same family

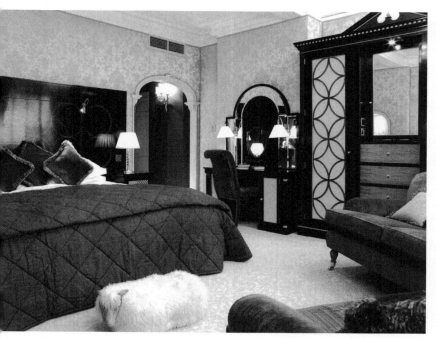

The Silk Room at the Goring offers classic luxury.

since 1910. Only one hosted Kate Middleton, the wife of a future king and mother of another, in her final night as a single girl before she walked down the aisle of Westminster Abbey. This is the Goring, classic but not self-importantly so, assiduously appropriate in style and rich in expensive fabrics, down to the Gainsborough silk on the walls, yet still goofy enough to put a stuffed sheep in every room and a statue of the founder in its huge back garden. The fleet of doormen wears bowler hats, and the signature canary-yellow china at its hotly pursued afternoon tea (4-month wait; p. 90) is made just for the hotel. The effect is something like an English country house, especially as you look out oversized windows at its blooming yard.

Beeston Place, SW1. www.thegoring.com. ℗ **020/7396-9000.** 69 units. Rooms £323–£840. Tube: Victoria. **Amenities:** Restaurant; bar; gym access; free Wi-Fi.

Hotel 41 ★★ A secret romantic nest only steps from Buckingham Palace, Hotel 41 is a hushed hideaway on the top floor of its moderate-priced cousin, The Rubens. You take a tiny private lift and tread a snug network of creaking corridors to reach its heart, a two-level, galleried conservatory bedecked like something to make Henry Higgins purr: Mahogany shelves, inviting seating, sculptural busts and an oversized globe, and a yawning skylight to let the light in. There, staff makes the rounds, quietly addressing guests by name and filling glasses with champagne and plates with an endless flow of scones and hors d'oeuvres. People forget to go outside and see London. The rooms are equally individualized and top-flight: done nearly entirely in black-and-white and lacking nothing. There's no on-site restaurant or spa and some rooms have no view to speak of—the focus is on intimacy, service, and discretion. The duplex Conservatory Suite, with a skylight over the bed, is popular with newlyweds and other nuzzlers.

41 Buckingham Palace Rd, SW1. www.41hotel.com. ℗ **020/7300-0041.** 30 units. Rooms £312–£500. Tube: Victoria. **Amenities:** Bar; free snacks; access to nearby gym; free Wi-Fi.

The Milestone Hotel ★★★ The Milestone steeps itself in all things Anglophilic. First is the location on the southern edge of Kensington Gardens—upper-floor rooms have a view of Kensington Palace itself. The hotel is actually three townhouses that have been combined, so each room is distinct in size and shape, and the furnishings—antique paintings, rich rugs, enormous beds, fat couches—make you feel like you're staying in a rich relation's country mansion rather than a citified hotel. You're awash in thoughtful amenities, from a welcome cocktail in the glass conservatory to a small bag of prunes and another of handmade hard candy waiting bedside at night. Staff, from the top-hatted doormen to the butler that attends to higher-level rooms, is alert yet unfussy. High tea in the plush lounge is a treat here as well.

1 Kensington Ct., W8. www.milestonehotel.com. ℗ **020/7917-1000.** 63 units. Rooms from £292. Tube: High St. Kensington. **Amenities:** Restaurant; tea room; welcome beverage; bar; conservatory; fitness center; spa; indoor resistance swimming pool; room service; free bottled water; free Wi-Fi.

St. Ermin's Hotel ★★ A decade ago, it was a package-tourist misery locals nicknamed "St. Vermin's." But with a new owner and much investment, glory has been restored to this handsome 1889 Queen Anne structure, a hotel since 1899. The lobby's latticed riot of plasterwork and sweeping Art Nouveau stairs is enough to make a tourist drop his baggage to soak in the London-ess of it all, but the history is just as rich: The premises were long used as a headquarters for British spy efforts—Ian Fleming, the creator of James Bond, was among those who worked here. Room sizes vary wildly, from puny to palatial, so you may need the guidance of a live person to get the right one, but they're all quiet and well-appointed by recent renovation—not five-star but solidly four. Children are emphatically welcomed (family rooms are available), and there's an agreeably pubby bar on premises; the Tube is on the same block and Westminster Abbey a 5-minute stroll east. The buffet breakfast is weak, but that can always be improved—precious Old World British vibrations such as these are to be protected and patronized.

2 Caxton St., SW1. www.sterminshotel.co.uk. ⓒ **020/7222-7888.** 331 units. Rooms £199–£459. Tube: St James's Park. **Amenities:** 2 restaurants, bar, fitness center, Wi-Fi (free).

Moderate

The Grosvenor Hotel ★ May we pause to celebrate the resplendent creation that was the English train station terminal hotel? The Grosvenor opened in 1862—it was the first hotel in town to install a lift—and although it's no longer at the top of the hospitality food chain, its wide corridors and sweeping staircases can still make you feel like you're the central character in a romantic novel. A recent £20 million renovation restored a once-timeworn lobby to grandeur and the first class railway lounge is now Réunion, a dusky cocktail bar overlooking the concourse of Victoria Station. While the common spaces are Victorian, the high-ceilinged rooms strike a modern tone. There's nothing dowdy about those: striped fabrics, metal- and earth-tone velour upholsteries, air conditioning, and Bose MP3 stations. Some rooms are on the small side, given that the place still uses the bones of the 1862 original and 1910 extension, but they're nice enough for that to be overlooked. For more space, simply upgrade to an Executive.

101 Buckingham Palace Rd., W1. www.guoman.com/grosvenor. ⓒ **020/7523-5055.** 345 units. Singles typically around £168, doubles £192, Executives £268. Cheaper on weekends. Tube: Victoria. **Amenities:** 2 restaurants; tea room; cocktail lounge; room service; fitness center; executive club; free Wi-Fi.

Lime Tree Hotel ★★ Matt and Charlotte Goodsall brightened a once-frumpy guesthouse into a place that feels as current as it is friendly. The conjoined brick town houses are historic, so no lift is permitted, but everything is updated with slate-and-white paint, fresh curtains, and touches such as bedside reading lights. If you have a first-floor room on the front, you'll have a small balcony over busy Ebury Street; in the quieter back, you'll overlook the cute flower garden. Only three rooms have their own bathrooms; the rest share. A basement room is larger than the others but has no view. The Lime Tree is popular so the owners have no need to discount for longer stays.

135–137 Ebury St., London SW1. www.limetreehotel.co.uk. ℂ **020/7730-8191.** 25 units. £120 single, £160–£210 double. Rates include full breakfast. Children 4 or under not permitted. Tube: Victoria or Sloane Square. **Amenities:** Free Wi-Fi.

Sanctuary House Hotel ★ Once, many pubs ran nondescript inns as sidelines. The pub here is just a so-so Fuller's location (there are hundreds of them), but the hotel upstairs is a creaking, well-tended reward unto itself for value and charm, and the staff is unusually responsive for such a small property. The look plays up its Victorian origins with faux-antique telephones and plenty of handsome wood trim, but the modernized bathrooms and soft beds betray the fact that it's the beneficiary of some recent renovations by intelligent hoteliers. Even more miraculously, it's so near Big Ben that you can hear the bell peal.

33 Tothill St., SW1. www.sanctuaryhousehotel.co.uk. ℂ **020/7799-4044.** 34 units. £155–£255 double, cheaper on weekends. Tube: St James's Park or Westminster. **Amenities:** Air conditioning; free Wi-Fi.

Inexpensive

Luna Simone Hotel ★ Because this prototypical townhouse budget B&B began as two hotels that were conjoined in the 1990s, you'll sometimes see it called the Luna & Simone. A protected building with old metalwork on the banisters and oddly sized guest rooms, it has kept up by way of inexpensive furniture and basic amenities, and consequently attracts many return guests. Eat quickly—the simple English breakfast ends early, at 9am. There's no lift or AC, but also no sharing of bathrooms. Cheap and cheerful, the way London used to do it—the owners have been at it since 1970.

47–49 Belgrave Rd., SW1. www.lunasimonehotel.com. ℂ **020/7834-5897.** Singles from £88, doubles £123–£151. Rates include breakfast. Tube: Victoria or Pimlico. **Amenities:** Free Wi-Fi.

Lynton B&B Hotel ★ Strictly old-school, the Lynton, close to Victoria Station, is the kind of prototypical family-run crash pad London has mostly stamped out. Brothers Mark and Simon Connor took it over from their nan, who ran it since the mid-'60s (it's been a guesthouse since after the World War II, but a century ago was the home of a local horse doctor). The Gentrification Fairy has not yet pummeled the Lynton with her merciless wand—it's pleasingly dog-eared, and the Connors, some of the last London-bred B&B proprietors left on Ebury Street, care deeply about their family tradition and dispense genial opinion at the slightest encouragement. Expect quarters that are entirely sufficient but hardly deluxe, for those who'd rather spend money on other things. There's no lift—the council won't allow one.

113 Ebury St., SW1. www.lyntonhotel.co.uk. ℂ **020/7730-4032.** 13 units. £65–£70 single, £80–£115 double. Rates include breakfast. Tube: Victoria. **Amenities:** Free Wi-Fi.

SHOULD I pack IT?

Mind the culture gap! Don't let these quirks take you by surprise:

- Although all hotels include towels and linens, at family-run places you'll find for the most part that travelers are expected to bring their own washcloths.
- Many beds have duvets but not top sheets. It's just a European style; locals would probably explain that the duvet cover *is* the top sheet.
- You may find that your bed is made each day, but your sheets aren't changed. This, too, is normal, and it saves on water, electricity, and detergent. If you want them changed, simply request it.
- In the budget category, nearly all rooms have TVs these days, but not cable, so expect only four or five broadcast (or "terrestrial") channels.
- Ask for a loaner hair dryer or curling iron because your non-British one probably can't handle the increased voltage. New non-British hair curlers fare better, although they may get hotter than they do back home.
- Not every small hotel stocks irons, sometimes for safety reasons.
- Family-run B&Bs can't afford a porter, but rare is the place that doesn't have at least one strong person to help with your baggage if asked.
- Many places don't have air-conditioning because before climate change, London didn't get that hot. If there's a heat wave, though, you'll be glad to have it.

The Nadler Victoria ★★   The emerging Nadler brand does "affordable luxury"—its phrase—and it's sharp about it, delivering value in easy limestone colors and amenities that strive to be intuitive. Each room, no matter the category, gives you a mini-kitchen with Nespresso machine and a tap with Brita water, 30 daily minutes of local/national phone calls, swanky hairdryers, and TVs that let you do everything—read the latest newspapers, listen to a free music library, even stream content from your own computer. The best value in room types, "Small Double," has a bed that's 4½ feet (135cm) wide, but categories scale up to Superior and Deluxe, with true 6-foot-wide (180cm) king beds. Right out the front door is the Buckingham Palace complex, so you'll be in the nearest hotel to the queen (and close to St. James's Park and Green Park). The Victoria area is a little dull but it's a nexus for bus lines, three Tube lines, and rail lines to the countryside.

10 Palace St., London, SW1. www.thenadler.com/victoria. ✆ **020/3697-3697.** 73 units. Rooms £120–£255. Tube: Victoria. **Amenities:** Free access to nearby gym; free Wi-Fi.

MARYLEBONE & MAYFAIR

For visitors who want a balance of central location and private residential vibe, Marylebone's the place. A 10-minute walk takes you to the "smart" end of Oxford Street and Mayfair to the south, or the wide-open fields of Regent's Park to the north.

Expensive

The Beaumont ★★★   The cheeky proprietors call this relative newcomer "American-style," but you might peg it for Art Deco; after all, its 1926 façade was once the garage of Selfridges' department store, the halls and lifts are full of glossy shots of bygone stars, and its bar and restaurant—serving duck egg hash at breakfast—strongly evoke a 1930s Los Angeles grill, like a Mayfair version of Hollywood's Musso & Frank. Or maybe they mean that it's friendly, not stuffy—after all, the top-hatted doormen welcome you by name whenever you return, such as from Selfridges itself, steps away. Either way, it's a five-star hotel that benefits from the fact its guts were custom-built a few years ago, meaning rooms could be customized to be cutting-edge (free streaming movies, free minibar, heated bathroom floors) and the staff, with no decades-old laurels upon which to rest like its neighbors, must double over in an effort to please you. The Beaumont is most noted for Antony Gormley's geometric sculpture of a brooding man perched on one of its outcroppings—inside is an arty wooden suite that's favored by society spenders—you're more likely to love a "Classic" room facing the courtyard or a "Superior" facing the quiet street and a pocket park.

8 Balderton St., W1. www.thebeaumont.com. ℅ **020/7499-1001.** 73 units. Rooms from £370. Tube: Bond St. **Amenities:** Restaurant; bar; fitness center with hamam; free local shuttle car; free local calls; free movies; free Wi-Fi.

Brown's Hotel ★   History is in every creak: The first-ever phone call was placed from its ground floor. While staying here, FDR and Eleanor honeymooned, Agatha Christie plotted murders, Rudyard Kipling finished *The Jungle Book,* and Stephen King started *Misery.* In 1907, Mark Twain scandalized the press by appearing in its lobby in his blue bathrobe. "Mark Twain exhibited himself as an eccentric today," tittered the *Times* on the front page, "and every staid Londoner who witnessed the exhibition fairly gasped." Brown's is still an upstart among dowagers: A contemporary update by Sir Rocco Forte exorcised fustiness, which in London means foreigners won't feel like fish out of water (at some expensive places, that counts for a lot). If you're staying elsewhere, you still can satisfy yourself with the servile atmosphere, dark woods, and live piano at its tea, one of London's better services (p. 90).

30 Albemarle St., W1. www.brownshotel.com. ℅ **020/7493-6020.** 117 units. Rooms £376–£703. Tube: Green Park. **Amenities:** Restaurant; bar; tea room; spa; gym; free local calls; free throttled Wi-Fi (£16/day unrestricted).

Claridge's ★★★   The red brick Claridge's is the quintessential luxury Mayfair hotel, proudly proclaiming good taste in discretion as administered through glittering Deco accents. The building dates to 1894 (when Gilbert & Sullivan's producer rebuilt it), but modern amenities are installed among the gilded plasterwork and (non-working) fireplaces—the fitness center and spa are huge and up-to-date, and neither floorboards nor exacting staff grumble. From the bathrooms (heated floors, high-tech toilet/bidets) to cavernous

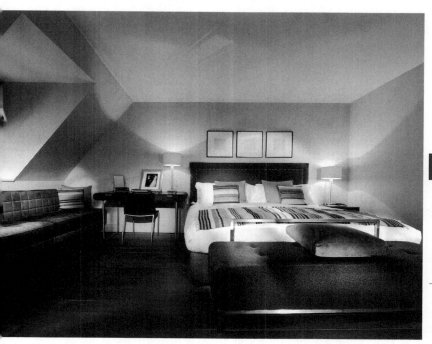

The King Room at Brown's Hotel, where foreigners are made to feel comfortable.

wardrobes and plump beds as wide as some studio apartments, there's not much to complain about. Its main lift is the last in Central London to be operated by hand—there's a sofa inside should you tire during your 5-level journey to the top floor—and its clubby cocktail bars and Fera restaurant are favored by modern-day fashion icons (your Von Furstenbergs, your Jaggers, your Eltons—wealthy Americans, in particular, love it, and so did the Queen Mum) who detest the snotty exclusivity that can make the Ritz such a drag.

Brook St., W1. www.claridges.co.uk. © **020/7629-8860.** 203 units. Rooms from £450. Tube: Bond St. **Amenities:** Restaurant; 2 bars; spa; fitness center; business center; free Wi-Fi.

The Lanesborough ★★★ I sneezed at the Lanesborough. Moments later, my butler—everyone has one here—flew to my side bearing a silver tray of hot tea, fresh-cut ginger on a porcelain plate, and Acacia honey. And so it should be at one of the finest hotels in which I hope you will ever be so lucky to stay, where guest needs are meticulously anticipated and fresh-cut blooms are delivered to your bathroom counter the moment your back is turned. A recent £80-million renovation tore out every fixture and fully recrafted the interior with gilt, made-to-measure Regency-style finery—like a mansion made of Wedgwood china, Corinthian leather, and canopy king beds. It's an English pastiche for the super-wealthy, but a pitch-perfect one, and honeymoon Nirvana. At the Lanes-borough, intense formality dwells discreetly with new tech: TVs repose behind false paintings in gilt frames. Downstairs, near two portraits that, though unremarked, are actually originals by Sir Joshua Reynolds, moneyed regulars sip glasses of port dating as far back 1778 and smoke £4,000 cigars in what many consider the world's best-stocked cigar lounge. Should the tariff at London's most expensive hotel understandably be out of your reach, at least stop by for the exquisite Afternoon Tea (p. 90).

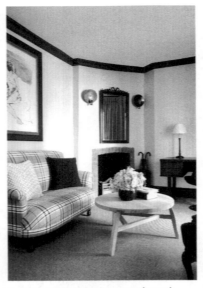

A sitting area in a guest room at the posh Lanesborough Hotel.

Hyde Park Corner, SW1. www.lanesborough. com. ℂ **020/7259-5599.** 93 units. Rooms from £766. Tube: Hyde Park Corner. **Amenities:** Restaurant; bar; cigar lounge; fitness center; complimentary chauffeured car; free land-line calls to US, Canada, and Europe; free Wi-Fi.

The Langham ★★   In 1863, while Americans were shooting each other in farmyards, London was assembling the first and most celebrated grand dame hotel in Europe. She survives, but it was touch and go during the 20th century, and now she's very nice in a generically luxurious way. The polished lobby is perfumed, the lifts swathed in leather, and each room a private cocoon of wainscoting and enveloping beds. In 2017, a new spa and gym was added. Its Palm Court has been serving high tea since 1865, and its frivolous cocktail menu is deemed one of the world's cleverest. It's a few short blocks from Oxford Street's best shopping.

1c Portland Place, Regent St., W1. www.langhamhotels.com. ℂ **020/7636-1000.** 380 units. Rooms £312–£444. Tube: Oxford Circus. **Amenities:** 2 restaurants; 2 bars; indoor pool; spa; fitness center; business center; free Wi-Fi.

The Stafford Hotel ★   Back when it opened in 1912, the intimate Stafford appealed to Americans on a European spree; it even named its yacht-clubby bar The American Bar. Today, renovated to business-class standards (its Mews outbuilding is a particular romantic zone, but all areas are quiet and have super-soft beds), this rambling hideaway down a cul-de-sac in St James's, a short passageway from Green Park, is not quite as in-demand as it once was. However, that means it can be your little secret, and it doesn't have to succumb to the arrogance rife in London's top-tier hotels. Having a subterranean wine cellar that's some 400 years old, which consequently empowers it to be the only hotel in London to retain its own Master Sommelier (only 247 people have ever attained that designation), goes a long way toward attracting

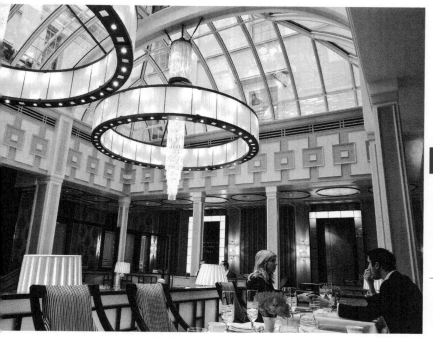

The Stafford Hotel adds modern British décor to a Victorian hideaway on a St. James cul-de-sac.

a discerning, but not snobby, clientele. There's still quite a bit that's old-fashioned about it—does anyone use an in-room CD player anymore?—but perhaps a lost hiccup-in-time is just what you need.

16–18 St James's Pl, SW1. www.thestaffordlondon.com. © **020/7493-0111.** 127 units. Rooms £200–£288. Tube: Green Park. **Amenities:** Restaurant; bar; fitness center; free Wi-Fi.

The Wellesley ★★★   A jewel box overlooking Hyde Park, the Wellesley, which despite its Art Deco panache opened only in 2012, caters to the ultra-top end of the market; with only 36 rooms, mostly suites, indulgence is held paramount. The tiny Oval restaurant alone is one of the prettiest dining nooks in the city. It's also London's only hotel that was a Tube station: The Hyde Park Corner ticket hall of the early Piccadilly Line once lay behind its iconic 1906 facade of arched oxblood-red tiles, although everything has been exquisitely rebuilt for your comfort and, it must be said, your ego. Your 24-hour butler, just a button's push away, heeds your every command. You might find some amenities feel like a contemporary satire of *The Great Gatsby:* a giant hotel cigar humidor and a Rolls-Royce (license plate: WEII SLY) that will chauffeur you anywhere nearby. Ask them to take you to McDonald's.

11 Knightsbridge, SW1. www.thewellesley.co.uk. © **020/7235-3535.** 36 units. Doubles £346–£560. Tube: Oxford Circus. **Amenities:** Restaurant; bar; cigar lounge and humidor; jazz lounge; Rolls-Royce shuttle; free Wi-Fi.

Moderate

22 York Street ★★   You might wonder at first if you have knocked on the door of a private home of some bohemian doctor or lawyer. Inside, Michael and Liz Callis (not always there; they have staff) are going for a farmhouse feel, with warm wooden floorboards, plenty of antiques and oriental rugs, and large bathrooms, almost all of which have tub/shower combinations. Guests are let loose to treat the five-level premises as their own, which includes plenty of tea, coffee, and biscuits. Adding to the homey feel, breakfasts are served in the kitchen at a communal country table where you meet your fellow guests. Although they're not explicitly banned, kids may not feel comfortable here. The top floor gets hot in the summer.

22 York St., W1. www.22yorkstreet.co.uk. © **020/7224-2990.** 10 units. Singles from £95, doubles from £150, triple £180. Rates include continental breakfast. Tube: Baker St. **Amenities:** Free Wi-Fi.

Grosvenor House, A JW Marriott Hotel ★   If you've got Marriott points to burn, you won't be sorry you chose it. It's a big early-20th-century edifice with corporate-hotel fallibility (rich bedding and an excellent Hyde Park–facing afternoon tea that score, sometimes-oversubscribed service and a rammed executive lounge that don't), but rooms are decently sized and undergoing a refreshment that includes such luxuries as the ability to stream your own entertainment to the TV. The position in far western Mayfair grants some

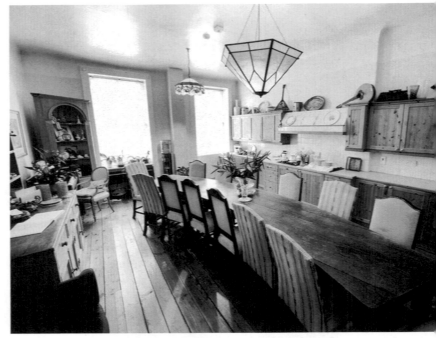

The kitchen and dining table at 22 York St. provide a homey feel to guests.

FINDING HOTELS online

You may be used to booking through sites such as Expedia, but when it comes to London, think again. Many London hotels, particularly the most affordable ones, are privately owned, and many of them are represented on the Web by third-party travel agents and booking engines that pad the price with a few extra bucks, which they'll skim off for themselves as commission. If you call the hotel directly for your bookings, you'll not only get the lowest price, but you'll also have the power of negotiation.

Another danger of making an online reservation: There are heaps of lousy budget hotels in London, particularly around Paddington and Earl's Court, that post misleading images on the Web, and it's easy to end up in a seedy one. This is why you trust a book like Frommer's—we have been to every single place we recommend.

Mobissimo.com, HotelsCombined. com, and **Kayak.com** are three "aggregator" sites that scan dozens of sites for deals and pull them all together. If you hit them, you don't need to hit Travelocity or the like, because it includes them in the search. Some major chains have teamed up to create **RoomKey.com,** which collects discounted rates from only their holdings.

Visit London, the city's official tourism office, has an area on its website (www.visitlondon.com) for discounted bookings, although it's maintained by LateRooms.com. **Lastminute.co.uk** is one of the most popular booking sites in the U.K., but its rates don't always represent savings, and the apps **Hotel Tonight** and **Hotels Now** sometimes bear cheap fruit. Other popular offshore hotel sites include **Booking.com, Euro cheapo.com, Agoda.com, Laterooms. com,** and **Venere.com. Priceline.com** and **Hotwire.com** operate here. And **Tingo.com** refunds the difference if a hotel price drops after you book. As with all bid-for-travel sites, you could end up with a deal, but remember that as hotels add star levels, they also add extra charges.

rooms winning park views, but it also means there aren't many shops and restaurants out the door and the Tube is 10 minutes in any direction. If you don't have your heart set on charm, it's sure to please.

86–90 Park Lane, W1. www.marriott.com. © **020/7499-6363.** 127 units. Rooms £200–£288. Tube: Marble Arch. **Amenities:** Bar/restaurant; fitness center; slow Wi-Fi free, fast Wi-Fi £5/day.

Hyatt Regency London—The Churchill ★★
A strong choice for those with Hyatt membership considerations, it's a 2-minute walk from the back door of Selfridges' department store, and many rooms recently received smart renovations with completely fresh bathrooms (robot toilets!) and truly well-selected art. Ten years ago, this circa-1970 building was a bit tired, but Hyatt has put the property on its front burner with millions of pounds in investment. Now it offers everything a 5-star should, like all-night room service, and even if the location is a little off the main, it's still near the Tube, unquestionably comfortable, and run with snap for such a large place.

30 Portman Square, W1. Londonchurchill.regency.hyatt.com. © **020/7486-5800.** 440 units. Rooms £288–£431. Tube: Marble Arch. **Amenities:** 2 restaurants, bar, fitness center, tennis and jogging track in adjoining square; Wi-Fi (free).

The Zetter Townhouse, Marylebone ★★★ In nearly every way, it plays the part of the curious abode of an eccentric "wicked uncle" who collects oddities and likes to drink—each room has its own quirky character of antique mismatched furniture, hand-hung wallpaper, vintage glass slides embedded in bathroom walls, and expensive punchbowl-set glassware. Yet the essence of this spot near Hyde Park and Oxford Street is fully modern, down to strong showers. Downstairs, the dusky, parlor-style lounge bar (Seymour's Parlour) keeps pouring coffees and well-made cocktails deep into the night. This is detailed luxury living with a frisky point of view, and it's a winkingly Londonish one at that; instead of a door hanger, you use a bowler hat painted with messages for the housekeeper ("NOT NOW"). There's another location in Clerkenwell, but this area has more going for it. *Tip:* The Studio Suite has a four-poster that could rival the Great Bed of Ware in the V&A, but the basement room has the least charm.

29–30 Seymour St., W1. www.thezettertownhouse.com/marylebone. ℗ **020/7324-4544.** 24 units. Rooms from £180. Tube: Marble Arch. **Amenities:** Bar/restaurant; free Wi-Fi.

THE SOUTH BANK, SOUTHWARK & BOROUGH

From medieval times until about 15 years ago, "respectable" Londoners wanted nothing to do with this once-industrial area. They wish they'd bought property now. It's actually a terrific place to dwell in good weather, when the area comes alive with walkers, booksellers, pub-goers, and playgoers reveling in the nearby re-creation of Shakespeare's Globe. Furthermore, moderate hotels are proliferating.

Expensive

Shangri-La Hotel at the Shard ★★ Staying here, on the 36th to 52nd floors of a glass-sheathed skyscraper, means that your room will be encased with floor-to-ceiling windows overlooking the city. You're a bird singing in a gleaming cage. When you take a bath (in your marble-coated washroom with heated floors), you may feel as if you're flying over the Tower of London, and when you swim in the horizon pool in the sky above St Paul's, the vista is so surreal that you may wonder if it's all a dream. Such glassy nirvana comes with Zen interiors to match: clean-lined, simple, and inflected by the Asian culture from which the Shangri-La brand hails (for example, in-room amenities might be stored in a bento-style box). Rates are higher than at other luxury hotels in town, but literally so are the rooms, and that seems to justify it to nearly everyone's satisfaction.

31 St Thomas St., SE1. www.shangri-la.com/london/shangrila. ℗ **020/7234-8000.** 202 units. King rooms from £375. Tube: London Bridge. **Amenities:** Restaurant; bar; indoor pool; fitness center in-room Nespresso coffee and tea; free Wi-Fi.

Moderate

London Bridge Hotel ★ A 1916 telephone exchange building wedged near the base of the Shard, steps from Borough Market and above a major Tube stop, has been gussied up into a recommendable mid-level hotel with a bar people actually visit after work. Snug standard rooms have flourishes such as suede headboards, and deluxe rooms come with a few blessings you don't find in many other London hotels, including occasional walk-in closets. It's not worth the £250-plus it sometimes asks, but on weekends, rates plummet to around £99, which is golden. *Note:* This is not the same property as the Mercure with the same name.

8–18 London Bridge St., SE1. www.londonbridgehotel.com. ✆ **020/7855-2200.** 138 units. £140–£350 double. Tube: London Bridge. **Amenities:** Restaurant; bar; gym; free Wi-Fi.

The Mad Hatter Hotel ★★ Decent pub hotels, which are hotels above pubs, are a dying breed. Here, sizable, good-value rooms feel like they were lifted from a business hotel, and there are no crowds (but also not many stores around). Think decent-size bathrooms with tub/showers, rose-colored bedspreads matching painted accent walls, a lift, and ice machines—rare as diamonds in the U.K. Rates rarely crack £200, which is a big deal for someplace so central: 5 minutes from the Tate Modern and just over Blackfriars Bridge from the City. Some rooms can be conjoined for families.

3–7 Stamford St., SE1 www.madhatterhotel.co.uk. ✆ **020/7401-9222.** 30 units. £86–£181 double. Rates include full breakfast. Tube: Southwark or Blackfriars. **Amenities:** Pub; free Wi-Fi.

Mondrian London ★ Not quite central, alienating at times, the Mondrian is still special in some ways because the vistas from its Thamesfront units have no competition; book one and you'll feel like you're on a ship at water—which happens to be the theme here, coppery nautical motifs and all. There are plenty of self-aware embellishments (a basement cinema, yoga in the rooftop Rumpus Room bar, the Dandelyan bar serving excessively bespoke no-ice cocktails for a nip less than £20 each), but although the Mondrian esteems itself in its ironic stylings, it's in fact at its best when you use it to simply welcome the skyline into your bedroom—the restaurant opens to the river, the famous riverfront path literally runs beside it. If you had to take a room that doesn't face the water, I wouldn't bother. Despite its hipster preening, it's decent for families, too, since so many room types interconnect.

20 Upper Ground, SE1. www.morganshotelgroup.com. ✆ **020/3747-1000.** 359 units. Rooms from £175. Tube: Waterloo or Southwark. **Amenities:** Restaurant; 3 bars; spa; fitness center; free Wi-Fi (slow), fast Wi-Fi £7–10/day.

Park Plaza Westminster Bridge London ★ This glassy mega-hotel looks like a carburetor on a curb, but you won't believe the view from the "Iconic View" rooms: straight down Westminster Bridge at the Houses of Parliament and Big Ben's tower, like a floor-to-ceiling fantasy. Otherwise it's a business-class formula that feels more like a convention center, and the

HOW TO GET YOUR HOTEL FOR free

What if I told you that you could spend 6 nights in London, airfare and hotel included, for $799 in winter and $1,149 in summer? It's called an **air-hotel package**, and it can cost about the same as airfare alone—except it also comes with hotel, breakfast, and often a tour or two thrown in. How do they do it? Contracted rates and bulk buying.

The lowest prices are from eastern American cities such as New York and Boston, but for a few dozen dollars more, you can leave from just about any other American city. You can also often extend the return by as much as a month without having to buy more hotel nights (but you can do that, too). The catch is this: Many of the least expensive hotel options are pillow mills that have seen better days. For a little more peace of mind, upgrade to a slightly more expensive property.

The king of affordable air-hotel deals is **Go-Today.com** (www.go-today.com; © 800/227-3235), which usually offers 4- and 6-night packages to London, sometimes paired with other European destinations, including local flights between the cities (as low as $800 for 6 nights). Others: **Virgin Vacations** (www.virgin-vacations.com; © 888/937-8474) and **Gate 1 Travel** (www.gate1travel.com; © 800/682-3333). Scrutinize the airline-run sales like **British Airways Holidays** (www.baholidays.com; © 877/428-2228), because those rates may not always be the cheapest.

cheapest "Internal Facing" atrium-view rooms (scrutinize the room description) are starved of natural light. Still, that means less-desirable rooms are discounted in low season. Studio rooms have microwaves, fridges, and pullout beds, and there's a dark and soothing indoor pool.

200 Westminster Bridge Rd., London SE1. www.parkplaza.com/westminster. © **0844/415-6780**. 1,019 units. £177–£339 double, "Iconic View" starting at £250. 3-night minimum in some periods. Tube: Waterloo or Westminster. **Amenities:** 2 restaurants; bar; indoor pool; fitness center; spa; free Wi-Fi.

Inexpensive

Captain Bligh House ★★★ For a delicious taste of local London life without venturing far from the center of town, the Bligh—where Captain William Bligh lived after that sordid mutiny affair—is a transporting choice. Artists Gayna and Simon approach their wee guesthouse, built in the 1780s (before the invention of the lift), as a quiet home from home: Units have little kitchens for cooking up market ingredients, but you also get a starter pack of breakfast supplies. Although the Imperial War Museum (p. 152) is across the street, it's not a neighborhood crawling with tourists, so you'll kick back at the local pub and jump the many bus lines that go past. The value is over-the-top.

100 Lambeth Rd., SE1. www.captainblighhouse.co.uk. © **020/7928-2735**. 5 units. £90–£125 double. Tube: Lambeth North. **Amenities:** In-room kitchen; free Wi-Fi.

THE CITY & EAST LONDON

Not long ago, the City went to sleep at 7pm. Now, with Shoreditch and Spitalfields revitalized, there's good reason for creative types to linger by night.

Some of London's prime party zones, straight and gay, are near hotels where rates bottom out on weekends. The Liverpool Street station area lacks character, but it's near things that ooze character, and it's also a nucleus of the Night Bus system. Just be wary of going *too* far east in East London: There are corporate choices in the Canary Wharf district and temptingly cheap rooms by the ExCeL convention center in the Docklands region, but they're intended for conference-goers, and from there it will take you 45 minutes to reach Piccadilly Circus by the Tube and DLR. If sightseeing is your aim, make Shoreditch your eastern cutoff.

Expensive

Andaz London ★★   The Great Eastern, once one of London's great train station terminal hotels that's practically atop the Liverpool Street station, was renovated beyond much Victorian evidence and is now one of the City's more pleasant hotel surprises, with rooms both decently sized and luxurious. The Andaz, owned by Hyatt, makes a point of offering service that mixes ultra-casual (there's no check-in desk; staff greets you with an iPad) with an attentiveness appropriate to the price point. It also piles on the freebies: You pay nothing extra for a minibar stocked with water and juices, snacks, in-room gourmet coffee, local calls, and Wi-Fi. Soak in the showpiece spaces: Breakfast is taken in a glorious restaurant capped with glass cupolas, and ask to see the astonishing Grecian Masonic temple, a once-secret space with £4-million inlaid marble floors. The Andaz is near only a few sights but it's extremely well connected by bus and rail, and a few blocks north and east, you'll find food and nightlife in Hoxton, Shoreditch, and Spitalfields.

40 Liverpool St., EC2. www.london.liverpoolstreet.andaz.com. © **020/7961-1234.** 267 units. £205–£285 double. Tube: Liverpool St. **Amenities:** 3 restaurants; pub; wine bar; champagne bar; gym; local calls; free in-room beverages and snacks; free Wi-Fi.

Four Seasons Hotel London at Ten Trinity Square ★★   This luxury newcomer (2017) is ideal for sinking deep into your bed and vanishing into the sanctum of your room—most don't have views, after all, despite the seminal location overlooking the Tower of London, so when you're here, you feel indulgently removed from the city. Your personal space is massive because this used to be a civil office building (the conversion created such a maze that even you will have a hard time finding your door), clad in the finest materials and swaddled with softness because, after all, this is the Four Seasons. Add to that the prestigious La Dame de Pic, a highly rated experimental French restaurant, and you've got a super-luxe escape that's so removed from the tourist cluster—the neighborhood virtually shuts down after dark and on weekends—that it creates its own world. For that reason, this is a good honeymoon choice.

10 Trinity Square, EC3. www.fourseasons.com/TenTrinity. © **020/3297-9200.** 100 units. Rooms from £177. Tube: Tower Hill. **Amenities:** 2 restaurants, fitness center, cocktail bar, spa, fitness center, free kids' amenities, indoor pool, free Wi-Fi.

South Place Hotel ★★★ Plugged-in, stylish, and sexy: That's the crowd this hotel goes for, and you'll feel that way, too. The first hotel to be built from the ground up in the Square Mile for a century, every inch was run through the design filter, and much of the art was commissioned by celebrated contemporary artists. Rooms, charcoal-grey with wool carpets, are large and hushed and fully up-to-date with luxury expectations, so you'll find plenty of outlets, AV connections, blackout blinds closed from a bedside panel, and a big bed you can flop around in. The two restaurants, the Michelin-starred Angler and 3 Bar & Grill, have lured both name chefs and some of the liveliest professionals from The City. On weekends, when the neighborhood is quiet but you're near the goodies in Shoreditch, rates can dip to £170.

3 South Place, EC2. www.southplacehotel.com. ℗ **020/3503-0000.** 80 units. Doubles from £213, £20 more for bathtubs. Tube: Moorgate or Liverpool St. **Amenities:** 2 restaurants; 3 bars; guests' lounge; gym; spa; business center; free Wi-Fi.

Moderate

Ace Hotel London Shoreditch ★★ If you've grown up enough to have some money, but not enough to demand much of hotel staff, the Ace can plug you in to Shoreditch Cool. A stay here isn't about service but about style, since the Ace's agreeable pretentions have become a "lifestyle brand" for the fashionably impressionable. Millennials tap away on laptops all day at the lobby workbenches and well-dressed revelers thump away in its basement club. It's just a converted mid-level business hotel, but rooms are cushy if you're a hipster (huge beds and bathrooms, room-width built-in window sofas) and styled with self-knowing false irreverence (instead of drawers, you use plastic crates, as if you were still in kindergarten, your bedspread is denim, and there's a guitar—an Ace signature). It's too much of a scene, perhaps, but fun.

100 Shoreditch High St., E1. www.acehotel.com/london. ℗ **020/7613-9800.** 97 units. £135–£279 double. Tube: Shoreditch High St. or Liverpool St. **Amenities:** Restaurant; rooftop bar; basement club; gym; free Wi-Fi.

Apex City of London ★★★ An excellent contemporary boutique brand from Scotland that appeals to high standards for space and style, Apex is a friendly and peaceful urban retreat that actually looks like its pictures. You'll find it literally steps from the Tower of London, and a few rooms glimpse the Tower Bridge—along with the balcony, worth the upgrade of £15 to £30. It's handsomely designed in hardwood and walnut, Nespresso pods instead of awful instant coffee, and bathrooms larger than many B&Bs' guest rooms, including walk-in power showers. The only downside is The City is deader than Old Marley in the off hours, which is why it can be a steal on weekends. The **Apex London Wall,** just as good, is on the side streets north of handy Bank station, and the **Apex Temple Court,** off Fleet Street, is also tops, but for the views and its affordable proximity to the river, this one is a solid choice.

No. 1 Seething Lane, London EC3. www.apexhotels.co.uk. ℗ **020/7702-2020.** 179 units. £140–£340 double. Tube: Tower Hill. **Amenities:** Restaurant; bar; gym; free local calls; free Wi-Fi.

Inexpensive

The Hoxton ★★ The advent of "the Hox" changed the way London thought of budget lodging: Chintz and linoleum went out, to be replaced by good-looking staff versed in local hotspots and compact rooms that pack in more style and cleverness than the low price would allow. You sleep on a platform bed under exposed brick walls and among set pieces like Union Jack pillows and steamer trunks for chests of drawers. You bathe under a rain shower in a futuristic cylinder. Your continental breakfast is delivered each morning via a bag you hang on the door, which can make you feel like a monkey at the world's most self-conscious zoo, and there's free water and milk for your little fridge and an hour of free telephone calls a day, even if you call internationally. Downstairs there's a grill, a bar, and coffee and free Wi-Fi flowing at all hours, make it as much a gathering place for disaffected Millennials as it is a way station for travelers. Book as far ahead as possible to keep the price under £200—you could get more space and service elsewhere for more than that.

1 Austin St., E2. www.hoxtonhotels.com. ⓒ **020/7550-1000.** 208 units. Rooms £99–£269. Tube: Aldgate or Tower Hill. **Amenities:** Restaurant; 1 hr. free calls; free Wi-Fi.

Qbic London City ★★ From a tiny affordable design hotel brand in Holland, Qbic is a wacky antidote to the formula budget hotels. Everything you need—bed, outlets, bathroom with a rain shower, TV—is a part of a pre-fabricated bed/bathroom structure that dominates the center of the room. The cheapest rooms, called "Smart," don't have a window—did you need one? It's not a capsule hotel, just one that came up with a multipurpose hospitality unit with plenty of room to walk around and stash your suitcase. Your lamp is made out of petrified garden hose, your clothing rack a strange ladder/planter of some sort—it's just fun. There are free coffee and tea machines on every floor and a preposterously funky lobby where organic continental breakfast is served. You'll be within walking distance to Spitalfields/Shoreditch (15 min.) and the Tower of London (15 min.). As a bonus, the staff gives good advice on local culture.

42 Adler St. E1. london.qbichotels.com. ⓒ **020/3021-3300.** 171 units. Rooms from £70 but usually more like £138. Tube: Aldgate East. **Amenities:** Lounge; free coffee; free Wi-Fi.

Shoreditch Inn ★★ Budget hotels are few and far between in this part of London, which now values caché above saving cash, but here you find a modern value-priced hotel that won't frighten you. Encumbered by none of the lifestyle-obsessed frills that its preening neighbors obsess over, it's simply clean and recently refit with the little touches that distinguish it as a standout of its price class: double-glazed windows (to muffle Shoreditch revelry), quality toiletries, roomy quarters, and enough selection at breakfast, even if said breakfast is taken in the basement. That it's in the middle of the action and front rooms that overlook a church from 1740 have me wondering when the dream will end and the owners will put the price out of reach. They could ask for more.

1 Austin St., E2. www.shoreditchinn.com. ℂ **020/3327-3910.** 14 units. £69–£149 double. Rates include continental breakfast. Tube: Bethnal Green. **Amenities:** Free Wi-Fi.

RENT A ROOM

Airbnb is old news in England: English-hosted accommodations were long one of the world's great travel bargains. Londoners have always been eager to make a few pounds by welcoming you into their homes, and as they vie for your business, they make for some great places to find cheap deals. One potential hidden advantage of this sort of stay comes if you've got a car—for example, if you're stopping in London during a drive round the island. Staying with a family in Zone 3 or 4 may enable you to park your car cheaply. What's included? At the minimum, a bed and breakfast. Everything else depends, since homestays are as unique as the hosts themselves. Your hosts may offer to show you the town or they may leave you in peace. They may have searingly fast Wi-Fi or they may think electric kettles are the cutting edge of technology. Armed with your wish list, these brokers, some of whom are truly Old School, should be able to pair you with suitable options:

o **At Home in London** (www.athomeinlondon.co.uk; ℂ **020/8748-2701**). Operating since 1986. Properties in West London, near the Tube: mid-£80s (central London) to £30 a night (Zones 2 & 3).

o **The Bed and Breakfast Club** (www.thebedandbreakfastclub.co.uk; ℂ **07879/661-346**). Operating since 1988. Upscale but not out of reach: from £80 to £125 with a cooked breakfast.

o **London Bed and Breakfast Agency** (www.londonbb.com; ℂ **01474/708-701**). Specializes in finding trustworthy hosts for single female travelers: between £70 and £120 in Zones 1 to 3.

o **London Homestead Services** (www.lhslondon.co.uk; ℂ **020/7286-5115**). Operating since 1985. Rooms in traditional homes found in commuter neighborhoods a good half-hour train ride from town: £18 to £40 for both doubles and singles.

o **Happy Homes** (www.happy-homes.com; ℂ **020/7352-5121**). Operating since 1989. Specializes in homestays in southwest London, about a 25-minute commute to the West End: £20 to £65, plus a one-time fee of £35 to £65 per room.

o **Annscott Accommodation Service** (www.holidayhosts.free-online.co.uk; ℂ **020/8540-7942**). Operating since the early 1990s. Rooms about 30 minutes by train from the city: £17 to £54 single, £34 to £90 double.

RENT A FLAT

If you don't want to rent a room in a home, rent a whole flat. When you arrive, you'll often find a folder that schools you in the best local shops and restaurants, and you may encounter neighbors keeping an eye on the place and on your welfare (at one property I know of, the owner herself pops round and pretends to be a helpful neighbor), which is an advantage if you want to learn more city secrets. Many properties have minimum stays of 5 to 7 nights. Renters such as **Airbnb.com, FlipKey.com,** and **Housetrip.com** (owned by the same company), and **VRBO.com** can charge as much as nice hotels. Those become a value when you've got a group. If you want a layer of protection, British-based **FG Properties** (fgproperties.com; © **020/3865-0596**) meets the hosts who list units on its database, which itself populates to Airbnb and HomeAway, and serves as a responsible intermediary for customers.

Because London apartments are in such high demand, there is little incentive for owners to upgrade facilities, so it's easy to rent a stinker. For higher-quality results, we recommend booking through a London rental specialist—one who has vetted the unit and has a relationship with its owner. Our favorite, for its interesting span of 60-odd homes from mid-range to fantasy, is **Coach House Rentals** (chslondon.com/london; © **020/8355-3192**), run by the passionate Harley Nott, who furnishes concierge services. It shines brightest in West London and Westminster. Large, well-appointed units go from around £115 to £300 a night—as much as hotels, but for places that sleep up to 10 people. Discounts kick in after 6 nights. It also operates a lovely B&B space near Balham, in residential South London (3- to 5-night minimum, depending on the season).

The highly recommended **New York Habitat** (www.nyhabitat.com; © **212/255-8018** in U.S.) represents hundreds of flats and has a licensed, U.S.-based office. Units for two range £80 to £250, but they come larger.

London Perfect (www.londonperfect.com; © **888/520-2087** from the U.S.) has class but isn't snooty and its flats, many of which look like spreads from lifestyle magazines, are extremely well-maintained; owners who let fittings get dated are cut from the roster. Someone meets you at the property when you arrive for the first time. Prices start around US$200 a night for studios and one-bedrooms sleeping up to 4 people, largely in tony neighborhoods like South Kensington and Chelsea. There's usually a 7-night minimum.

Loving London Apartments (www.lovinglondonapartments.com; © **800/961-8138** from the U.S.), a clearinghouse for flats, vets every property. What began in 2003 for Spanish vacation villas spread to London in 2005. You can find late-breaking "hot deals" on its site; using those, £100 a night is an advance-booking standard.

Set up in 1995, **Outlet 4 Holidays** (www.outlet4holidays.com; © **07974/729-099**) has flats better located for tourists than perhaps any other firm's. Locations are around Soho's cafe-and-club scene, smack in the West End. £130 a night is the norm, but there are extra fees for checking in outside of business hours or anytime on Sunday. Should trouble arise, its representative is in Soho, so you won't have far to go for assistance.

A high-end renter, **One Fine Stay** (www.onefinestay.com; © **7826/529-286** in the U.K., **855/553-4954** in the U.S.) shoots its flats as if it's photographing a fashion spread, which tells you something about its target market. Central

London digs are over £200 a night, with impeccable design and service to match.

Citadines (www.citadines.com; © **011-33-141-/05-79-05**) runs corporate-style hotel rooms fitted like little apartments, and it has five locations city-wide. In order of centrality: Trafalgar Square, The Cavendish, Holborn, South Kensington, and Barbican (cheapest, from £87).

HOME EXCHANGES

You'd be surprised how many Londoners are dying to visit your own stomping grounds, and if you make contact with the right people, you can swap homes (sometimes simultaneously). It sounds strange, but nothing tends to get stolen because swappers often become good friends. Not just that, but neighbors will often pop by to check up on you, so you have a built-in source of insider advice.

So which club should you choose? Here are the biggies, in alphabetical order:

HomeExchange.com (© **800/877-8723**): This slick service claims 65,000-plus listings in 150 nations. This is important because the more members, the more potential swaps. Results can be broken down by interest. It costs $150 a year for Americans to list.

Homelink.org (© **800/638-3841**): Popular with British and Australian travelers (with reps in 27 countries), this service costs $95 per year.

Intervac (www.intervacus.com; © **866/884-7567**): Intervac has been around for 6 decades and its claim to fame is that some 80% of its listings are international (30,000 families are represented), which means (as it puts it), "you compete with fewer Americans for overseas properties." Access to all listings is $99 a year, but you can take a limited 20-day trial for free.

Additional exchange sites include **SabbaticalHomes.com,** catering to academics; and **HomeAroundtheWorld.com,** for gays and lesbians (£45 for a year). Or you could roll the dice with a website like **CouchSurfing.com,** on which folks (generally younger) offer spare space to visitors. That's free, but there is no vetting system, so consider the risks before taking an offer.

CHEAP DORM ROOMS

Staying in a college room in holiday periods is an ideal budget saver for visitors of any age. Reservations are accepted starting in spring. At all of them, expect a wood-frame bed with linen, a desk, a dresser, an in-room sink, the possibility of an equipped kitchen (although it might be shared), an en suite bathroom (usually), laundry facilities, breakfast (often at a reasonable charge), Wi-Fi, and phones in the room or in the hall.

London School of Economics (www.lsevacations.co.uk; © **020/7955-7676**): Check these out first. Its eight properties are in terrific condition, with the dignity that you'd expect of a school that trains the world's power players in business. Rooms rent cheaply (£45–£150) for July, August, and the first chunk of September. A few rooms may be available at Christmas or Easter, too.

Some single "private accommodation" rooms at **City University London** (www.city.ac.uk/accommodation; © **020/7040-7040**) are available from early July to early September. Prices are around £210 a week.

University College London (www.ucl.ac.uk/residences; © **020/7631-8310**): Its dorms, clustering in Bloomsbury, are less prestigious than LSE's, but they aren't depressing. From late June to September, 10 residences are available at £37 to £57, but only five properties have private bathrooms.

King's College (www.kingsvenues.com; © **020/7848-1700**): As of 2017, five halls are available for short rental from late June through mid-September. The candidates have kitchens but not utensils and cost £45 to £65.

International Students House (229 Great Portland St., W1; www.ish.org. uk; © **020/7631-8300;** Tube: Great Portland St.): Part dorm, part subdued hostel, in two buildings. Ballpark per-person rates are mid-£20s in a gender-separated dorm, £50 single, £37 twin, £30 quad (cheaper if booked by mid-May). Bathrooms are shared, and some are co-ed but partitioned. Other academic rooms are more private. Breakfast is included.

WHERE TO EAT

I n 1957, Arthur Frommer visited London for his seminal *Europe on $5 a Day*. His report was gloomy: "With great despair, this book recommends that you . . . save your money for the better meals available in France and Italy. Cooking is a lost art in Great Britain; your meat pie with cabbage will turn out just as tasteless for 40¢ in a chain restaurant as it will for $2 in a posh hotel." The report today is happily quite different: Bon appétit!

4

As it turns out, good English cooking wasn't a lost art at all. True, there are still plenty of places you'll find a crap meal, but cabbage is no longer the national affliction, as it was in the days of rationing. Now that London swarms with people from across the world, you'll find nearly every style of cuisine—ask any Londoner for their favorite restaurant and it's bound to be a foreign food. In the past 40 years, British consumption of sugar, potatoes, and flour have halved. Countless restaurants now serve ingredients fresh from the farm. Fish and chips, for a time relegated to the suburbs, made a comeback, and Indian restaurants, or "curry shops," now serve the country's unofficial comfort food. Thai food and burgers are more common than them all. Even most of the major museums (listed starting on p. 109) run cafes that, surprisingly, more than pull their weight.

Don't like meat? London's greenie culture thrives, and virtually every menu will have plenty of dishes for vegetarians to eat. The situation for vegans isn't quite as obvious, but most kitchens understand vegan dietary requirements. The news is just as good for people with **food allergies:** A majority of potentially irritating ingredients are marked when you buy pre-made food at the major shops.

Beware of relying on Yelp, Google, or Apple Maps to find places. Online inventory is often vastly incomplete, opening hours are often way off, and the results favor chains, so you'll miss a lot of good things. You can sometimes find some meal deals on **Open Table.co.uk** and **SquareMeal.co.uk.** And here's an insider tip: By law, restaurants must charge you a higher tax rate if you eat on premises, so take-away is always cheaper.

Each convenient place in this book was chosen to say something about London of the moment—you'll taste what it's like to eat like a Londoner today.

BLOOMSBURY, FITZROVIA & KING'S CROSS

These areas north of the central tourist district are more residential and consequently less of a scene than other parts of town can be, but now that the hip developements around Granary Square, north of King's Cross, are coming on line, the scenesters are beginning to follow.

Expensive

Dabbous ★★★ INTERNATIONAL   Dabbous (the S is silent) shines through arty, crisp dishes using local and seasonal ingredients. The setting is kind of ugly, all concrete and exposed ducts, and the words on the menu give no hint of the inventiveness to follow; the fun is putting yourself in Chef Ollie Dabbous' hands and seeing what inventions he's come up with: coddled egg with smoked butter, then returned audaciously to the shell? Popcorn ice cream? Rather than over-salt or heavily spice, he'll lightly char something or create a suspended emulsion of another thing. Downstairs in Oskar's Bar, cocktails are made with homemade infusions and there's a shortened menu of barbecued meat. More, please.

Tipping & Prices
Price categories are based on a typical main course.
o **Expensive** £17 +
o **Moderate** £10 to £17
o **Inexpensive** under £10
Doggy bags are frowned upon and most restaurants expect you to give up your table after 90 minutes to 2 hours. Always check the bill to see if service is included. If it is, you don't have to tip. If not, 10% to 15% is customary.

39 Whitfield St., W1. www.dabbous.co.uk. © **020/7323-1544.** Set 4-course lunch menu £36; 4-course dinner menu £59; 7-course tasting menu £75. Tues–Fri noon–2:30pm and 5:30–11:30pm; Sat noon–2:30pm and 6:30–11:30pm. Reservations required. Tube: Goodge St.

Moderate

Bill's ★★ INTERNATIONAL   A 5-minute walk from the British Museum and handy for many uses—big breakfasts, lunches, dinner, tea with scones and clotted cream, feeding kids, or downing cheap cocktails—this casual spot is part of an affordable small group of restaurants that started as a greengrocer (they're rigorous about quality ingredients). In few other London establishments will you find mac and cheese, burgers, pecan pie, and Caesar's salad on the same menu. It's a lifesaver when you're in need of drama-free grub served briskly, which is why you'll be glad to hear there are also locations near Piccadilly Circus (36–44 Brewer St., W1), off the Long Acre shopping street (St Martin's Courtyard, WC2), in Southwark (Victor Wharf, Clink St., SE1) and in Greenwich town. The afternoon tea is around £10 and not half bad, plus there's free Wi-Fi.

42 Kingsway, WC2. www.bills-website.co.uk. © **020/2742-2981.** Main courses £9–£13. Mon–Sat 8am–11pm; Sun 9am–10:30pm. Tube: Holborn.

London-Wide Restaurants

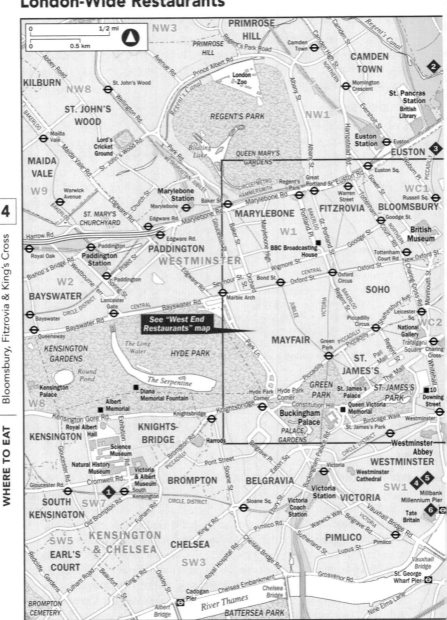

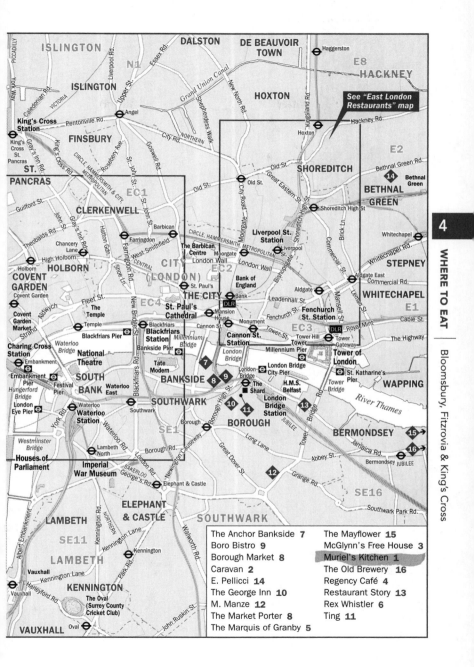

The Anchor Bankside **7**   The Mayflower **15**
Boro Bistro **9**   McGlynn's Free House **3**
Borough Market **8**   Muriel's Kitchen **1**
Caravan **2**   The Old Brewery **16**
E. Pellicci **14**   Regency Café **4**
The George Inn **10**   Restaurant Story **13**
M. Manze **12**   Rex Whistler **6**
The Market Porter **8**   Ting **11**
The Marquis of Granby **5**

West End Restaurants

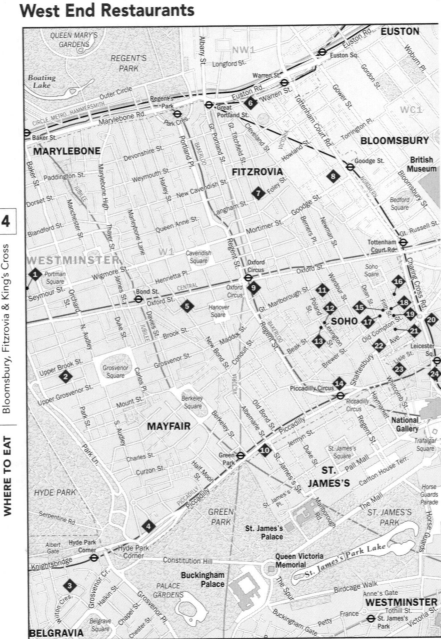

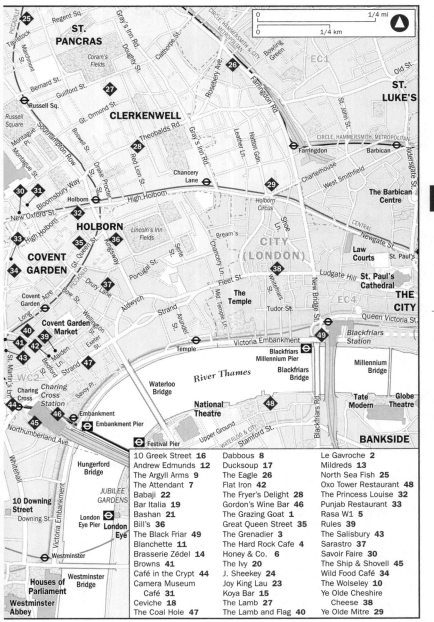

10 Greek Street **16**	Dabbous **8**	Le Gavroche **2**
Andrew Edmunds **12**	Ducksoup **17**	Mildreds **13**
The Argyll Arms **9**	The Eagle **26**	North Sea Fish **25**
The Attendant **7**	Flat Iron **42**	Oxo Tower Restaurant **48**
Babaji **22**	The Fryer's Delight **28**	The Princess Louise **32**
Bar Italia **19**	Gordon's Wine Bar **46**	Punjab Restaurant **33**
Bashan **21**	The Grazing Goat **1**	Rasa W1 **5**
Bill's **36**	Great Queen Street **35**	Rules **39**
The Black Friar **49**	The Grenadier **3**	The Salisbury **43**
Blanchette **11**	The Hard Rock Cafe **4**	Sarastro **37**
Brasserie Zédel **14**	Honey & Co. **6**	Savoir Faire **30**
Browns **41**	The Ivy **20**	The Ship & Shovell **45**
Café in the Crypt **44**	J. Sheekey **24**	Wild Food Café **34**
Camera Museum	Joy King Lau **23**	The Wolseley **10**
Café **31**	Koya Bar **15**	Ye Olde Cheshire
Ceviche **18**	The Lamb **27**	Cheese **38**
The Coal Hole **47**	The Lamb and Flag **40**	Ye Olde Mitre **29**

Caravan ★★ INTERNATIONAL   The redevelopment of the 67-acre post-industrial void north of King's Cross station will take a decade, but the chic energy is already here, and Caravan, in the old Granary building, is a big reason why. So basic and industrial-feeling (long blond-wood tables, canvaslike sheets for window shades, plain metal racks for bar shelves) that it feels like it could be converted to a ceramics shop overnight, Caravan is always busy but glows with *joie de vivre* on days when its front patio is open. The place roasts its own coffee, bakes its own goods—the jalapeno cornbread is moist and kicky—and pushes its tapas-size dishes into fun flavor realms like coconut lime chicken salad, salt beef terrine, and chipotle ricotta in edible zucchini flower. After dinner, kick back in its front yard in an amphitheater overlooking the Regent's Canal. Another, newer location is found a few streets behind the Tate Modern (30 Great Guilford St., SE1; ℂ **020/7101-1190;** Southwark or London Bridge tube).

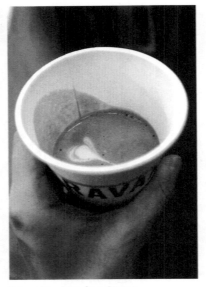

Enjoy a Macchiato from Caravan.

1 Granary Sq., off Goods Way, N1. www.caravanrestaurants.co.uk. ℂ **020/7101-7661.** Small plates £5–£7; pizzas £7–£9. Mon–Fri 8am–10:30pm; Sat 10am–10:30pm; Sun 10am–4pm. Reservations recommended (but not accepted Sat–Sun daytime). Tube: King's Cross St Pancras.

The Eagle ★★ TRADITIONAL BRITISH   By now, the gastropub trend is so widespread the term is meaningless, but foodies note: It began here in 1991 (or so most agree), in Clerkenwell, a then-ungentrified area between Bloomsbury and Islington. Loft-dwellers and design firms have since taken over, but The Eagle remains, and on its own terms. Behind the bar of a bare-to-the-wood corner saloon, the sometimes-surly staff prepares a changing selection of about a dozen flavorful dishes a day, from the likes of pork loin salad to pan-roasted sole to the house specialty, the insidiously spicy Bife Ana steak sandwich dripping with marinated garlic and onion. Tables are shared (it's bad for groups), menu by blackboard only (preview today's on Instagram: @eaglefarringdon), furniture reassuringly shabby and mismatched, and foodie crowds reliably in force—come early to ensure your share. Order at the bar and relax with a beer, because here, the food's the thing, and it arrives on its own schedule.

159 Farringdon Rd., EC1. www.theeaglefarringdon.co.uk. ℂ **020/7837-1353.** Main courses £8–£18. Mon–Sat noon–11pm; Sun noon–5pm. Tube: Farringdon.

Bloomsbury, Fitzrovia & King's Cross

WHERE TO EAT

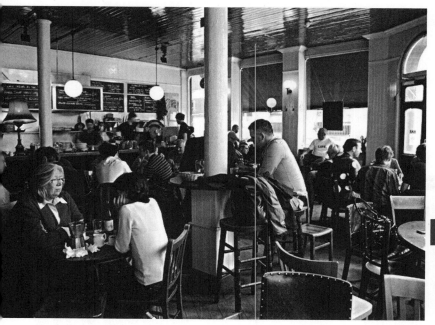

The Eagle gastropub.

Honey & Co. ★★ MIDDLE EASTERN   It's packed for good reasons. First, the food brilliantly adapts Middle Eastern dishes to London palates. Spectacular lamb schwarma is tender as brisket and spiked with pomegranate and mint, and is served in a little pot with hot and soft pita. Chicken dumplings come in a broth that smells like love. The "strawberry spliff" dessert proves that berries, phyllo, mint, and olive oil go well together. The other reason this place is packed is it's knee-knockingly tiny: 20 table seats and 4 in the window, so make a reservation or miss out on this assured, sometimes revelatory, meal.

25a Warren St., W1. www.honeyandco.co.uk. ℃ **020/7388-6175.** Main courses £8–£15. Mon–Fri 8am–10:30pm; Sat 9:30am–10:30pm. Tube: Warren St. or Great Portland St.

North Sea Fish ★★ SEAFOOD   Don't expect a linoleum-lined chippie, but a classy fish market-cum-restaurant, hidden on a lost-in-time side street. Every hotel manager within a walkable radius recommends it. Portions are huge, and there's always a selection of fresh fish (sole, salmon, halibut, and so on). If you need a healthier option, you can also get your fish grilled. Try the terrific homemade tartar sauce, or, for fans of little fishies, sample grilled sardines with salad. Keep in mind that take-away is about half the price of sitting down to eat.

7–8 Leigh St., WC1. www.northseafishrestaurant.co.uk. ℃ **020/7387-5892.** Main courses £11–£20. Mon–Sat noon–2:30pm and 5–10:30pm; Sun 5–9:30pm. Tube: King's Cross St Pancras or Russell Square.

Savoir Faire ★★★ FRENCH   After braving the rummage sale of mediocre gastronomic clip joints around the British Museum, patrons are known to smugly proclaim this their "discovery"—omitting the reality that it's been presenting what it correctly terms "affordable gourmet" since 1995. How could anyone have ignored this traveler's gift, where nothing is processed and everything is made-to-order? Meals are more than reliable; in this area, they're miracles on plates. Baguette sandwiches and burgers are under £9, but upgrade: Lunch prix-fixe is £16 (dinner £25) and might include ample portions of nimbly executed dishes like red-wine-braised duck legs, bouillabaisse, tequila-lime chicken, or beef daube so tender you wonder if they've got Julia Child's ghost back there.

42 New Oxford St., WC1. www.savoir.co.uk. ℂ **020/7436-0707.** Main courses £5–£15; 2-course set menu £16–£25. Daily noon–4pm and 5pm–10:30pm. Tube: Holborn or Tottenham Court Rd.

4 | Inexpensive

The Attendant ★ CAFE   A unique one for the coffee culture fans. They only serve light meals here, but they roast their own beans and the setting is worth a detour: a gourmet coffee/loose-leaf tea cafe in an underground men's toilet in Fitzrovia. The facilities had been abandoned for 50 years; the conversion was so artful you might not realize it at first: Eight elaborate Doulton & Co. Victorian porcelain urinals are now individual coffee-sipping bays, and an overhead water tank became an unexpected planter. If you're hungry, try the sea salt caramel brownies or bacon on sourdough with tarragon butter. The coffee's so good, Attendant has added more locations, but those lack the charm of being in a loo.

27a Foley St. at Great Titchfield St., W1. www.the-attendant.com. ℂ **020/7637-3794.** Sandwiches and baked goods £3–£5. Mon–Fri 8am–6pm; Sat 9am–6pm, Sun 10am–6pm. Tube: Oxford Circus or Goodge St.

Camera Museum Café ★ INTERNATIONAL   There aren't many cheap, non-chain, easy options near the British Museum, but if you don't need much, check out this spot squirreled away in a camera shop specializing in Hasselblad lenses; walls are decorated with shots taken by local artists and there's a small display of antique cameras. Food is on-the-go simple (sandwiches, juices, and homemade soups of the day) but there are lots of coffee-table books on art and Britain to read, plus Wi-Fi and outlets for foot-resting and further planning.

44 Museum St., WC1. www.cameramuseum.uk. ℂ **020/7242-8681.** Light meals £4–£7. Tues–Fri 11am–7pm; Sat noon–7pm, Sun noon–6pm. Tube: Tottenham Court Rd. or Holborn.

The Fryer's Delight ★★ TRADITIONAL BRITISH/TAKE-AWAY   In this age, no one would dare name their joint something as hydrogenated as The Fryer's Delight. Fortunately, this joint is not of this age. It's a true old-world chippy, where the fry fat is from beef drippings, chips come in paper

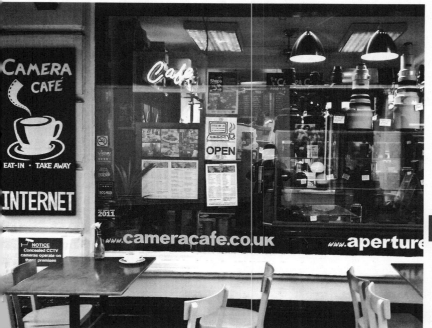

Camera Café offers simple food, handily near the British Museum.

wrappings, the wooden booths and checkered floor date to the lean postwar years, and the men behind the counter are almost callously gruff. Prices are anachronistic, too: Nothing's more expensive than £7. Order yours with mushy peas. It's a 10-minute walk east of the British Museum; look for the logo of a codfish tipping his bowler hat (seriously). If you like fish and chips more upscale, try **Bonnie Gull** in Fitzrovia (21 Foley St., W1; www.bonnie gullseafoodshack.com; ✆ **020/7436-0921;** £15 at dinner) or **Golden Union** in Soho (38 Poland St., W1; www.goldenunion.co.uk; ✆ **020/7434-1933;** £12).

19 Theobald's Rd., WC1. ✆ **020/7405-4114.** Main courses £5–£6. Mon–Sat noon–10pm. Tube: Holborn or Chancery Lane.

SOHO & LEICESTER SQUARE

Visitors spend much of their time around here, the dining and entertainment hub of London. So a miasma of dining also-rans, from junky steam-table buffets to overpriced bistros, sponge off tourists. Soho's southern fringe hosts a meager Chinatown in the neon-tinted 2-block section between Leicester Square and Shaftesbury Avenue. I don't think many of its restaurants are distinguished enough to single out. Many of them use MSG, too, despite public health currents.

Expensive

The Ivy ★ TRADITIONAL BRITISH   A West End tent-pole for 101 years, from Coward to Cumberbatch, this is where London thespians pretend to slum it, eating hamburgers even as they lift cognac beneath its iconic wood paneling and harlequin mullioned windows. "The Ivy is like a safari park in which the rare and exotic creatures are nurtured," wrote the *Guardian*. A 2015 renovation didn't shuck its caché, although it did add a sumptuous flatiron bar—you can eat at it—where spotting celebrities, should there be any (try after 9pm), is made all the more subtle. The menu of Ivy classics (lobster macaroni, shepherd's pie) has been embellished with Asian-ish notions (barbecued squid salad, Togarashi popcorn rock shrimp), which only increases the bohemian affect. From the glass jug on the bar, order a "100 Year Legacy," which is a never-ending cocktail—a Martinez, an archaic variation of a Manhattan made with gin—dispensed from a communal spout and added to as time goes on. It's an experiment that only began in 2017, but if anyplace has the wherewithal to nurture an eccentric quirk into long tradition, it's The Ivy.

1–5 West St., WC1. www.the-ivy.co.uk. ⓒ **020/7836-4751.** Main courses £15–£20. Set menu (Mon–Thurs 2:30pm–6pm and all day Sun) 2 courses £24, 3 courses £28. Mon–Wed noon–11:30pm, Thurs–Sat noon–midnight, Sun noon–10:30pm. Tube: Leicester Square or Covent Garden.

The Ivy restaurant offers a mix of new fare and classics.

Moderate

10 Greek Street ★★★ CONTEMPORARY EUROPEAN   Sometimes, restaurants get it so right—from friendly and knowledgeable staff to unfussy surroundings (chalkboard, mirrors) to pure, clean, well-made food—that you

LONDON food chains I RECOMMEND

London, like so many other cities, is experiencing an economic shift that squeezes out mom-and-pop establishments in favor of better-heeled chains; you'll see these mid-priced, kid-friendly names on storefronts wherever you go. They're delicious and most are English-owned, so rely on them as well:

- **Benito's Hat:** Like competitior Tortilla, it's a worthy Chipotle imitator.
- **Busaba Eathai:** Peppy noodles and Asian dishes at communal tables.
- **Carluccio's:** New York–style Italian. Tile walls, pasta, fish, meats, coffees.
- **Giraffe:** Every kind of comfort food, extremely family-friendly, can get noisy.
- **Leon:** Free-trade, organic alternative to fast food includes "hot boxes" of Moroccan meatballs,

halloumi wraps, and "superfood" salads.

- **M&S Simply Food:** Marks & Spencer's (p. 205) stand-alone shops for sandwiches, hit-or-miss ready-made dishes, and well-selected inexpensive wines.
- **Ping Pong:** Chinese dim sum in a vibrant, hip environment, plus cocktails.
- **Pizza Express:** Artisan-style pie. No one pays full price; see www.pizza-express.com/latest-offers for consistent discounts such as 25% off.
- **Simit Sarayi:** Turkish coffee, stuffed buns, sandwiches on seeded bread.
- **Wagamama:** Hearty noodle bowls eaten at shared long tables.
- **Wahaca:** Substantial Mexican done well with British-grown ingredients.

Wagamama serves patrons at shared tables.

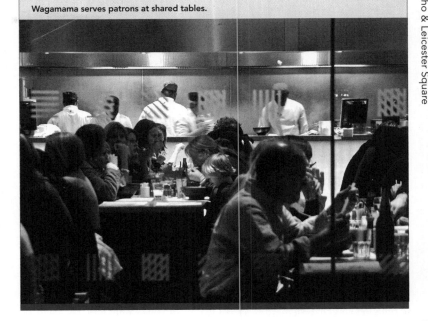

wonder why they can't all be this way. The menu, all choices a top value for the money, changes but the impeccable standards don't: Frequent standouts include whole lemon sole with samphire (an edible coastal plant) and artichokes, Brecon lamb, Gloucester Old Spot pork, elderflower sorbet, a continuous trickle of fresh-baked breads, and an affordable wine list chosen with as much care as the fish and meat cuts. If there's a downside, it's that they only take reservations for lunch (noon–2:30pm), which means you risk missing out on dinner if you don't come early. Or just sit at the tiny bar.

10 Greek St., W1. www.10greekstreet.com. ℗ **0209/7734-4677.** Main courses £12–£19. Mon–Sat noon–11pm. Tube: Tottenham Court Rd.

Andrew Edmunds ★★★ BRITISH   The relaxed, townhouse-style storefront, a study in natural woods and candle-lit purity, has been going for 30 years, enduring most likely because it hasn't caved to Soho trendiness and its stupendous wine list is priced fairly. Chairs don't match, staff isn't in uniform, and the menu is hand-scribbled daily with a haste that belies the effort the chef puts into sourcing farmhouse meats and preparing seasonal ingredients. Expect choices along the lines of skate wing with cauliflower and capers, free-range Aylesbury duck breast, and artichoke spaghetti with wild garlic and almond pesto, plus the occasional nose-to-tail adventure. Superb dessert cheeses are selected from area farms. It's very London, and the slick crowd can't commandeer it because bookings are only accepted a week out. The lunchtime pasta of the day is £7, and a lunch set menu goes for £15.

46 Lexington St., W1. www.andrewedmunds.com. ℗ **020/7437-5708.** Main courses £13–£23. Mon–Fri noon–3:30pm and 5:30–10:45pm; Sat 12:30–3:30pm and 5:30–10:45pm; Sun 1–4pm and 6–10:30pm. Reservations essential. Tube: Piccadilly Circus or Oxford Circus.

Bashan ★★ ASIAN   Set away from Chinatown's rabble of late-night steam-table chow, this Hunan establishment on a corner in lower Soho costs a touch more than its Gerrard Street rivals, but the trade-off is it's spicier (British kitchens are usually terrified to turn up the heat) and more reminiscent of actual Chinese cooking. This is not to say it's fully authentic, but it's a lot closer than its competition. In other ways, it hews to the Chinatown experience: dauntingly long menu, somewhat transactional service, a hearty welcome that extends only as far as your spending. Speaking of that: In the U.K., rice is usually an extra charge.

24 Romilly St., W1. www.bashanlondon.com. ℗ **020/7287-3266.** Main courses £11–£25. Daily noon–11pm. Tube: Piccadilly Circus or Leicester Square.

Blanchette ★ FRENCH   Divinely assembled tasting plates, which change with seasons, focus on ingredients: things like grilled flavor-rich beef *onglet* (hanger steak) with snails or mushrooms, grilled asparagus with aged Comté cheese, hot bread delivered in a brown paper bag with soft butter spread with a wooden paddle. The food may be crafted, but there's no fussiness in the welcome. The look is much like a casually urbanized French farmhouse of rough wood and exposed brick; a long bar under caged light bulbs is ideal for

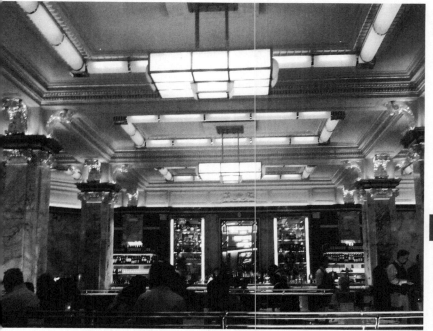

The dining room at Brasserie Zédel features gilt and marble.

tasting charcuterie, cheese, and sipping wine. The pre-theater menu brings three courses for under £20.

9 D'Arblay St., W1. www.blanchettesoho.co.uk. © **020/7439-8100.** Small plates £3–£8, larger plates £9–£14. Mon–Sat noon–11pm; Sun noon–5pm. Tube: Oxford Circus.

Brasserie Zédel ★★★ FRENCH   When you enter via its grand staircase, you feel like Toulouse-Lautrec in search of tonight's muse: The gilt-and-marble cellar dining room, awash in fin-de-siècle statements like platter mirrors and vested waiters, is a perfect piece of Paris off Piccadilly. This is not a crusty holdover but a pitch-perfect recreation out of what was once the Regent Palace Hotel, which in 1915 was the largest hotel in Europe. Menu choices are as authentic as Pernod, pastis, oysters, quiche Lorraine, and sublimely seasoned steak tartare (often, the first thing I order upon returning to town). The adjoining **Bar Américain,** a 1930s Art Deco treasure by an architect survivor of the *Lusitania,* does indulgently uptight cocktails and champagne, while its 80-seat cabaret, **Live at Zédel,** is an elegant venue that does matinees and evening shows (£15–35, no drink minimum). This bit of the Continental high life is not nearly as expensive as it looks, and its Gallic poise only adds to the deliciousness.

20 Sherwood St., W1. www.brasseriezedel.com. © **020/7734-4888.** Main courses £13–£15; 2 courses £10; 3 courses £13. Mon–Sun 11:30am–midnight (Sun 11pm). Tube: Piccadilly Circus.

Ceviche ★★★ PERUVIAN   This is my firm favorite in Soho. Owner Martin Morales quit his job at Disney's European music division to pursue his true passion: food. Now he is a TV personality, a cookbook author, and runs this hopping, cheerful Peruvian hangout that pours the best pisco sour in town. Flavors are indescribably punchy, citrusy, and unrepeatable anywhere else you've eaten. Favorite small plates include the *don ceviche* sea bass made with *limo chili* tiger's milk, and the succulent *corazón mío* of beef skewers marinated in *panca chili anticuchera*. Once your tongue tastes its first vibrant zip, you'll feel compelled to come back. They now give diners a spoon to lap up leftover tiger's milk—probably because I kept asking. A second, spacious location is just north of the Old Street Tube stop (2 Baldwin St., EC1), while the owner's similar **Andina** is in Shoreditch (1 Redchurch St., E2; www.andinalondon.com; ✆ **020/7920-6499;** Shoreditch High St. or Liverpool St. tube stops).

17 Frith St., W1. www.cevicheuk.com. ✆ **020/7292-2040.** Small plates £7–£12. Daily noon–11:30pm (Sun until 10:15pm), hot kitchen closed Mon–Thurs 3pm-5pm. Reservations suggested. Tube: Piccadilly Circus or Tottenham Court Rd.

Ducksoup ★★ INTERNATIONAL   The sort of invisible hidey-hole you have to be told about, Ducksoup is barely marked. Indeed, when you first open its old door, the first thing you see is a stack of LPs and a record player, the sole sound system, that might be playing Grace Jones' "Nightclubbing" or Toots & the Maytals' "Funky Kingston." The day's menu changes. The metal grille on the windows and life-beaten walls make it look like a greasy cafe that would sling a fry-up at you, but instead, there's a funky wine list and solid, whole-food selections, which change daily, such as grilled artichoke with lemon and capers, rabbit pappardelle, and chargrilled bream. The room feels like a London that went out with Thatcher, but dishes sit solidly within London's 21st-century gustatory passions.

41 Dean St., W1. www.ducksoupsoho.co.uk. ✆ **020/7287-4599.** Main courses £8–£18. Mon–Sat noon–10:30pm, Sun noon–5pm; bar open later. Tube: Tottenham Court Rd.

Koya Bar ★★ JAPANESE   A queue for a quick and cheap bowl of noodle soup? Well, ordinary soup wouldn't merit it. But this stuff is no mere soup. The dining room is plain, bearing nothing more special than wood stick chairs, cheap chopsticks in cups, menu boards, and rows of metal coat hooks, and staff will rush you. Even the menu of *udon* (wheat flour noodles) and more *udon* would appear to have no tricks. But then the finished product arrives in several parts, ferried by impish waitresses, for you to mix yourself, and the fog lifts. Noodles are made fresh each day using traditional methods. The walnut miso enchants. The pork *udon* is made of spring onion, salty roast pork crumble, a mystically *umami* (savory taste) broth base, and 6 ounces of pure Colombian cocaine. I'm not actually sure about that last ingredient, but it would explain a lot. You will drink the dregs from the bowl.

50 Frith St., W1. www.koyabar.co.uk. ✆ **020/7434-4463.** Main courses £7–£14. Daily noon–3pm; Mon–Weds 8:30–10:30pm, Thurs–Fri 8:30am–11:30pm, Sat 9:30am–11pm, Sun 9:30am–10pm. No reservations. Tube: Tottenham Court Rd.

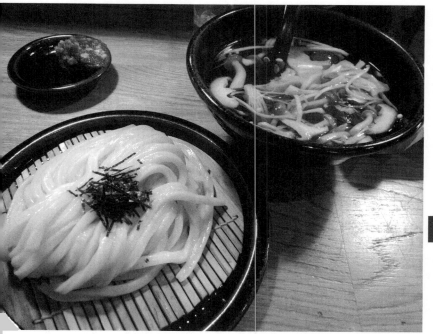

Udon at Koya features Japanese cuisine worth waiting in line for.

Mildreds ★ VEGETARIAN   Usually packed, it's where vegetarians with palates go. The menu is ever-changing but always assembled with more care than the usual beans and tofu: Sri Lankan sweet potato and lime cashew curry, tortelloni with pumpkin and ricotta, and risotto cake with grape mustard sauce are three samples from its internationally derived menu. Big bowls and plates, appetizing presentation, and a vibe like a contemporary home have secured Mildreds a following even among carnivores—it even got a cookbook published. Save room for the peanut butter chocolate brownie—you won't believe it's gluten-free.

45 Lexington St., W1. www.mildreds.co.uk. © **020/7494-1634.** Main courses £9–£12. Mon–Sat noon–11pm. No reservations. Tube: Tottenham Court Rd.

Inexpensive

Babaji ★ TURKISH   When you need a decent pre-theater nosh, Shaftesbury Avenue mostly offers only tourist rubbish and coffee shops hawking pre-fab sandwiches. The exception is here, where casual but well-made Turkish food is doled out in a two-level brass-and-tile shop with great windows for people-watching (although it's often so busy you won't be encouraged to linger). The specialty is almost a dozen types of *pide*—oblong Turkish pizzas, the best filled with meat, cooked in a big oven on the ground floor. You'll also love the watermelon lemonade, oven-baked halloumi cheese, and honey-and-chestnut filled desserts. If it seems more swish than your typical baklava slinger, you're right: It's by Alan Yau, who created Wagamama (p. 79) and Busaba Eathai. Be warned: Unlike in Turkey, you'll be charged for your accompanying cup of tea.

52 Shaftesbury Ave., W1. www.babaji.com.tr. © **020/3327-3888.** Main courses £8–£10. Mon–Thurs noon–11pm, Fri–Sat noon–11:30pm, Sun noon–10pm. Tube: Piccadilly Circus or Leicester Square.

Bar Italia ★★ COFFEE/ITALIAN   Italians settled Soho in the 1940s, and before they decamped for the suburbs, they installed a set of mod, gleaming coffee bars and cafes. This straggler from 1949 is a haunt of slumming celebrities and artists, yet modest enough for the rest of us. While this institution is busy all day—making simple sandwiches, delivering pastries—it swells with revelers after midnight. Even Rome doesn't have bars that steam, press, and shuffle coffee across such defiantly worn '50s linoleum with such gusto. "Like everything in this city that Londoners really enjoy, it reminds us of being abroad," quipped the *Guardian*. Whatever; it practically leaks hipness.

22 Frith St., W1. www.baritaliasoho.co.uk. © **020/7437-4520.** Coffee £3–£4; pizza £10–£11; panini £7. Mon–Sun 6:30am–4:30am (Sun 2am). Tube: Leicester Square.

Café in the Crypt ★ INTERNATIONAL   Super-central and unquestionably memorable, it's the tastiest graveyard in town! Under the sanctuary of the historic St Martin-in-the-Fields church at Trafalgar Square, atop the gravestones of 18th-century Londoners, one of the West End's sharpest bargains is served. The menu at this dependable 200-seat cafeteria changes monthly, but the large portions always include a few hot meat main dishes, a vegetarian choice, soups, salads topped with meats, and sweet apple crumble with custard; there's also fish and chips on Friday. The church keeps the wine and draft beer flowing, and afternoon tea is but £10. Bottom line: It's fun, delicious, central, and a budget savior.

Trafalgar Sq., WC2. www.smitf.org. © **020/7766-1158.** Main courses £6–£9. Mon–Tues 8am–8pm; Wed 8am–10:30pm (with 8pm jazz for ticket holders only after 6:30pm); Thurs–Sat 8am–9pm; Sun 11am–6pm. Tube: Charing Cross.

Gordon's Wine Bar ★ INTERNATIONAL   The atmosphere is matchless at London's most vaunted and vaulted casual wine bar. It was established in 1890 (when Rudyard Kipling lived upstairs) and, thank goodness, hasn't been refurbished since—look in the front display window and you'll see some untouched champagne bottles intentionally left to grow furry with dust. These tight, craggy cellars beneath Villiers Street are wallpapered with important newspaper front pages from the 20th century—Thatcher's resignation, the death of King George VI—while ceiling fans threaten to come loose from their screws. Everything is suffused in a mustardy ochre from more than 42,000 past evenings of indoor tobacco smoke (no longer legal). Tables are candlelit, music is not played—not that you could hear it over the din of conversation. Dozens of wines and sherries by the glass are around £5, and you

KEEPING THE BILL low

If you're watching your money, bear in mind these cultural differences:

Avoid soda: It costs more than £2, and often for a puny glassful, no refills.

Avoid over-tipping: Credit card slips may have a line for a tip, even if the tip was already built in. Only tip (10%–20%) if the menu says "service not included" or similar.

Avoid rice dishes: It's customary to pay £2 to £3 for a side dish of plain rice, even if you think it should come with what you ordered.

Avoid eating in: Establishments are obliged by law to charge 20% in tax if you decide to eat your purchases there.

Avoid water: Well, avoid it bottled. If you just order "water," waiters may bring expensive bottled water, so if you want it for free, specify "tap water."

Avoid starters: Even where mains are £7, starters can be £4 to £6.

Avoid cocktails: Mixed drinks can cost a dizzying £8 to £11, and they're all the same middling strength because of measure standardization. If you do drink, stick to beer (£3–£4 a pint) or wine (around £5 a glass).

can select from a marble display of English and French cheeses or a steam table of hot food. In good weather, the event expands outside along Embankment Gardens with casual alfresco meals such as stuffed peppers and marinated pork loin. (The stone arch was built around 1625 as a palace gate on the Thames, but its mansion is long gone and the river moved 46m/150 ft. south.) Come down well before offices let out to secure seating; it won't accept bookings.

47 Villiers St., WC2. www.gordonswinebar.com. © **020/7930-1408.** Main courses £7–£10. Mon–Sat 11am–11pm; Sun noon–10pm. Tube: Charing Cross or Embankment.

Joy King Lau ★ DIM SUM   For those who insist on eating with the tipsy Soho revelers in Chinatown, there's this long-termer with multiple levels, perpetually packed on weekends and bank holidays. Décor? Tired. Service? Robotic. Food quality? Swings between crapshoot and rapture. Customers who aren't used to the brisk attitude of servers in a Chinese food hall like this may grumble, but there's something invigorating about joining the carnival and slurping down whatever they place in front of you. Sticking to the dim sum menu from noon to 5pm (and not springing for the Cantonese set menu) satisfies most people. Always remember: You're in London, not China.

3 Leicester St., WC2. www.joykinglau.com. © **020/7437-1132.** Main courses £8–£19. Daily noon–11:30pm (Sun until 10:30pm). Tube: Leicester Square.

COVENT GARDEN

The area was once more interesting, but CAPCO, which governs the leases, has adopted a policy of squeezing out oddballs in favor of imported brands such as Shake Shack, Le Pain Quotidien, Apple, and Balthazar. The food within the market is tourist-priced, but if you simply must eat there, head to the lower level where you'll find £6 *tartines* (open sandwiches) at **Chez Antoinette** and good cheese at the **Crusting Pipe** wine bar.

Expensive

J. Sheekey ★★ SEAFOOD   Smartly turned-out waiters prep you with so many strange fish-eating utensils that your place setting starts to look like a workstation at Santa's workshop. Such presentational flourishes are appropriate to theaterland, where this has been a bistro-style classic for years, and although prices aren't generous, portions and quality are. The least expensive main dish, fish pie, is fortunately its trademark, but there are plenty of other choices, from shrimp-and-scallop burgers to a delectable lemon sole, plus a changing slate of game and meats for the fish-averse. Despite all the fuss, children are welcomed.

28–32 St. Martin's Ct., WC2. www.j-sheekey.co.uk. © **020/7240-2565.** Main courses £18–£44. Weekend lunch set menu: 3 courses £29. Mon–Fri noon–3pm and 5pm–midnight; Sat–Sun noon–3pm and 5:15pm–midnight (Sun until 10:30pm). Reservations recommended. Tube: Leicester Square.

Rules ★★ TRADITIONAL BRITISH   For a high-end kitchen that takes British cuisine seriously, go with an icon. Rules is London's oldest restaurant

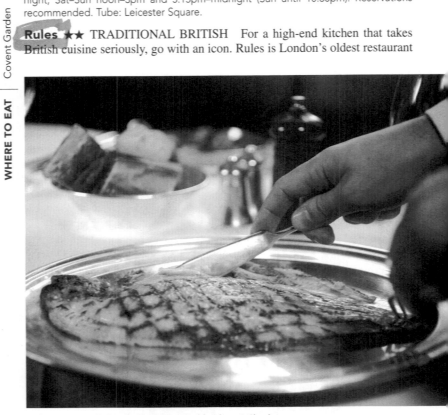

A classic Dover sole is expertly deboned tableside at J. Sheekey.

(est. 1798), and its patrons have included Graham Greene, Charles Dickens, Evelyn Waugh, and Edward VII, who regularly dined here with his paramour Lillie Langtry. (The management is less than discreet about it; the nook they used is named for him.) Being a major stop on the tourist trail has gone slightly to its head and it's steeped in its own hype; beer comes in a "silver tankard," for example, and the landmarked rooms are an overdressed mélange of yellowing etchings, antlers, and rich red fabrics. But what's on the table is indisputably high-class: English-reared meat like roast loin of roe deer, whole roast squab or grouse (it serves 18,000 game birds annually), and cocktails like that famous one made of tonic, juniper, and quinine. Its nearest rival, **Simpsons-in-the-Strand** at the Savoy hotel (p. 43) has been going since 1828, but in 2017, it stopped trying to keep up and modernized with a new menu.

35 Maiden Lane, WC1. www.rules.co.uk. © **020/7836-5314.** Main courses £22–£35. Daily noon–11:45pm (Sun until 10:45pm). Tube: Covent Garden.

Sarastro ★ MEDITERRANEAN What if Mozart went insane on hollandaise sauce? He'd open this flamboyant paean to the opulence of opera. In a design that must give the fire marshal sleepless nights, Sarastro's every cranny has been gilded, sheathed in shimmering fabric, or filled with erotic statuary (enjoy the self-pleasuring Diablo). Along the walls, 10 intimate opera boxes, reached up precarious stairs, survey the silliness, which is often embellished by musicians. The menu—like it matters amid such foppery—is Turkish, though not as fun as the setting, with lots of meats (mixed grill, "Sultan's Delight" diced lamb) and no shyness about the sauces. Many nights, opera singers serenade diners. It's not dead cheap, but it's an event. And not only tourists come—locals celebrate here too, albeit slightly sheepishly, which is also how I suggest it here.

126 Drury Lane, WC2. www.sarastro-restaurant.com. © **020/7836-0101.** Main courses £17–£25. Daily 12:30pm–midnight. Tube: Covent Garden.

Moderate

Browns ★ TRADITIONAL BRITISH In London, there's a Browns for fashion, and a Brown's Hotel, but Browns the spacious brasserie is the Browns you can afford. Installed in the former Westminster County Courts, this high-quality, Brighton-based English chain serves updated English food and imported beer. The globe lanterns, enormous mirrors, and staff buttoned into crisp white oxford shirts impart the sense of a Gilded Age chophouse. Expect lots of indulgently hearty dishes such as lobster risotto, steak and Guinness pie, fish and chips, or a nice fat burger with Irish cheddar. A sense of tradition—starchy but the kind that's welcoming to tourists—is the main product here.

82–84 St. Martins Lane, WC2. www.browns-restaurants.com. © **020/7497-5050.** Main courses £9–£15; Sunday roast £11–£15. Mon–Fri 8am–10:30pm (Fri until 11pm); Sat 10am–11pm; Sun 10am–10:30pm. Tube: Leicester Square.

Flat Iron ★★★ STEAK   For a mere £10, you get an absolutely perfect 200g steak or steakburger, a cup of salad, a serving of beef-dripping popcorn, and on the way out the door, a cone of caramel ice cream topped with shavings from a block of dark chocoloate. No wonder there's a queue at peak hours. The menu is focused—no chicken, no pork, and sorry, vegetarians—plus good cocktails and well-suited side dishes. Specializing makes the cooking expert and the juicy meat is over-the-top delicious. The beef comes from a herd of cows in Yorkshire "cared for by third-generation beef farmer Charles Ashbridge," and each week, 7 tons of it are served at Flat Iron's several locations (others include 9 Denmark St., off Tottenham Court Rd., and 17 Beak St., off Carnaby St.). This version by Covent Garden is the best for killing time before your table is ready.

17/18 Henrietta St., WC2. www.flatironsteak.co.uk. No phone. Mains £10. Daily noon–midnight (Sun until 11pm). No reservations. Tube: Covent Garden or Leicester Square.

Great Queen Street ★★★ TRADITIONAL BRITISH   Here, the people behind the seminal **Eagle** (p. 74) present the essence of gastropub cuisine in the more convenient environs of Covent Garden and with showier meats. There's a pub feel with scuffed wood floors, burgundy walls, and sconces capped with fringed mini-shades. The slow-cooked dishes are clean and reassuringly ingredient-proud. Offerings (they change) may include Old Spot (a breed of pig) pork chops with sticky shallots, Hereford beef, griddled quail with celery salt. One menu regular is lamb's shoulder cooked for 7 hours and accompanied by *gratin dauphinoise* (potatoes in crème fraîche)—that one feeds four, which hints at the social atmosphere encouraged here. The Cellar Bar (open until midnight Tues–Sat) serves the cold dishes from the same menu.

32 Green Queen St., WC2. www.greatqueenstreetrestaurant.co.uk. © **020/7242-0622.** Main courses £16–£34. Mon–Sat noon–2:30pm and 5:30–10:30pm; Sun noon–3:30pm. Tube: Covent Garden or Holborn.

Wild Food Café ★★ VEGAN   Upstairs in the Granola Triangle of Neal's Yard, beside the excellent homeopathic dispensary Neal's Yard Remedies, this popular and packed place serves plant-based fare that's truly flavorful at prices Covent Garden left behind: olive and shiitake burgers, pine-nut quinoa with horseradish tahini, and raw chocolate as a component in some very impressive desserts. At peak mealtimes, there's always a bunch-up of punters at the door. Don't be daunted; wait to get the next available communal seat whether it's at the bar or at a table. It's some of the best vegan food you'll find in the city, but even usual meat eaters depart stimulated and satisfied.

First Floor, 14 Neal's Yard, WC2. www.wildfoodcafe.com. © **020/7419-2014.** Main courses £8–£13. Summer daily 11:30am–11pm; rest of year Tues–Thurs 11:30am–9pm, Fri–Sat 11:30am–10pm, Sun11:30am–7pm. Tube: Covent Garden.

Inexpensive

Punjab Restaurant ★★★ INDIAN   Ignore that it looks like every other hack kitchen sponging off the Covent Garden tourist trade—this place predates the recent curry trend, which is why it survived the crest of the popularity wave. Punjab has been cooking since 1947, when it was opened by Gurbachan Singh Maan, a wrestler, and moved to this location in 1951 to serve the bureaucrats of the India High Commission during a tumultuous political period. Now, his fourth generation runs it with striking professionalism. It proclaims itself the oldest North Indian restaurant in the U.K., and staff have worked here, beneath the gold silk wallpaper, for decades. Cooking is light on the oil and *ghee* (clarified butter). Meats and tandoori (the oven was installed in 1962) are well marinated, and so they arrive tender. The menu is cheeky, too: "If you have any erotic activities planned for after you leave us, perhaps you should resist this sensational garlic *naan*." On a recent visit, two diners at a neighboring table ribbed each other about who had been coming here longer; the winner got hooked in 1987—40 years into the story. Reserve ahead on weekends.

80 Neal St., WC2. www.punjab.co.uk. © **020/7836-9787.** Main courses £8–£13, sometimes a £15 per person minimum. Mon–Sun noon–11pm (Sun 10pm). Tube: Covent Garden.

MAYFAIR & MARYLEBONE

It's hard to find a dining establishment in these high-toned hoods that isn't overpriced, swooning with self-importance, and wooing a clientele that's better-connected than you are. The "in" spots seem to change with the tides, but you may rely on—and be welcomed by—these stalwarts.

Expensive

Le Gavroche ★★★ FRENCH   There are always newcomers in Mayfair hoping to capture the vanity crowd, and trendy styles with fresh young chefs rise and burn out, but Le Gavroche remains the top choice for classical French cuisine. Its leader, Michel Roux, Jr., is the son of the chef who founded the restaurant in 1967. The famous cheese soufflé is still there after all these years. Also on the menu: lobster with lemongrass and coconut-infused *jus,* roast suckling pig, and roast Goosnargh duck, plus desserts including apricot and Cointreau soufflé. The cheese board is exemplary. It's all beautifully presented and served with style. The wine list is a masterclass in top French wines, and is kind to the purse as well on lesser-known varieties. It all takes place in a comfortable, conventional basement dining room that may be too old-fashioned for some, but is endearingly classic to those who have cherished this place for a half century.

43 Upper Brook St., W1. www.le-gavroche.co.uk. © **020/7408-0881.** Main courses £35–£60, set lunch £66; tasting menu £150 (without wine). Weds–Fri noon–2pm and 6pm–10pm; Tues and Sat 6pm–10pm. Reservations required. Tube: Marble Arch.

The Wolseley ★★★ CONTEMPORARY EUROPEAN   "No Flash or Intrusive Photography please," chastises diners in a footnote on the menu. That's because this opulent bistro in the Grand European style, posing with every polished surface to appear like something Renoir would want to paint, is home base for celebrities and power lunchers. Built as a luxury car dealership for a doomed manufacturer, then used as a bank, a decade ago it became a caviar-scooping, oyster-shucking, tea-pouring hotspot, convincing nearly everyone who sips its pea-and-lettuce soup that it's always been this way. Waiters are unattainably attractive and look down their noses as they gingerly place salad Niçoise and Swiss souffle, enacting the calculated Continental crispness we crave.

160 Piccadilly, W1. www.thewolseley.com. ℗ **020/7499-6996.** Main courses £15–£20; sandwiches £11. Mon–Fri 7am–midnight; Sat–Sun 8am–midnight (Sun until 11pm). Tube: Green Park.

Moderate

The Grazing Goat ★ BRITISH   A block north of Oxford Street, this farmhouse-style gastropub (light wood, bare tables, a bar presiding over the conversations, strong but casual service) attracts a varied crowd for wine or a locally brewed pint, quality house-cured meats, and classic British proteins such as rotisserie beef, venison, chicken, fish and chips, and the title character served with a raisin mustard jus. The all-day Sunday Roast (beef, pork, or lamb) with all the trimmings is swishier than what a pub serves, but a tonic for feet run weary by shopping at nearby Selfridges. Hidden gem alert: It also has eight country-house-inspired B&B rooms, each with a king bed and free Wi-Fi (from £210).

6 New Quebec St., W1. www.thegrazing goat.co.uk. ℗ **020/7724-7243.** Main courses £14–£22. Daily noon–10pm (Sun until 9:30pm), kitchen closes 1 hr prior. Tube: Marble Arch.

The Hard Rock Cafe ★ AMERICAN   You'll find one in every city from Key West to Kuwait. Its burgers (though excellent) nudge £20, it's cramped, and much of the so-called memorabilia consists of instruments played once and tossed aside. Waiting up to 90 minutes for a table chews up time that could be used for real sightseeing. But this Hard Rock was the world's first, opened in 1971, so there is a grudging authenticity. And you don't have to eat here to take a free tour of its cellar museum, The Vault, packed with historic guitars.

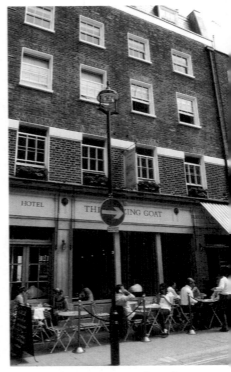

The Grazing Goat attracts a varied crowd.

150 Old Park Lane, W1. www.hardrock.com. ☎ **020/7514-1700.** Main courses £12–£17. Mon–Sun 9:30am–11:30pm (Sun until 11pm). Reservations recommended. Tube: Hyde Park Corner.

Rasa W1 ★ INDIAN   Oxford Street is for corporate stores and predictable chain food—you can do better. This kicky Indian alternative, which shines a light on the fun flavors of southwest India, lies off a quiet side street just southeast of the Bond Street station. It may be casual like a standard Indian joint (pinkish walls, tablecloths too nice for its price point), but even everyday items are pumped up—what's just "coconut rice" on the menu is in fact blended with cashews, a leading crop of Kerala. The crab *thoran,* crab meat stir-fried with coconut, mustard seeds, and ginger, is touted as an owner's grandmother's recipe. And imagine this: mangoes and green bananas cooked in yogurt with green chilis, ginger, and fresh curry leaves. That's the sweet-and-sour *moru kachiathu,* and it's a menu highlight.

6 Dering St., W1. www.rasarestaurants.com. ☎ **020/7629-1346.** Main courses £11–£16. Mon–Sat noon–3pm and 6–11pm, Sun 1pm–3pm and 6pm–9pm. Tube: Bond St. or Oxford Circus.

KENSINGTON & WESTMINSTER

South Kensington near the museums is a particular quandary; the museums offer insultingly overpriced food services while most nearby establishments would not be the culinary highlight of any city. If you must eat in South Ken, scout around the cafés at Exhibition Road near the Tube stop; look into **Orsini** (8A Thurloe Place; www.orsinicaffe.co.uk; ☎ **020/7581-5553**), serving competent Italian; or **Franco Manca** (91 Old Brompton Rd.; www.francomanca. co.uk; ☎ **020/7584-9713**), a local chain that does pizza on sourdough crust. Otherwise, the pickings are ripe with the usual chains.

Expensive

Rex Whistler ★★ BRITISH   Should one find oneself in a parlor conversation about dining history, one could validly submit that the Rex Whistler, opened in 1927 within the Tate Britain, began the trend of fine dining inside great museum institutions. Back then it was a bit of a lark, encircled by Whistler's whimsical mural *The Expedition in Pursuit of Rare Meats,* in which a food-finding expedition travels on bicycle through lands populated by unicorns and truffle dogs, but in years since, the restaurant has garnered serious appreciation for its rich wine list—the sommelier will even consult with you before you arrive. Today's menu champions British cooking using fresh seasonal produce, from Scottish salmon to Yorkshire mutton to succulent guinea fowl.

Tate Britain, Millbank, SW1. www.tate.org.uk. ☎ **020/7887-8825.** 2-course meals from £30, 3-course meals from £36. Daily 11:30am–5pm; frequent evening openings to coincide with popular exhibitions. Reservations essential. Tube: Pimlico.

STEEPED IN TRADITION: afternoon tea

Afternoon tea is an overpriced tourist's pursuit, to be sure, but that doesn't mean it's not delightful to pass the time by pretending to be fancy. Arrive hungry and you'll be served a never-ending banquet of scones, clotted cream, pastry, light sandwiches, and a bottomless brewed torrent. Dress up, if you please, and be discreet about photos. Hundreds of places throw teas, but these are among the most transporting, legendary, or best-located. Most places will add champagne for £5 to £20 more.

Brown's Hotel This Mayfair institution, open since 1837, offers exacting execution and a handsome paneled room but is not overly snooty. It veers trendy: "Tea-Tox" is its lower-fat, lower-carb version. www.roccofortehotels.com. ℓ 020/7518-4155. Noon–6:30pm; £55. Tube: Green Park. Also see p. 52.

Fortnum & Mason The venerable department store on Piccadilly has sold tea for 3 centuries, so naturally in its Diamond Jubilee Tea Salon, nibbling off duck-egg-blue china and serenaded by grand piano, you choose from 150 tea types, many of which are supplied to the other hotels on this list. The crowd can be touristy. www.fortnumandmason.com.

ℓ 020/7734-8040. £44. Tube: Green Park. Also see p. 203.

The Goring Near Buckingham Palace, it serves on its own bespoke canary-yellow china in your choice of the blood-red lounge, the airy conservatory, or the garden. Book at least 3 months ahead, but sit as long as you want once you're there. ℓ 020/7396-9000. 3–4pm; from £49. Tube: Victoria. Also see p. 47.

Great Court Restaurant, The British Museum Enjoy more sensibly priced scones under the courtyard's central glass canopy. It's a gorgeous but casual setting you're sure to visit anyway. www.britishmuseum.org. ℓ 020/7323-8990. 3–5:30pm; £20. Tube: Russell Square. Also see p. 113.

Houses of Parliament Take tea overlooking the Thames in the modern Terrace Pavilion rooms behind the House of Commons. www.parliament.uk/visiting. ℓ 020/7219-4114. Generally 2pm and 3:45pm; £29 plus price of tour. Tube: Westminster. Also see p. 130.

The Lanesborough Dazzling in every way, from the delicacy of the pastry to the airy Regency frills of the

Inexpensive

Muriel's Kitchen ★★ AMERICAN/INTERNATIONAL The window is a fantasia of icing-blobbed, fruit-topped, sugar-dusted pastry temptation, but the real reason to step inside this rustic-style, casual restaurant is locally grown, organic comfort foods such as beef lasagna, five-spice marinated pulled pork, chili con carne, and creamy chicken and apricot curry. The high, wooden tables feel like something from an American farmhouse even as they look out on the neighborhood's French residents and the families on their way to the big Kensington museums around the corner. Being one of the few non-corporate choices in South Ken has brought success; other locations are at 36–38 Old Compton Street in Soho and on the north side of Leicester Square. 1–3 Pelham St., SW7. www.murielskitchen.co.uk. ℓ 020/7589-3511. Main courses £10–£16. Mon–Sat 8am–11pm; Sun 9am–10pm. Tube: South Kensington.

conservatory glass overhead, for cozy class this Knightsbridge hotel institution defeats The Ritz by a strong scone's throw, I'd say. lanesborough.com. *©* **020/7259-5599.** Weekdays 2:30pm–4:30pm, weekends 3pm–4:30pm; £48. Tube: Hyde Park Corner. Also see p. 53.

The Langham The first London hotel to initiate the custom (in 1865) is still top quality, but it's also one of the most commercial, having branded itself with a Wedgewood partnership. This Oxford Circus tradition is particularly popular with Asian tourists. palm-court.co.uk. *©* **020/7636-1000.** 5 seatings 12:15pm–5:30pm; £49. Tube: Oxford Circus. Also see p. 54.

The Milestone The antiqued, library-like Park Lounge overlooking Kensington Gardens is your stop if you're near Kensington Palace. It doles out 11,000 doggy boxes a year for guests who can't finish—a courtesy that's uncommon at teas. www.milestonehotel.com. *©* **020/7917-1000.** 3 seatings 1–5pm; from £40. Tube: High St. Kensington. Also see p. 48.

The Ritz The only way most of us can afford the formal gilding, mirrors, and boisterous floral arrangements of the Ritz, at 150 Piccadilly, is to submit to the machinelike attentions of the servile waiters in its Palm Court (1906), who process 400 people daily during hours the gentry would find unseemly for tea. It's fancy but not cuddly. No jeans or sneakers, with jacket and tie required for men. Book 6 to 8 weeks ahead. www.theritzlondon.com. *©* **020/7300-2345.** 5 seatings 11:30am–7:30pm; £54 adults, £30 children. Tube: Green Park.

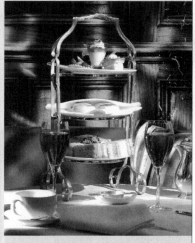

Tea at Brown's Hotel is a Mayfair institution.

Regency Café ★★★ TRADITIONAL BRITISH The midcentury "caff" diner, once a staple of London life, is rapidly being swept into Formica heaven by trendy bistros. Among the few holdouts still doling out classic English breakfasts all day is the 1940s Regency, a discount-Deco elegy to another age in yellowed white tiles and bolted-down plastic chairs. This isn't a gastronomic treasure (the fryer is in heavy use, white bread heaped high, sausage a food group); it's an anthropological one. Big-value food including £3.50 burgers or homemade meat pie is prepared with lightning speed, and your order is jarringly bellowed so that you can come fetch it. For another marvelous "caff," see E. Pellicci (p. 100).

17–19 Regency St., SW1. www.regencycafe.co.uk. *©* **020/7821-6596.** Main courses £3–£8. Mon–Fri 7am–2:30pm and 4–7:30pm; Sat 7am–noon. Tube: Pimlico or Westminster.

THE SOUTH BANK & THAMES

For a casual street food meal, head behind the South Bank Centre for the South Bank Market, a collection of changing food stalls cooking up curries, duck confit burgers, sausages, and other cheap and ready-to-eats. It runs Friday through Sunday, starting around noon and wrapping up by about 8pm.

Expensive

Oxo Tower Restaurant, Brasserie & Bar ★ INTERNATIONAL   The Oxo commands a gratitude-inducing panorama of St Paul's and the City from Southbank, which despite the overpriced aspirations of the menu is really why you come here. The Brasserie, which has live music in the evening, does only moderately ostentatious food such as seared tuna and spring chicken for about £4 less per main course than the main, special-occasion Restaurant. You may soon forget the food (it's delicious, but so is the food at many places), but you won't forget the view. Put your glad rags on and make a night of it.

22 Barge House St., SE1. www.harveynichols.com/restaurants. ℗ **020/7803-3888.** Main courses £20–£38; 3-course lunch £37. Mon–Fri noon–3pm and 6–11pm; Sat noon–3pm and 5:30–11pm; Sun noon–3:30pm and 6:30–10pm. Reservations recommended. Tube: Blackfriars or Waterloo.

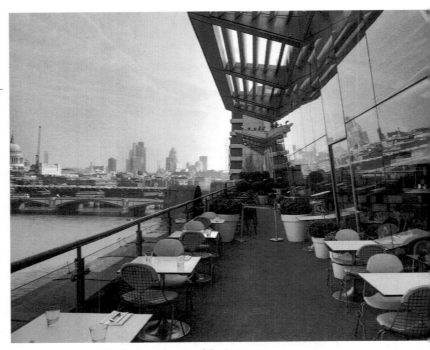

Oxo Tower Brasserie offers a spectacular view of the City.

THE world COMES TO LONDON

Those fortunate enough to have traveled broadly know how sadly rare it is to find places where people of wildly different colors, religions, and nationalities can live together in relative harmony. London, though, like New York City, Toronto, or Sydney, is certifiably multi-ethnic, with some 300 languages and 45 distinct ethnic communities. (By 2030, it's predicted, half the city's population will be foreign-born.) It's a fine opportunity for some culinary world travels of your own. Here are the Tube or rail stops for some of the major concentrations:

Bangladesh: Bethnal Green, Whitechapel

Caribbean: Brixton, Willesden Junction

Egypt: Shepherd's Bush

Ghana, Nigeria, Congo, West Africa: Seven Sisters, Hackney Central, or Hackney Downs (National Rail)

India, especially northern: Southall (National Rail)

Ireland: Kilburn

Kenya: Barking

Kurdistan: Manor House

Lebanon: Shepherd's Bush

Nigeria: Peckham Rye (National Rail)

Persia: Edgware Road

Poland: Hammersmith, Ealing Broadway

Somalia: Streatham (National Rail)

Sri Lanka and South India: Tooting (National Rail)

Syria: Shepherd's Bush

Turkey: Dalston Kingsland and Stoke Newington (National Rail)

Vietnam: Hackney Central or Hackney Downs (National Rail), Old Street

Restaurant Story ★★★ MODERN BRITISH The moment you sit, your server lights a white taper and you slide your menu from the leaves of *Sketches by Boz* by Charles Dickens, who lived nearby in his penniless youth. By the time a fusillade of about six *amuse-bouche* "snacks" hits you (paper-thin cod skin studded with emulsified cod roe, a sweet black eel mousse "Storeo"), your candle has melted, you're told that the wax was actually beef fat, and you're handed a leather pouch of fresh-baked bread to sop up the rich drippings. The tale may differ when you come, but there will be 10 more frivolously surprising, small-plate courses to go in this 3- to 4-hour Michelin-starred odyssey. The dramatic and whimsical delights are by hot young talent Tom Sellers, and his prix-fixe menu, which never stops amusing and dazzling with flavor duets, speaks of London cooking both old and new: scallop carpaccio with cucumber balls rolled in dill ash; Jensen's gin (Sellers loves gin) and apple consommé topped with garlic blossoms; and "Three Bears" porridge—one sweet, one salty, one just right.

201 Tooley St., SE1. www.restaurantstory.co.uk. © **020/7183-2117.** 5-course lunch £45 (Tues–Thurs), lunch menu £80, 10 courses £120. Tues–Sat noon–2pm and Mon–Sat 6:30–9:30pm. Reservations essential. Tube: London Bridge or Bermondsey.

Moderate

Boro Bistro ★★ FRENCH/ALGERIAN Tucked downstairs in the brick vaults under a building on the west side of Borough High Street, just east of

Southwark Cathedral, this French-with-a-pubby-twist bistro tends to be a fast favorite with first-time visitors. Lit by candles that have accumulated wax over countless nights—the Romanesque ambience makes even old friends feel like they're on a date—you dine at funky beaten wood tables on craft beers, shared platters (truffle sausage, baked Camembert), burgers (grilled Montbeliard sausage with shallot marmalade), and French tapas (buttered baby artichoke with black pepper mayo). In nice weather, the terrace is ideal for a drink (in cold weather, there are heaters and fleece blankets) or to get off your feet after a day walking the Thames or at Borough Market, both just steps away.

Inexpensive

M. Manze ★★ TRADITIONAL BRITISH If you're truly fearless, brave the classic East End dishes of jellied or stewed eels. But if not, there's still a reason to come here: a jewel box of a shop, serving since 1891, with green glazed Victorian tile and wooden benches, which is in such rare condition it's protected by the government. In fact, when it was awarded its historic plaque, no one could figure out how to mount it to the wall without breaking preservation laws. Manze also does meat or vegetarian pastry pies—which to be fair, most customers prefer—as it has done since the days when it fed dockworkers and laborers. The parsley-made "liquor" sauce doesn't really taste like much, but the gravy and mash taste like nostalgia itself.

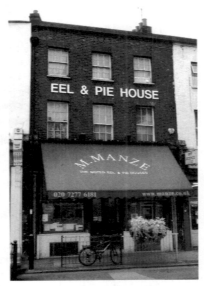

M. Manze offers Cockney classics like meat pies and jellied eels.

87 Tower Bridge Rd., SE1. manze.co.uk. (© **020/7407-2985.** Main courses £3–£6. Mon 11am–2pm; Tues–Thurs 10:30am–2pm; Fri–Sat 10am–2:30pm (Sat until 2:45pm).

EAST END & DOCKLANDS

Much of the city's most exciting cooking for a fun night out has migrated to Shoreditch and Spitalfields, leaving Mayfair to cater to the expense-account gourmets and Soho to feed the beery hordes.

Expensive

Lyle's ★★ BRITISH The kind of place where chefs like to eat, where the dishes appear simple and fluid and yet require authority to accomplish, Lyle's

BOROUGH market

A chronicle of overstimulation, this popular market combines Victorian commercial hubbub with glorious, farm-fresh flavors, rendered as finger food for visitors. About a dozen greenmarket vendors sell their country meats, cheeses, and vegetables beneath its metal-and-glass canopy all week long, but the market really blooms Thursday through Saturday, when more than 100 additional vendors unpack and the awe-inspiring scene hits its swing. The least crowded time is Thursday between 11am and noon; Saturdays are plain nuts. It's best to pay with cash—most dishes are around £6–7—and you'll eat standing up.

If there's any country that has farming down, it's England, and this market is its showplace. Follow the crowd across Bedale Street, past the artisan cacao at **Rabot 1745,** to the **Green Market,** along the fence by the cathedral. **Roast Hog** (www.roasthog.com) slices pig off a turning spit; **Greedy Goat** scoops lactose-free goat milk ice cream.

Under the Victorian glass canopy of Three Crown Square, **Le Marché du Quartier** (www.marketquarter.com) does duck confit sandwiches. Sample never-exported cheeses like melt-in-your-mouth **Bath soft cheese** (www.parkfarm.co.uk) or aromatic unpasteurized **Gorwydd Caerphilly** (www.trethowansdairy.co.uk). **Shellseekers,** the fishmonger in the center, is known for hand-dived Devon scallop, served in its own shell and topped with a bacon and sprout stir-fry; a bathub-big pot of paella bubbles at its neighbor **Bomba.** Buy a flute of Prosecco from one of the vendors selling it and feel your palate lighten.

Roast (www.roast-restaurant.com), which runs an expensive restaurant upstairs, has a stall for rich meats such as roast pork belly with crackling, or Bramley applesauce and beef with horseradish cream. **Padella** does succulent and savory pasta small plates. At **Maria's Market Café,** the second-generation proprietor slaves over a stove making fresh bubble (a mushy version of home fries) for vendors and visitors alike.

The **Brindisa** booth (www.brindisa.com), facing Stoney Street, feeds a steady line of punters its grilled chorizo sandwich with oil-drizzled pequillo peppers from Spain. Outside on Stoney and Park streets, by the well-stocked **Market Porter** pub (p. 104) and casual sit-down restaurant **Elliot's,** are more finds: **Kappacasein** dairy from Bermondsey (www.kappacasein.com), which melts great wheels of Ogleshield cheese into decadent *raclette* or goopy grilled cheese; **Monmouth Coffee Company** (www.monmouthcoffee.com), one of London's most revered roasters of single-farm beans; **Gelateria 3bis,** with its ultra-creamy *fior di latte* gelato and a warm chocolate fountain for pre-filling cones; and **Neal's Yard Dairy** (www.nealsyarddairy.co.uk), the gold standard for English cheese, tended by clerks in caps and aprons.

It's all food you can only enjoy in London. You may locate all of none of these delicacies among the clamor; this overstimulation of the senses is an individual game.

8 Southwark St., SE1. www.boroughmarket.org.uk. (©) **020/7407-1002.** Mon–Wed 10am–3pm; Thurs 11am–5pm; Fri noon–6pm; Sat 8am–5pm. Tube: London Bridge.

has a short, changing New British-meets-Nordic menu, but it runs deep with inventiveness and delicacy: lemon sole with buttermilk and sea aster (a salt marsh plant), raw beef with mussels that's actually chopped beef with shellfish emulsion, soured cream with chocolate as a dessert. Dishes are neatly

THE HEIGHTS OF cuisine

London's skyscrapers are shooting up like bamboo, and with them, dining aeries to be remembered. The city's taste buds are too sophisticated to tolerate a top-floor restaurant with bottom-feeder grub—these places compete with terrific cuisine that's a pleasure to eat. Only the prices could be considered unpleasant. Reservations are suggested for all of them.

Duck & Waffle *The scene:* All day and night—yes, it's 24 hours, and doubles as a skilled *cocktailerie*—it cycles through shared-plate menus that lean toward richness, including foie gras crème brûlée, braised cuttlefish, barbecue crispy pig ears, and the namesake dish with mustard maple syrup. *The view:* It's a little inland from the Thames, so the nearest views are of the Gherkin and the City. 40th Floor, 110 Bishopsgate, EC2. www.duckandwaffle.com. ✆ **020/3640-7310.** Sharing plates £9–13. Tube: Liverpool St.

Darwin Brasserie *The scene:* The multistory atrium atop the "Walkie-Talkie" is like an upscale mini-mall of evening pursuits, including thump-thump-thump beats at Sky Pod bar and a seafood place, Fenchurch Seafood Bar & Grill. Our choice, Darwin, has an honest menu (Cornish lamb, Scottish rib-eye, fish and chips) on an elevated floor where some of the horizon may be obscured by the tower's drooping-eyelid roofline, but it's still spectacular. (Soak in the panorama from elsewhere in the atrium after dinner.) The airport-style security queue downstairs can be a drag but it thins out after sunset. *The view:* the Tower of London, the Thames, the Shard, and beyond. Sky Garden, 36th Floor, 20 Fenchurch St., EC3. skygarden.london/Darwin. ✆ **0333/772-0020.** Dinner main courses £17–£26. Breakfast Mon–Fri 7–10:30am, Sat 8–10am. Lunch Mon–Fri 11:30am–4pm, Sat–Sun 11:30am–3:30pm. Dinner Mon–Sat 5:30–10:30pm, Sun 5:30–10pm. Tube: Monument or Bank.

Ting *The scene:* Much more romantic than Duck or Darwin, the principal dining room of the Shangri-La hotel (p. 58) does exquisite but unadventurous classics like monkfish, slow-roasted piglet belly, Cotswold free-range chicken, and steak. Pair it with cocktails on the 52nd floor at **Gong,** the hotel's tight little bar. *The view:* sweeping eastern panorama from Southwark, including London Bridge Station, the Tower of London, and Tower Bridge. 35th floor, The Shard, 32 London Bridge St., SE1. www.gong-shangri-la.com. ✆ **020/7234-8108.** Dinner main courses £23–38. Daily 6:30–10:30am, noon–2:30pm, and 6–11:30pm. Tube: London Bridge.

creative, but flavors remain clean, even if the blank loft space in which they're served is a bit factory-like. If things are busy, you can always sit at the bar. Tea Building, 56 Shoreditch High St., E1. lyleslondon.com. ✆ **020/3011-5911.** Main courses £13–£29; 3-course set dinner £39; small plates £4–£8. Mon–Fri 8am–11pm; Sat noon–11pm. Reservations recommended. Tube: Shoreditch High St. or Liverpool St.

Moderate

Jones Family Project ★★ BRITISH   If you love beef, the way JFP's Josper grill can almost mystically seal in the flavors of its Yorkshire Longhorn could blow your mind, but then again, the burger topped with oxtail-stock mayo might also do it. It's not just about beef, though; fish, duck, and pork (that's cut like beef) are also knowingly prepared in generous portions—most proteins come from The Ginger Pig, a network of principled farmers. Sides such as truffled mac and cheese and tomato salad underscore the traditional cuisine goals, but the friendly, groovily '70s downstairs dining space makes a convivial hideaway, good for conversation and stretching out when you're in Shoreditch. It's an especially good stop on Sunday afternoons for its weekly roast, and the upstairs bar is open until midnight Monday to Saturday.

78 Great Eastern St., EC2. www.jonesfamilyproject.co.uk. © **020/7739-1740.** Main courses £14–£27. Mon–Sat noon–midnight; Sun noon–6pm. Tube: Old St.

Poppies ★★ SEAFOOD   Big crispy portions flopping on big oval plates eaten with a big knife and fork to big 1950s sock-hop music: The franchise-ready Poppies does for British fish and chips what peppy jukebox diners have done for midcentury American food. Amusingly, it wraps its chips in custom-printed newspaper since it's now illegal to use the chemical-laden real thing. For all its plastic theatricality, it hews to authenticity: The chief dish, cooked to order, is sustainably caught and sourced from third-generation fishmonger T. Bush at Billingsgate Market, and even the uniforms worn by the "Poppettes" waitresses—a red sailor frock with a jaunty, bellhoppy cap—come from Collectif in Camden's Stables Market. For those whose palates swerve differently, there's also chicken, the chance to try jellied eels, and Minghella ice cream hailing from the Isle of Wight. There's a West End location in Soho (55 Old Compton St., W1; © **020/7734-4845;** same hours).

6–8 Hanbury St., E1. www.poppiesfishandchips.co.uk. © **020/7247-0892.** Main courses £10–£12. Mon–Thurs 11am–11pm; Fri–Sun 11am–11:30pm (Sun until 10:30pm). Tube: Shoreditch High St. or Liverpool St.

Rochelle Canteen ★★ BRITISH   A sublime secret is hidden away, discovered only if you ring a doorbell beside a green door in a brick wall. You'll pass through the grassy yard of an 1880s school, and in the old bike shed, join

---

Brick Lane: 24-Hour Playground

Brick Lane, named for its medieval status as a source for bricks, was once a Jewish area but has become so strongly identified with immigrants from the Indian subcontinent that its name has transcended geography to become a shorthand term for England's South Asian population. In the span of just a few blocks, most of which have signage in both English and Bengali, lines of Indian restaurants jockey for business. No discerning Londoner would claim that any serve the city's best Indian cuisine, and most of them are in fact run by Bangladeshi or Pakistani entrepreneurs catering to a milder English notion of northern curries. (If you want something more modernized, try **Gunpowder** [gunpowderlondon.com], 1 block east on Commercial Rd. at Fashion St.). But it's nonetheless a fun place to stroll, leverage competition, and sit down for a bargain meal in a happening hood. (Bring your own wine, though, since most are run by Muslims who don't sell alcohol.) By day, the connecting Dray Walk is a short block of sophisticated boutiques and laid-back cafes. On weekends, it hosts blocks upon blocks of markets for vintage clothes, books, food, and art—Sundays are good for hours of browsing and noshing (www.bricklanemarket.com).

a daytime garden party. The changing menu is rigorously British, high-quality and fresh, yet without flourish: green pea soup, roast sirloin, cuttlefish ink stew, leek and wigmore tart, fish and chips, loose-leaf tea. Your companions will be high-functioning artists, designers, and professionals, many of whom now lease space in the former school, plus the occasional kid, if they behave as well as a Victorian child. In fine weather, it's easier to find a seat because dining spills outdoors, the better to enjoy jugs of rhubarb and ginger fizz.

Rochelle School, Arnold Circus, E2. www.rochelleschool.org. © **020/7729-5677.** Main courses £13–£15. Mon–Fri 9am–2:30pm (spring–summer to 3:30pm), Thurs–Sat 6pm to 10pm; closing changes seasonally. Reservations suggested. Tube: Shoreditch High St.

St John Bread & Wine ★★ TRADITIONAL BRITISH   Hand-in-hand with the gastropub trend is "nose-to-tail" eating. That's a polite way to say your chef doesn't waste a single morsel of the animal, resulting in tastes that were commonplace to his agrarian English forefathers (heart, cockscomb, marrow, whole pigeon) but are new to most North American tongues. Most places charge, um, an arm and leg for it, but you can sample it at this lower-priced offshoot of the influential St. John restaurant (still running in Smith-field), which in the 1990s brought back British cooking in a big way. Walls are simple white, chairs are plain wood, and the kitchen staff is serious about food, no matter its form. Experience dishes like cold lamb with chicory and anchovy, smoked sprat (sardines) with horseradish, and laver bread (made with seaweed) with oats and bacon. A meal here can be an adventure (ever eaten dandelion?).

94–96 Commercial St., E1. www.stjohngroup.uk.com. © **020/7251-0848.** Main courses £7–£10 before 6pm, around £15 after 6pm. Mon–Fri 8am–4pm and 6–11pm, Sat 8:30am–11pm, Sun 8:30am–9pm. Reservations recommended. Tube: Aldgate East or Shoreditch High St.

Inexpensive

Beigel Bake ★★ BAKERY   The city's most famous bakery, Jewish or otherwise, never closes but there's often a line. The queue moves quickly here even if time doesn't—signs still post an area code that hasn't been active since 2000. The patronage is a microcosm of London, ranging from bikers to hipsters to arrogant yuppies to the homeless. Its beigels (*bi*-gulls) are not as puffy or as salty as the New York "bagel" variety, and they even come filled for under £2—the same price, astonishingly, as a half-dozen plain ones. Its pastries are gorgeous, too: The chocolate fudge brownie, less than £1, could be nursed for hours. Watching the clerks slice juicy chunks of pink salt beef in the window, then slather it onto a beigel with nostril-clearing mustard from a crusty jar, is an attraction unto itself. Londoners complain it's gotten touristy, but what tourist trap serves tea for just 60p, I ask you?

159 Brick Lane, E1. © **020/7729-0616.** Daily 24 hr. Tube: Shoreditch High St.

E. Pellicci ★★★ TRADITIONAL BRITISH   London's tradition of mid-century diners, or "caffs," is quickly being gentrified into nostalgia, but this fry-up on deeply authentic and unflashy Bethnal Green Road has been run by the affable Nevio family since 1900. Some of them were born upstairs, and the matriarch of the family has commanded the kitchen since 1961. The Deco interior, a greasy spoon fantasia of sunburst icons, chrome, and primrose, was carved by a regular in 1946 and is now protected by law. You'll be boisterously welcomed with open arms—Mama, cooking Italian specialties such as cannelloni, may wave to you from the kitchen—and you'll spend a happy meal sharing a table with locals ("Where are you from?" "Looks like rain tomorrow"), sipping the best cuppa 70p tea you ever had. As proof of your acceptance by the regulars, after you're done you may be sent out with a parting gift of homemade cake. There's no more iconic "caff" in town, certainly none happier.

332 Bethnal Green Rd., E2. epellicci.com. ✆ **020/7739-4873.** Main courses £2–£8. Mon–Sat 7am–4pm. Tube: Shoreditch High St. or Bethnal Green.

20 PUBS YOU'LL LOVE

Pubs are the beating heart of British life, as they have been for centuries. Your neighborhood hangout is called your "local," but many of the oldest premises have been so well-loved (or so well-bombed) that their original features are gone. Most are now company-owned, depressingly standardized, and modern-looking—how many British pubs have stripped out ceilings and carpeting to expose ductwork and wood in a feeble attempt to look modern? The following pubs, however, all centrally located, should do you right. All of them serve food of some kind (burgers, meat pies, and the like) for at least part of the day; you usually order at the bar, where you receive a numbered tag for your table so that servers can find you.

Pubs commonly charge around £5 for a pint of the favored serving size—about 20 American ounces—and the ABV percentage tends to be strong. A good cask ale is a specialty you must try while you're in England. Cask ale is not refrigerated because it's stored in the cellar, where the temperature is right for the fermentation process to continue until the drink hits your glass. Cask ale is drawn using stiff hand-pumped taps, and it only stays fresh for a short time, like bread or pastry—so don't be surprised if the beer you select has already run out. To find pubs that persevere in the dying art of pouring old-fashioned cask ales, visit the **Campaign for Real Ale** (www.camra.org.uk). Mixed drinks are also served, but mixers are charged extra and don't expect a generous pour because measures are standardized. They'll have bottled beer and cider, too. When the bell is rung, it's last call—as early as 11pm—and the landlord *will* turf you out.

The Anchor Bankside ★★   This Thameside patio in sight of St Paul's dome is perhaps the most agreeable (and popular) spot in London at which to sit with a fresh-pulled pint. There's been a tavern here at least since the 1500s, when Londoners ferried to Southwark for bear baiting, gardens, brothels, and Shakespeare (the playwright surely would have known the place). Diarist and royal confidant Samuel Pepys is said to have watched London burn to the ground from the safety of this shore in 1666. The industrial Anchor brewery that subsumed it for 200 years was cleared away in the 1980s, and a spacious (but always crowded) riverside terrace was added. Beer snobs kvetch that it's become a tourist draw, but that's all right with me; pubs have always been hangouts for the common man. Few pubs so perfectly meld abundant history with an enviable location.

34 Park St., SE1. www.taylor-walker.co.uk. © **020/7407-1577.** Mon–Weds 11am–11pm, Thurs–Sat 11am–midnight, Sun noon–11pm. Tube: London Bridge.

The Argyll Arms ★★   Having a beer in here can feel like drinking in a bejeweled red velvet box, thanks to the acid-etched glass screens that subdivide the busy bar into dignified drinking areas. Originally installed in 1895 to prevent brawls between the working and middle classes (at a time when even subway rides were segregated), the screens somehow survived the 20th century. Drinks are £1 more than they should be, but it's one of the prettiest pubs in London, and its location southeast of Oxford Circus makes it an easy stop.

18 Argyll St., W1. www.nicholsonspubs.co.uk. © **020/7734-6117.** Mon–Thurs 10am–11:30pm, Fri–Sat 10am–midnight, Sun 10am–11pm. Tube: Oxford Circus.

The Black Friar ★★★   Deservedly protected by landmark status, this 1904 Art Nouveau masterpiece (also spelled the Blackfriar) is as jolly as the fat friars that bedeck it in bronze, wood, and glass. A short walk from St Paul's, it was once snuggled down a few dark alleys, but neighboring demolitions liberated it; now it's blessed with a noisy outdoor patio and walls of windows bathed in afternoon sunshine from over the Thames. The back saloon was designed for the upper classes, hence its exceptionally overbaked interior in marble and bronze; the undulating front bar, where pop music plays and pub crawls frequently pass through, is extraordinarily well-stocked with a range of cask ales and cider. Pricey food is shuttled from the upstairs kitchen via a hand-cranked dumb waiter.

174 Queen Victoria St., EC4. www.nicholsonspubs.co.uk. ℗ **020/7236-5474.** Mon–Fri 10am–11pm, Sat 9am–11pm, Sun noon–10:30pm. Tube: Blackfriars.

The Coal Hole ★ A onetime haunt of actor Edmund Kean, who drank himself to an early curtain, was rebuilt in 1904 in the Arts and Crafts style and is still a hangout for performers at the adjoining Savoy Theatre. Use the entrance in back, by the stage door, to access the clubbier lower level. The antique street lamp on the Strand is a vestige of an experimental gaslight piping system that burned off sewage gases before the farty stink could overcome citizens. Bottoms up!

91 Strand, WC2. www.nicholsonspubs.co.uk/thecoalholestrandlondon. ℗ **020/7379-9883.** Sun–Weds 10am–11pm, Thurs 10am–11:30pm, Fri–Sat 10am–midnight. Tube: Charing Cross or Embankment.

The George Inn ★★★ Unquestionably one of the most important ancient pubs still standing, the George traces its lineage to at least 1542, when a map of Southwark first depicted it; the Tabard Inn, where Chaucer's pilgrims gathered in *Canterbury Tales,* was then a few doors south (it's gone now). Shakespeare knew it (check out Pete Brown's 2012 book *Shakespeare's Local*), and Dickens memorialized it in *Little Dorrit.* The oldest section, a galleried wood-and-brick longhouse, dates to 1677, built after a horrific fire swept the district. It later functioned as an 18th-century transit hub, its courtyard encircled with a tavern, a hotel, stables, wagon repair bays, and warehouses; the rise of a railway nearly destroyed it, and only one side of the complex survives. (The National Trust now protects it.) Sip ale in the low-ceilinged timber-and-plaster chambers, or sit in the cobbled courtyard, in the Shard's shadow, and soak up the fading echoes of history.

75–77 Borough High St., SE1. www.nationaltrust.org.uk/george-inn. ℗ **020/7407-2056.** Mon–Sat 11am–11pm; Sun noon–10:30pm. Tube: London Bridge.

The Grenadier ★★★ They say this was the Duke of Wellington's local bar and the unofficial clubhouse for his regiment, hence the battlefield artifacts on display; they also say someone was beaten to death here for cheating at cards, hence the routine ghost sightings. This tiny plank-floored, currency-festooned pub/restaurant, pretty as a picture in a cobbled mews, comes off like a boozer in some upcountry village, with only 15 places at its pewter-topped island bar. Once a haunt for servants of the surrounding townhouses, clientele these days skews toward an international mix of students and businessmen. The pub is also said to be known for its Bloody Marys (I think they're overrated). To find it, head down Grosvenor Crescent from Hyde Park Corner station, hang a hard right just before Belgrave Square onto Wilton Crescent, and take your first right onto Wilton Row.

18 Wilton Row, SW1. www.taylor-walker.co.uk. ℗ **020/7235-3074.** Daily noon–11pm. Tube: Hyde Park Corner.

The Lamb ★ Quiet, not too touristy, this east Bloomsbury choice (where Ted Hughes took Sylvia Plath on their early dates) is representative of a neighborhood local that still has some prime Victoriana from the old days. Check out the rare sunburst etched-glass snob screens obscuring the bar, built so you don't have to look the help in the eye. Or put 50p in the polyphon in the corner—that's a musical metal disc that works like a music box and was the gramophone of a century ago. The carpet is a tired tartan, the walls lined with sepia photographs of long-forgotten stage actresses, and the cask beers are out-of-the-ordinary enough to intrigue.

94 Lambs Conduit St., WC1. www.thelamblondon.com. ☎ **020/7405-0713.** Mon–Wed 11am–11pm; Thurs–Sun 11am–midnight, Sun noon–10:30pm; food served until 9:30pm. Tube: Russell Square.

The Lamb and Flag ★★ Too tiny and thronged after work to supply much respite, it is nonetheless the epitome of a city pub, tucked down an atmospheric brick alley and blessed with an original fireplace. It has been known throughout its 380 years as both the Coopers Arms and the Bucket of Blood (the latter because it hosted illegal prizefights in the early 1800s), and its building is said to be Tudor in origin. No one can prove it, since it was heavily rebuilt in the 1890s. You'll find it on a lane just east of the intersection of Floral and Garrick streets, near Covent Garden. But you probably won't find a place to sit unless you start drinking after lunch, which the regular drinkers on its memorial wall surely did.

33 Rose St., WC2. www.lambandflagcoventgarden.co.uk. ☎ **020/7497-9504.** Mon–Sat 11am–11pm; Sun noon–10:30pm. Tube: Covent Garden or Leicester Square.

The Market Porter ★ Facing the gastronomic mayhem of Borough Market, this lovely old timber-beamed boozer is a fine place to drink in any time of the week. In fact, more times than most pubs, because its location earned a special license to open at 6am when vendors are working. Sundays and off-hours are pleasant for sitting by a double-sided fire drinking one of its nine traditional ales (choices change) or eating upstairs—ingredients all come from the market. It can also act: It appeared as the Third Hand Book Emporium in the third Harry Potter film.

9 Stoney St., SE1. www.markettaverns.co.uk. ☎ **020/7407-2495.** Mon–Fri 6–8:30am and 11am–11pm; Sat–Sun noon–11pm (Sun until 10:30pm). Tube: London Bridge.

The Marquis of Granby ★ Amusingly, some pubs near the Houses of Parliament are equipped with a "division bell," which rings—rather like a fire alarm—to warn socializing MPs they have only 8 minutes to scurry back to vote. Other pubs with division bells—St. Stephens Tavern on Bridge Street across from Big Ben, the Red Lion on Whitehall—are cloyingly touristy, but not The Marquis. A single-room pub with bare floorboards and high wood

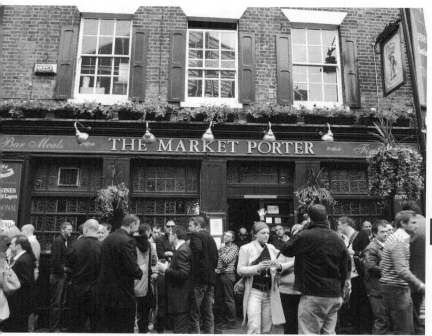

Crowds spill onto the sidewalk at beloved "locals" like The Market Porter, handy to Borough Market.

walls, it's a hangout for government types and prides itself on real hand-pumped ale.

41 Romney St., SW1. www.nicholsonspubs.co.uk. © **020/7227-0941.** Mon–Fri 11am–11pm, Sat noon–9pm. Tube: Westminster or Pimlico.

The Mayflower ★ The story goes that in 1620, local resident and sea captain Christopher Jones was recruited by some dissenters, who boarded his ship the *Mayflower* alongside this pub (then it was the Shippe; the current building is from the 1700s) to set sail to Southampton and thence to the New World. It's hard to imagine, and otherwise it's a fairly traditional pub (oak beams, wood paneling) with real ales and a fire. The tiny backyard on the Thames is a worthy place to raise a pint and survey your personal slice of the river on a summer day. Would the Pilgrims have called that a sin? Surely, but you're more fun than they were.

117 Rotherhithe St., SW16. www.themayflowerrotherhithe.com. © **020/7237-4088.** Mon–Sat 11am–11pm; Sun noon–10:30pm. Tube: Rotherhithe.

McGlynn's Free House ★ McGlynn's isn't hundreds of years old, or even important, but it fulfills the image of a "local" where neighborhood folks hang out and the landlord welcomes new faces. Its coal-blackened brick corner building, painted in old-fashioned green and red trim, is hard to find (it's southwest of Argyle Square in King's Cross), which accounts for some of its appeal. It's the sort of place with a few "pokie" gambling machines jangling in the corner, and a rugby or football game on the TV every afternoon.

1–5 Whidborne St, WC1. www.mcglynnsfreehouse.com. © **020/7916-9816.** Mon–Sat 11am–11pm; Sun noon–10:30pm. Tube: Russell Square or King's Cross St Pancras.

The Old Brewery ★★ In 2010, a new microbrewery named Meantime took up residence in Sir Christopher Wren's palatial Old Royal Naval College (a stately UNESCO World Heritage site where the Paris scenes in 2012's *Les Misérables* were shot), which sits on the Thames in outlying Greenwich. It occupied the very brewery building that once furnished Napoleonic War veterans with their three daily pints. Now, the Old Brewery, run by respected British beermaker Young's, serves drinks on a large outdoor patio, and seasonal English fare inside. The beer selection isn't as rewarding as it once was, but on a sunny day, there are few places more dreamy for a pint in Maritime Greenwich (p. 27).

The Pepys Building, Old Royal Naval College, SE10. www.oldbrewerygreenwich.com. © **020/3437-2222.** Mon–Sat 10am–11pm; Sun 10am–10:30pm. Tube: Cutty Sark DLR.

The Pride of Spitalfields ★★ Lovingly shabby, with a tired floral carpet and weary red upholstered banquettes, the backstreet boozer east of Brick Lane is the embodiment of a homey pub pulling pleasing pints. The upright piano is rarely played (recorded classic punk is preferred), the sewage system is finicky, the beer bottles are dusty, but the goings-on are lively and neighborly. Unlike in some neighborhood joints, they understand tourists, so if you're friendly, you'll have fun. In the afternoon, you can get cheap salt beef for a few pounds. Jack the Ripper suspect James Hardiman, a "cats meats vendor," drank here when it was called the Romford Arms; today, however, a cat runs the place—the entitled rescue house cat, Lenny, who has his own Twitter account (@LennyThePubCat). He's the only pretentious one here.

3 Heneage St., E1. © **020/7247-8933.** Mon–Sat 11am–11pm; Sun noon–10:30pm. Tube: Aldgate East.

The Princess Louise ★★★ This Victorian fantasia just south of the British Museum is worth a visit even if you don't drink. Its lost-in-time feeling begins with the proud signage, a traditional marquee of gold lettering on black. The 1891 interior has been miraculously maintained in mint condition: Morris & Son etched glass, mirrors, mahogany privacy screens, cast-iron bar, Corinthian columns, Simpson & Son mosaic tile floor—even the men's room marble urinals are legally protected from alteration. There's no music, no TVs, and all of the libations are by the resolutely old-fashioned Samuel Smith, which has been brewing since 1758 in Yorkshire and still draws its water from its original well.

208 High Holborn, WC1. www.princesslouisepub.co.uk. © **020/7405-8816.** Mon–Fri 11am–11pm; Sat–Sun noon–11pm (Sun 6:45pm). Tube: Holborn.

20 Pubs You'll Love

WHERE TO EAT

The Salisbury ★ The Covent Garden/Leicester Square location is unbeatable, and the ornate exterior and interior are unmistakably Victorian—ostentatious, just-how-drunk-was-the-designer Victorian, to be precise. Thrill to the Grecian urns in the brilliant-cut glass, the pressed-copper tables, and the nymphs entwined in the bronze lamps. Long a haunt of the city's theatrical community, it's now a suitable pit stop for any West End exploration. It does burgers and fish and chips, too, albeit by the corporate recipes of the Taylor Walker pub company. Theater fans should check out the cellar, which is papered with posters, many of them rare, from '80s and '90s shows.

90 St Martin's Lane, WC2. www.taylor-walker.co.uk. (C) **020/7836-5863.** Mon–Wed 11am–11pm, Thurs 11am–11:30pm; Fri 11am–1am, Sat noon–1am, Sun noon–10:30pm. Tube: Leicester Square.

The Ship & Shovell ★★ One of the most endearing configurations for any pub you'll ever see, it's cleft in two by an alley trod by commuters on their way to Charing Cross. On the north, there's a traditional Victorian-style space, and on the south, a cozier room with a languidly sloping floor and private snugs. A cellar links the halves. The bewigged tubby chap on the swinging sign is Admiral Cloudesley Shovell who, in 1707, wrecked his ship and drowned 800 sailors, which certainly gives the interior's nautical theme an ignoble context. It's special for another reason, too, being one of the few pubs in town to pour Dorset ales from Hall and Woodhouse brewers, a family brewer dating to 1777.

1–2 Craven Passage, WC2. www.shipandshovell.co.uk. (C) **020/8391-1311.** Mon–Sat 11am–11pm. Tube: Charing Cross or Embankment.

The Ten Bells ★ It's said that Annie Chapman, one of Jack the Ripper's victims, downed her last beer at this Spitalfields boozer, while another, Mary Kelly, picked up her clients outside; for an icky period in the '70s, the pub capitalized on infamy by being renamed for their slayer. These days, the toilets are a bigger threat to health and safety than Jack the Ripper ever was. The pub's Victorian tilework has been restored, and a mural was added to celebrate the new artistic vitality of the neighborhood. It's a busy local waterhole where the clientele is young and friendly, the furniture casually mismatched, and the partying ever more intense as the evening advances. Nicholas Hawksmoor's Christ Church, which towers next door, silently observes the latest mortals at play.

84 Commercial St., E1. www.tenbells.com. (C) **020/7247-7532.** Mon–Wed noon–midnight; Thurs–Sat noon–1am; Sun 1pm–midnight. Tube: Liverpool St.

Ye Olde Cheshire Cheese ★★★ Just the sort of rambling, low-ceilinged tavern you imagine London is full of (and was, once), it was built behind Fleet Street in the wake of the Great Fire in 1666; steady log fires and regularly strewn sawdust make it still smell like history hasn't finished passing it by. In later generations, it played regular host to Dr. Samuel Johnson (who lived behind on Gough Square), Charles Dickens (who refers to it in *A Tale of Two*

Cities), Yeats, Wilde, and Thackeray. You can get pretty well thackered yourself today: There are six drinking rooms, but the cozy front bar—of pallid light, candles in the fireplace, and antique paintings of dead fish—is the most magical. Observe the stuffed carcass of Polly the Parrot, enshrined above the bar since 1926: Her "adept use of profanity would have put any golfer to shame," according to her obituary in the *New York American*. **Note:** Don't confuse this place with the Victorian-era Cheshire Cheese pub at Temple.

Wine Office Ct., off 145 Fleet St. ℂ **020/7353-6170.** Mon–Sat 11am–11pm. Tube: Blackfriars, Temple, or Chancery Lane

Ye Olde Mitre ★★★ Suspended in a hidden courtyard and seemingly between centuries, this enchanter—no televisions, no music—was once part of a great palace mentioned by Shakespeare in *Richards II* and *III*. The medieval St Etheldreda's Chapel, the palace's surviving place of worship, stands outside. This extremely tiny pub (established in 1546 but built in its present form in 1772) has two entrances that feed either side of the bar. The one on the left grants you access to "the Closet," a fine example of a semiprivate sitting area called a "snug"; the one on the right brings you face-to-face with a glass case containing a blackened stump, said to be part of a cherry-tree maypole that Elizabeth I danced around. (Yeah, right, drink another one.) Suck down one of the house specialties: pickled or Scotch eggs. To find the pub, look for a little alley among the jewelry stores on Hatton Garden, between 8 and 9 Hatton Garden.

1 Ely Ct., off Ely Place, EC1. www.yeoldemitreholborn.co.uk. ℂ **020/7405-4751.** Mon–Fri 11am–11pm. Tube: Farringdon or Chancery Lane.

EXPLORING LONDON

Engand has been a top dog for 500 years, and London is where it keeps its bark. Many of the world's finest treasures came here during the Empire and never left. Most cities store their best goodies in one or two top museums. In London, riches hide everywhere. The major attractions could by themselves occupy months of contemplation. But the sheer abundance of history and wealth—layer upon layer of it—means that London boasts dozens of exciting smaller sights, too. You could spend a lifetime seeing it all, so you'd better get started.

Sightseeing discounts, such as 2-for-1s, are sometimes offered at **LastMinute.com** (click on the Experiences tab). The heavily promoted **London Pass** (www.londonpass.com) gets you into a bevy of attractions and a Golden Tours sightseeing bus for a fixed price (such as £64 a day or £86 for 2 days), but is unlikely to pay off in the small amount of time you're given to use it. Only the version that lasts 6 days (£139 adult, £126 child) would potentially pay off, but still only *marginally* and only if you barely pause to eat.

Historic Royal Palaces operates The Banqueting House (p. 138), Hampton Court (p. 179), Kensington Palace (p. 144), Kew Palace (p. 183), and the Tower of London (p. 164). An annual membership pass will possibly save you money if you plan to see several of them; do the math (www.hrp.org.uk; ✆ **0844/482-7788;** £50 one adult, £77 two adults, £66 for one adult plus up to six children, £93 two adults plus up to six children).

BLOOMSBURY, FITZROVIA & KING'S CROSS

The British Library ★★★ MUSEUM One of the planet's most precious collections of books, maps, and manuscripts, the British Library holds approximately 150 million items and adds 3 million each year, so when it puts the cream (about 200 items) on display, you will be positively astounded. The **Treasures of the British Library,** at the Sir John Ritblat Gallery, displays these in a

London-Wide Attractions

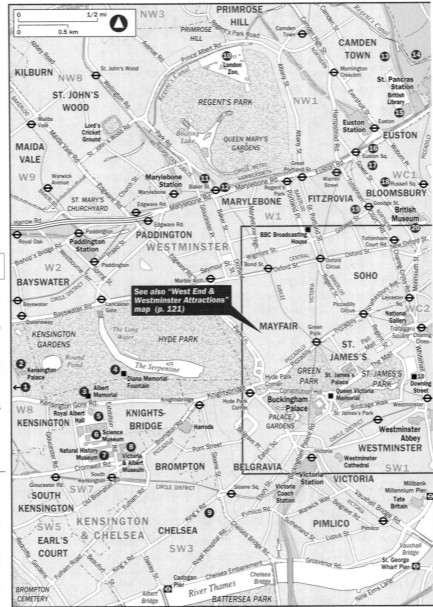

See also "West End & Westminster Attractions" map (p. 121)

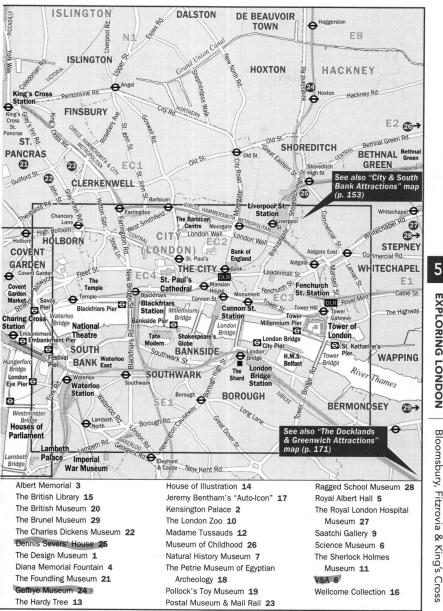

Albert Memorial **3**	House of Illustration **14**	Ragged School Museum **28**
The British Library **15**	Jeremy Bentham's "Auto-Icon" **17**	Royal Albert Hall **5**
The British Museum **20**	Kensington Palace **2**	The Royal London Hospital
The Brunel Museum **29**	The London Zoo **10**	Museum **27**
The Charles Dickens Museum **22**	Madame Tussauds **12**	Saatchi Gallery **9**
Dennis Severs' House **25**	Museum of Childhood **26**	Science Museum **6**
The Design Museum **1**	Natural History Museum **7**	The Sherlock Holmes
Diana Memorial Fountain **4**	The Petrie Museum of Egyptian	Museum **11**
The Foundling Museum **21**	Archeology **18**	V&A **8**
Geffrye Museum **24**	Pollock's Toy Museum **19**	Wellcome Collection **16**
The Hardy Tree **13**	Postal Museum & Mail Rail **23**	

Children's prices generally apply to those 15 and under. To qualify for a **senior discount,** usually you must be 60 or older. **Students** require ID for discounts. Some places offer **Family Tickets** with discounts for up to 3 kids with adults. Museums may post prices that include a voluntary **"gift aid"** donation, but you may ask to have it removed.

In addition to closing on public holidays and on December 25 and 26 (Boxing Day), some heritage properties open only in the summer.

cool, climate-controlled suite of black cases and rich purple carpeting. It ought to be mobbed, but isn't. The trove changes, but it has included:

o Two of the four known copies of the **Magna Carta,** 800 years old in 2015

o The **Gutenberg Bible** from 1455

o The Beatles' first lyric doodles: "A Hard Day's Night" on Julian Lennon's first birthday card (with a choo-choo on it) and "Yesterday"

o The **Diamond Sutra,** the oldest known printed book, which was found in a Chinese cave in 1907 and was probably made by woodblock nearly 600 years before Europeans developed similar technology

o The *Codex Sinaiticus,* one of the two oldest Christian Bibles (the Pope has the other) and illuminated manuscripts from Buddhism, Jainism, and Islam

o Jane Austen's diary and writing desk

o Alexander Fleming's handwritten discovery of penicillin from 1928

o Michelangelo's letter to his dad telling him he had finished the Sistine Chapel and pages from **Leonardo da Vinci's notebook,** in mirror writing

o Works in the hand of Mozart, Handel (his *Messiah*), Beethoven, Dickens, Trollope, Charlotte Brontë, and more.

o An 11th-century copy of *Beowulf* on vellum, in Old English; it's the only surviving manuscript, written when Ethelred the Unready was king.

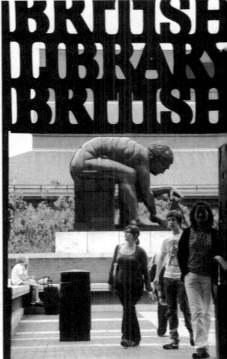

Entrance gate to the British Library.

Many of London's biggest museums are free to enter, but there's a catch: To make up the cash they miss out on, they find lots of other revenue streams. Many institutions charge £1–£2 for **maps** (to get around that, take a digital photograph of the posted floor plan in the lobby and use that as a guide). They also charge £12 or more for the most interesting **temporary exhibitions;** the most popular ones sell out ahead, so do some advance planning. Many will also loan out their star works to other institutions for money, so a marquee work named in this guide may be temporarily on vacation. Fortunately, the new British funding model also gives museums an incentive to operate superlative shops, publish wonderful keepsake guidebooks, and run gorgeous **cafes** that even attract people off the street—you'll never go hungry at the major attractions.

The King's Library, some 85,000 tomes assembled by King George III, floats in a glassed-in central tower and forms the core of the collection, like Thomas Jefferson's library does for Washington's Library of Congress—which means that the King who lost America and a principal engineer of that loss provided the seeds for their respective nations' libraries. The hall contains the **Philatelic Exhibition,** 500 drawers containing thousands of rare stamps.

You can't handle books unless you're a scholar, but the Library encourages anyone to hang out in its public spaces. In addition to the Treasures, the Library presents about 150 annual talks featuring celebrities and historians and some strong temporary exhibitions (about £12; check www.bl.uk/whats-on), including recent ones on Gothic horror, punk, and comic books. An exhibition on the Magna Carta marked the first time Thomas Jefferson's handwritten copy of the Declaration of Independence was displayed in London, the city at which it was originally targeted. That's curator clout. Twice a day, you can book an £8 tour of the superlative facilities.

96 Euston Rd., NW1. www.bl.uk. ⓒ **01937/546-546.** Free admission. Mon and Fri 9:30am–6pm; Tues–Thurs 9:30am–8pm; Sat 9:30am–5pm; Sun 11am–5pm. Tube: King's Cross St Pancras.

The British Museum ★★★ MUSEUM   Founded in 1753 and first opened in 1759 in a converted mansion, the British Museum is as much a monument to great craftsmanship as it is to the piracy carried out by 18th- and 19th-century Englishmen who, on their trips abroad, plundered whatever goodies they could find and then told the bereft that the thievery was for their own good. Yet the exquisite taste of these English patriarchs is unquestionable, and now the British Museum may be the museum to beat all the rest. In fact, it's the top attraction in the country—6.9 million people a year now. Put on your walking shoes because it's not the king of museums for nothing.

If you don't know what to look for, the Museum will be a stupefying series of rooms of urns notable mostly for the zombified tourists staggering through them. Rather than forcing enthusiasm with dutiful, intellectual numbness, do what you can to understand what you're seeing. Check the schedule of daily talks and exhibitions either online or by the pillar to the right as you enter the Great Court. These include a bevy of freebies: 15 daily **Eye-Openers,** focused on particular rooms; 45-minute **Lunchtime Talks** with guest curators (Tuesday–Friday at 1:15pm); 20-minute **Spotlight tours** about major holdings on Friday evenings; and **Hands On,** which allow you to touch some things. The website also has some suggested **"object trails"** for what to look for if you have limited time—useful because the staff rarely knows about anything except crowd control.

Consider renting a hand-held audio/video tablet (£6, both adult and kids' versions) that spotlights 200 of the best objects. From 10:30am to 3pm on weekends, you can also borrow free kids' backpacks that include discovery maps. Maps range from £2 to £6 depending on the level of guiding information you want (for a free one, print floor plans from the website).

Dominating the glass-roofed **Great Court** like a drum in a box, the cream-and-gold round **Reading Room,** completed in 1857, was once part of the British Library containing King George III's exemplary book collection. Patrons had to apply for tickets, and they included Lenin and Karl Marx, who developed their political theories here; other habitués included Bram Stoker, Sir Arthur Conan Doyle, and Virginia Woolf, who wrote upon entering "one stood under the vast dome, as if one were a thought in the huge bald forehead which is so splendidly encircled by a band of famous names." The **Great Court Restaurant** above the Reading Room serves full afternoon tea from 3pm for just £20—a bargain (reserve online or at © **020/7323-8990**). The Reading Room is closed to the public, but don't miss the paneled King's Library rooms (1827), now known as the **Enlightenment Gallery** and brimming with cabinets of curiosities retrieved from the ends of the Earth by the likes of Captain Cook himself.

Other holdings are grouped in numbered rooms by geography, with an emphasis on the Greek and Roman Empires, Europe, and Britain. Don't miss:

o The museum's most famous, and most controversial, possessions are the so-called **Elgin Marbles,** gingerly referred to as the **Sculptures of the Parthenon** (rooms 18 and 19) to disguise imperialist provenance. These slab sculptures (called friezes and Metopes), plus some life-size weathered statuary, once lined the pediment of the famous Parthenon atop Athens' Acropolis. After being defaced (literally—the faces were hacked off) in the 500s by invading vandals (okay, not the East Germanic Vandal tribes—these guys were Persian), the sculptures suffered further indignities in a 1687 gunpowder explosion before being sawed off and carted away by Lord Elgin. They're laid out in the gallery in the approximate position in which they appeared on the Parthenon, only facing inward so you can admire them. Greece begs ceaselessly for their return, but the British have argued that they're better cared for in London. The smog-burnt portions left behind in Athens, despite their glossy new galleries, make a muddy issue of conservation and politics even murkier.

British Museum

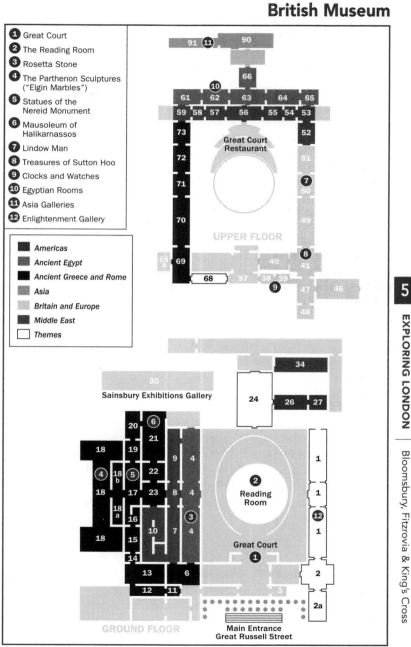

- **1** Great Court
- **2** The Reading Room
- **3** Rosetta Stone
- **4** The Parthenon Sculptures ("Elgin Marbles")
- **5** Statues of the Nereid Monument
- **6** Mausoleum of Halikarnassos
- **7** Lindow Man
- **8** Treasures of Sutton Hoo
- **9** Clocks and Watches
- **10** Egyptian Rooms
- **11** Asia Galleries
- **12** Enlightenment Gallery

Americas
Ancient Egypt
Ancient Greece and Rome
Asia
Britain and Europe
Middle East
Themes

UPPER FLOOR

Great Court Restaurant

Sainsbury Exhibitions Gallery

Reading Room

Great Court

GROUND FLOOR

Main Entrance
Great Russell Street

- Fragments of **sculptures from the Mausoleum at Halikarnassos,** one of the lost Seven Wonders of the Ancient World, loom in room 21. They're colossal in the original sense—one horse's head measures 2.1m (7 ft.) long.
- The pivotal **Rosetta Stone** (196 B.C.), in room 4, is what helped linguists crack hieroglyphics, and its importance to anthropology can't be exaggerated. Napoleon's soldiers found it in Egypt in 1799, but the British nabbed it in 1801. Consider it his first Waterloo. It now adorns everything from handbags to socks in the gift shops; free museums have to profit *somehow.*
- The grisly array of **Egyptian Mummies** in rooms 62, 63, and 64 petrify living children, and on your visit these galleries will probably be thronged as usual. In addition to the wizened, raisinlike corpses, there are painted coffins; the hair and lung of the scribe Sutimose, dating to 1100 B.C.; and scarabs galore. In room 64, check out the body from 3400 B.C., found in a fetal position without a coffin, which was preserved by dry sand. Beside it is another one, 400 years younger, that rotted to soil because it was laid to rest in a basket.
- Kids also stare moon-eyed at crumpled, leather-faced **Lindow Man** in room 50; he was discovered, throat slit, in a Cheshire bog nearly 2,000 years after his brutal demise. Preserved down to his hair and fingernails, he looks like he could spring to life and pound the glass of his case. Nearby (room 49) is the **Mildenhall Treasure,** a hoard of new-looking silver Roman tableware unearthed by Gordon Butcher, a Suffolk farmer, as he plowed fields in 1942; the saga of how Butcher was cheated of his fortune was chronicled by writer Roald Dahl. (Yes, pillage is something of a hidden theme in this place.) The **Lewis Chessmen** (room 40), made from walrus ivory, are whimsical favorites.
- Room 70, on the upper floor, contains many remarkable holdings: the bronze **head of Roman Emperor Augustus,** found in the Sudan and unsettlingly lifelike (it still has its eyeballs of glass and stone); the **Portland Vase,** a black, cameo-glass jug that would be very difficult to make even today; beside that, the historically important **Warren Cup,** a 1st-century silver chalice graphically depicting homosexual sex in relief; and a 3rd-century Roman **crocodile-skin suit of armor.**

Great Russell St., WC1. www.thebritishmuseum.org. © **020/7323-8299.** Free admission. Sat–Thurs 10am–5:30pm; Fri 10am–8:30pm. Tube: Tottenham Court Rd. or Holborn or Russell Square.

Other Bloomsbury Area Attractions

The Charles Dickens Museum ★ MUSEUM   Although Dickens moved around a lot, his last remaining London home, which he rented for £80 a year when he was 30, is now his testament. A museum since 1925, and restored to a period look in 2012 (when the attic and kitchen were opened for the first time), these four floors don't exude many Dickensian vibes; after all, he departed in 1839 after staying less than 2 years. It could be anyone's

JEREMY BENTHAM'S "auto icon"

England's own Ben Franklin, **Jeremy Bentham** (1748–1832) was a philosopher, a progressive, a subversive, a prison reformer, supporter of suffrage and the decriminalization of homosexuality, educator, and pen pal of U.S. president James Madison. Bentham worked to enable equal access to courts and schools, and he coined the words *international, maximize*—he codified *codification* itself.

He was so ahead of his time that he refuses to stay in the past: His will stipulated eternal access to his corpse—the gift that keeps on giving, really. Starting years before his death, he purportedly carried around a pair of glass eyes that were intended for his future "Auto Icon" (auto = self, icon = image), which would represent him forever. After he expired, his body was dissected for students. In 1850, a colleague dressed his remains and Bentham's severed head was placed between his own feet. There his remains remain, in a lobby at University College London. His skeleton is under his original clothing and gloves. Unfortunately, his noggin was clumsily preserved and kids kept swiping it (in 1975, some hooligans held it for a £10 ransom), so today, it's stashed in the vaults, staring blankly with those long-pocketed blue eyeballs. You can see the real head on an electronic display. "Some visitors find it disturbing to look at," warns the caption after you're already recoiling at the sight of the leathery thing. His new lifelike, doughy face sagely observes the current scholarly crop at UCL from beneath a straw hat. You'll find this freak show on the east side of Gower Street between University Street and Grafton Way, opposite the red-brick Cruciform Building. Go in the gates, veer right, and enter the door marked South Cloisters. Then hang a right and head for the stone lions (Tube: Euston Square).

humble home. Still, his celebrity got a kick-start while he lived here: *Oliver Twist* and *Nicholas Nickleby,* arguably his biggest hits, were written while he was in residence. As you inspect his desk, his razor, bars from a prison where his spendthrift dad was locked up, an unpleasant realization sets in: Charles Dickens was a brilliant storyteller, one of the most gifted in the history of the English language, but also a jerk. Tough on his kids and unfaithfully cruel to his wife, his other great talent seems to have been for ego.

48 Doughty St., WC1. www.dickensmuseum.com. ✆ **020/7405-2127.** Admission £9 adults, £7 seniors and students, £4 children 6–16. Tues–Sun 10am–5pm, last admission 1 hr before closing. Tube: Chancery Lane or Russell Square.

The Foundling Museum ★★ MUSEUM Small but devastating, it tracks the history of the Foundling Hospital, which took in thousands of orphans between 1739 and 1953. This was a period in which kids were treated like rubbish: For example, in 1802 a law was passed limiting the time children could work in mills—to 12 hours a day. By that measure, the benefactors were actually helping kids by locking them in this borderline prison. Don't miss the heartbreaking cases of tokens that mothers left at the doorstep with their babies. These tiny objects, into which a lifetime of hopes was imbued, never made it to their children lest they compromise anonymity. Also take the time to listen to the oral histories by some of the last kids to be raised by the

Hospital; at the time of recording, they were elderly but still obviously quite shaken. Upstairs is a modest but respectable collection of 18th-century English works (Hogarth, Reynolds, Gainsborough), which believe it or not was one of the first permanent art exhibitions in the world. Even today, the museum also brings in temporary exhibitions exploring the relationship between adult artists and children. The composer Handel loved the Hospital: He wrote his *Messiah* as a benefit for the facility in 1754 (a score is on display) and there are sometimes exhibitions about his work. The former exercise grounds, now called Coram's Fields, are still fittingly the domain of the child; adults are not permitted to enter without a kid in tow.

40 Brunswick Sq., WC1. www.foundlingmuseum.org.uk. © **020/7841-3600.** Admission £8 adults, £5 seniors and students, free for children 15 and under (higher posted prices include a "voluntary donation"). Tues–Sat 10am–5pm; Sun 11am–5pm. Tube: Russell Square.

The Petrie Museum of Egyptian Archeology ★★ MUSEUM   Britain made a lot of mistakes when it comes to Egypt, and not just with Suez. Almost as soon as "explorers" could break into ancient tombs, they would lose track of thousands of things they discovered or leave poor information about how they found it. Since the 1800s, University College London has worked to properly collect, identify, and date more than 80,000 artifacts; roaming its treasure-crammed cases, some of which are stocked with items that still stump scholars, can be awe-inspiring. From the cotton Tarkhan dress last worn 5,000 years ago to Roman funerary portraits painted in beeswax, the things one finds in these stacks could blow a mind.

Malet Place, University College London, WC1. www.ucl.ac.uk/culture/petrie-museum. © **020/7679-2884.** Free admission. Tues–Sat 1–5pm. Tube: Goodge St.

Pollock's Toy Museum ★ MUSEUM   Eddy Fawdry (and his wee dog Haggis) preside over this strange secret world of vintage toys, which he inherited from his grandparents and they from the Hoxton-based Pollock family, which made famous toy theaters. In room after creaky room, history stares back at you with doll's eyes: puppets, Gollywogs, the 1921 forerunner to G.I. Joe (Swiss Action Man), doll's houses, mechanical cast-iron banks, 1950s rocket toys, a board game based on the Falkland Islands invasion that was banned for being in poor taste. Stories are everywhere and the kitsch factor is through the roof, which brings us to the quirky, spirited building, which has been left leaning and unrestored since its erection in the 1780s (but received a new roof after the Luftwaffe blew off the original one). The ground-floor shop stocks unusual, hard-to-find toys that don't cost much, including handmade items and cardboard theaters—the original inspiration for this one-of-a-kind time warp.

1 Scala St., W1. www.pollockstoys.com. © **020/7636-3452.** Admission £6 adults, £5 seniors and students, £3 children 3–16. Mon–Sat 10am–5pm; last admission 4:30pm. Tube: Goodge St.

The Hardy Tree

In 1866, as laborers dug their way through his churchyard to create the new St Pancras Station, the Vicar of St Pancras noticed with horror that they were tossing aside thighbones and skulls. His cemetery contained the remains of Mary Wollstonecraft, J.C. Bach, Sir John Soane, and Ben Franklin's son, the last colonial governor of New Jersey, so the Vicar assigned a young architecture student named Thomas with the unenviable task of overseeing the relocation of some 8,000 bodies. As he worked, Thomas carefully arranged their discarded headstones around a tree. The tree survives, and today its trunk grows around the markers. Now it is called the Hardy Tree—you see, young Thomas, who created this eerie living monument, was about to become the famous novelist Thomas Hardy. (St Pancras Old Church, Pancras Rd., NW1; www.posp.co.uk; © **020/7424-0724;** King's Cross St Pancras tube.)

Wellcome Collection ★★ MUSEUM   Once upon a time, there was a very strange Midwestern pharmacist named Henry Wellcome. Henry got very wealthy and developed a taste for hoarding medical oddities, such as Napoleon's toothbrush, hair from George III, oil paintings of childbirth, and Japanese sex toys. When he died, he bequeathed a flashy museum for them, which now makes for a highly amusing hour's visit. Besides the permanent collection, there's always an offbeat temporary exhibit or two, pertaining to the human body and its uses—recent ones were on sex research and corpse forensics. It's always one of the most compelling museums in town, and its sizable shop is one of the more intellectual.

183 Euston Rd., NW1. www.wellcomecollection.org. © **020/7611-2222.** Free admission. Tues–Sun 10am–6pm (Thurs 10pm); Sun 11am–6pm. Tube: Euston Square, Warren St., or Euston.

SOHO, COVENT GARDEN & WEST END

The Courtauld Institute of Art Gallery ★★★ MUSEUM   Art historians consider the Courtauld one of the most prestigious collections on Earth, yet the tourist masses don't visit it, which makes for a very pleasant viewing experience. The small two-level selection is supreme, with several masterpieces you will instantly recognize. Among the winners are Manet's then-scandalous *Le déjeuner sur l'herbe,* depicting a naked woman picnicking with two clothed men, and his *A Bar at the Folies-Bergère,* showing a melancholy barmaid standing in front of her disproportionate reflection. There are multiple Cézannes, Toulouse-Lautrecs, and Tahitian Gauguins. Degas' *Two Dancers on a Stage* is iconic, as is Van Gogh's *Self-Portrait with Bandaged Ear.* Especially rare is a completed Seurat, *Young Woman Powdering Herself,* which depicts his mistress in the act of dressing and initially included his own face in the frame on the wall—he painted over it with a vase of flowers to avoid ridicule. Nearly every day at 1:15pm, there's a free lunchtime talk

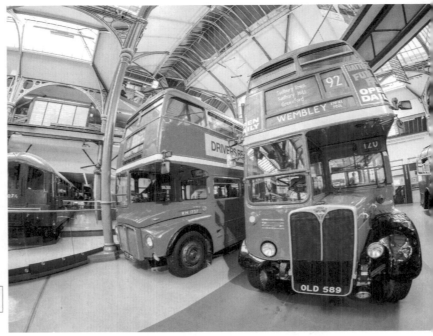

London Transport Museum.

focusing on one of the works. **Somerset House,** its home, was once a naval center and later was where Londoners came to settle taxes and research family history. The central courtyard, beneath which lie the foundations of a Tudor palace, has a grove of 55 ground-level fountains that delight small children; it's the scene of popular summer concerts and a winter ice rink, plus a cafe by the popular charcuterie-bakery Fernandez & Wells. Check out the changing free exhibitions at the **East Wing Galleries** and see if anything interesting is showing at the **Embankment Galleries,** which charges £10 adults, £8 seniors/students, depending on what's on display. The terrace overlooking the Thames (from across the street) can be enjoyed for free.

Somerset House, Strand, WC2. www.courtauld.ac.uk. ℭ **020/7848-2526.** Admission £9.50 adults, £8.50 seniors and students, free for children 18 and under (higher posted prices include a "voluntary donation"). Daily 10am–6pm, last admission 5:30pm. Tube: Temple.

London Transport Museum ★★ MUSEUM   Try to imagine London without its wheeled icons: the red double-decker bus, the black taxi, and the Tube, which are the best of their kind in the world and a draw for visitors. In Covent Garden's soaring cast-iron-and-glass 1871 flower-selling hall (Eliza Doolittle would have bought her flowers here), the vehicles' development and evolution are traced with excellent technology (lots of ambient sounds and video displays, although some are getting grubby or outdated) and detail

West End & Westminster Attractions

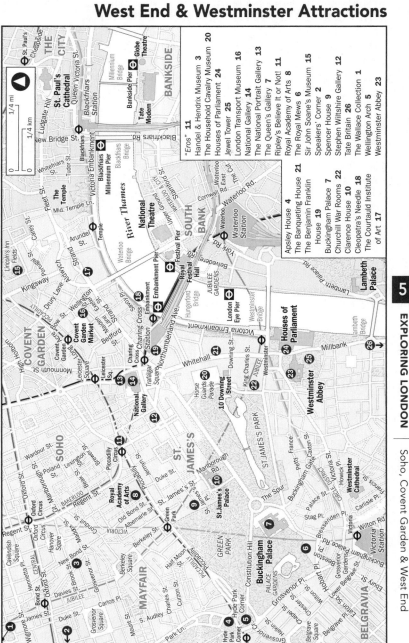

"Eros" **11**
Handel & Hendrix Museum **3**
The Household Cavalry Museum **20**
Houses of Parliament **24**
Jewel Tower **25**
London Transport Museum **16**
National Gallery **14**
The National Portrait Gallery **13**
The Queen's Gallery **7**
Ripley's Believe It or Not! **11**
Royal Academy of Arts **8**
The Royal Mews **6**
Sir John Soane's Museum **15**
Speakers' Corner **2**
Spencer House **9**
Stephen Wiltshire Gallery **12**
Tate Britain **26**
The Wallace Collection **1**
Wellington Arch **5**
Westminster Abbey **23**

Apsley House **4**
The Banqueting House **21**
The Benjamin Franklin House **19**
Buckingham Palace **7**
Churchill War Rooms **22**
Clarence House **10**
Cleopatra's Needle **18**
The Courtauld Institute of Art **17**

(there are even fake horse apples beneath the antique carriages). You can board a fleet of intact landmark vehicles, such as Number 23, a steam locomotive that powered the Underground in its most unpleasant days ("a form of mild torture," wrote the *Times* then); also on display are plenty of the system's famous Edwardian and Art Deco posters, many of which are art unto themselves. Designers will appreciate the background on Johnston, the distinctive typeface created in 1916 for the Underground by Frank Pick, which could now be considered London's unofficial font. Along the way, you'll learn a great deal about shifts in London life; you may even feel a twinge of embarrassment about the state of your own town's public transportation. It's a must for fans of London history and a good place to entertain children—but if you're childless, you'll need patience. The gift shop, which doesn't require a ticket, is exemplary.

Covent Garden, WC2. www.ltmuseum.co.uk. ② **020/7565-7299.** Admission £18 adults, £15 seniors and students, free for children 17 and under. Sat–Thurs 10am–6pm; Fri 11am–6pm; last admission 45 min. before closing. Tube: Covent Garden.

National Gallery ★★★ MUSEUM   When the bells of St Martin-in-the-Fields peal each morning at 10am, the doors promptly open on one of the world's greatest artistic fireworks shows—each famous picture follows an equally famous picture. Few museums can compete with the strongest, widest collection of paintings in the world—one of every important style is on display, and it's almost always the best in that genre. There are 2,300 Western European works, which is plenty to divert you for as long as you can manage. Six million visitors are drawn here every year, although most of them just wander around without getting properly close to the brushwork. Be different.

This stupendous museum is unfortunately marred by lazy presentation; it's very difficult to find the works you want to see. The map (£1) is a poor value since it omits major works. Directional signs lack room numbers, and the staff cares mostly about controlling visitors, not edifying them. It's almost like they want you to wander confused and unenriched. (To find a specific painting, track down a staffer wearing a lime green shirt—there's usually one in the Trafalgar Square lobby.) Mostly, they tell you to use your smartphone to look things up on the museum's website, using the museum's Wi-Fi, which may not work. (You can recharge your phone in the downstairs Espresso Bar if you have a cord.)

Posted signs are awfully straight-laced. Comprehensive audio tours covering 1,200 of the works are £4 and leaflets guide you to a subset of them in themed varieties (impressionists, technique, etc.). A $2 app catalogs more than 1,500 paintings—if there's a symbol by the work, you can look it up on the app—and a free version supplies 183 highlights. The website has some touring trail suggestions, but your visit would be best illuminated by some expert input. Check the info desk for events, such as the **10-Minute Talks** about a single work (Mon–Fri at 4pm); 45-minute **Lunchtime Talks** (1pm) about a specific work or artist; storytelling for kids; or the few hour-long

surprised how the best works capture the sparkle of life behind these charismatic shapers of history. Here, the names from your high school textbook flower into flesh-and-blood people, and the accompanying biographies are so sublimely evocative (Samuel Johnson is described as "massive, ungainly, plagued with nervous tics") that subjects come alive.

The ancient kings and queens have the most heft, partly because it's hard to wrap your brain around the fact that in many cases, the actual people posed alongside these very canvases. One of the most instantly recognizable paintings is the **Ditchley portrait of Elizabeth I** (room 2), in which the queen's jeweled gown spreads like wings and Her Majesty firmly glares at the viewer under stormy skies. Right away, it becomes clear that many artists are slyly commenting on the disposition of their sitters. The troublesome **Henry VIII** is shown in several likenesses. One is a delicate 1537 paper cartoon by Hans Holbein the Younger (for a mural at Whitehall—a rare survivor from that palace), in which the king suspiciously peers with flinty grey eyes—hinting at a shiftiness that His Majesty probably couldn't recognize in his own likeness, but that all who knew him feared (room 1). One painting of **King Edward VI,** painted when he was 9, is executed in a distorted perspective (called anamorphosis) that requires it to be viewed from a hole on the right side of its case (room 1). You'll also find **George Washington** (he was born an Englishman, after all), and one of the only authoritative images of **Captain James Cook** (room 14), who was so pivotal in colonial expansion. In room 12, look for the newly acquired **Chevalier D'Eon,** a male diplomat and fencing champion who lived as a woman in the late 1700s; in room 10 for the adorable little nose of William Hogarth in his terra-cotta bust; and in room 18, for the sketch of **Jane Austen** by her sister Cassandra—friends said it stank, but here it is. The **Brontë Sisters** appear together in an 1834 portrait found folded atop a cupboard in 1914; their alcoholic brother Patrick Branwell Brontë painted himself out but his ghostly image is eerily re-appearing (room 24).

Fortunately, the portraits don't stop when cameras were invented. **Margaret Thatcher,** imperiously glaring over the grey gunwale of a dais at the Conservative Party Conference in Brighton, is Paul Brason's fearsome and not-very-fond representation of the Iron Lady (1982, room 32); Paul Emsley's warm oil-on-canvas of **Catherine, HRH The Duchess of Cambridge** makes her look like she's 40 (2012, room 39); there's even a video of **David Beckham** sleeping in 2004 (room 38a). In contrast, Sir James Gunn's 1950 sitting-room portrait of **Queen Elizabeth II** with her parents, **King George VI** and the **Queen Mum** (room 31) mines Rockwell-esque imagery (Mum's about to pour tea, Dad's smoking) to make the Royal Family seem as normal and as middle-class as the Cleavers. Modern portraits tend to change often because there's simply not enough room to show everything. Just about everything can be photographed without a flash, and just about everything can be purchased as a poster in the gift shop, which is an unexpected trove of hard-to-find biographies.

Take the escalator to the top and work your way down (it'll take about 2 hours). The oldest works (Tudors, Jacobeans, Elizabethans) come first, and you'll progress forward in time, coming to photography just about when canvas fatigue sets in. Frankly, it helps to know a little history so these pictures ring some bells, so consider visiting near the end of your trip, when many of these names will be fresh in your mind from your tours. The £3 audio/video guide starts out dull, but by the end, it uses archival recordings, which is cool, and there's a $2 smartphone app (there's free Wi-Fi) of the highlights. Bring kids; the desk lends free discovery trails for them.

Late Shift evenings (Thursday and Friday 6–9pm), with DJs, talks, live music, and sketching sessions, are great fun and a smart way to free up daytime hours to see more attractions. Also consider the pre-theater menu (£20 for two courses, £24 for three) served from 5:30 to 6:30pm in the rooftop Portrait Restaurant (☎ 020/7312-2490), which has a breathtaking view of Nelson's Column and Big Ben's tower—it's better than the National Gallery's.

St Martin's Place, WC2. www.npg.org.uk. ☎ 020/7312-2463. Free admission. Daily 10am–6pm (Thurs–Fri until 9pm); last admission 45 min before closing. Tube: Leicester Square.

Sir John Soane's Museum ★★ MUSEUM   A doorman will politely request that you deposit your bags. With good reason: These two town houses on the north side of Lincoln's Inn Fields (fresh off a £7 million expansion that opened up closed rooms) are so overloaded with furniture, paintings, architectural decoration, and sculpture, that navigation is a challenge. The Georgian architect, noted for his egotistic neoclassicism (the Bank of England) as much as for his aesthetic materialism, bequeathed his home and its contents as a museum for "amateurs and students," and so it has been, looking much like this since 1837. It's as if the well-connected eccentric had just popped out to purloin another Greek pilaster, leaving you to roam his groaning wood floors, sussing out the *objets d'art* from the certifiable treasures. His oddball abode, which his will decreed must be left precisely as it was on the day he died, is a melee of art history in which precious paintings and sculpture jostle for space like baubles in a junk shop. Ask to join a tour of the **Picture Room,** built in an 1823 expansion, so you can watch its hidden recesses be opened, revealing layer upon buried layer of works (such as William Hogarth's eight-painting *The Rake's Progress,* a documentary of dissolution), filed inside false walls. Look sharp for Canalettos (which often fetch £9 million at auction) and a J. M. W. Turner (ditto). Curation appears convoluted and haphazard: The guides swear that although sunshine appears to pour onto the masterpieces through skylights, there are UV filters—yet architectural fragments from Whitehall Palace are plainly betrayed to the elements in the courtyard ("It was never covered because that's the way he wanted it," a guide says). You have to wonder how Soane could legally acquire antiquities such as the sarcophagus of Seti I, carved from translucent limestone but stockpiled for £2,000, and you won't know because nearly nothing is marked. (Just how the Hogarth hoarder wanted it, too.) Surf the simulated museum at explore.soane.org to get pre-acquainted, or take a guided 1-hour tour (£10): 11am and noon Tuesday and Saturday, also noon Thursday and Friday). Mostly, a visit reminds you of the unseemly way in which privileged Englishmen used to stuff their homes with

CLEOPATRA & "eros"

Two monuments in the West End have been enchanting visitors for years. When he finished his legendary fountain in the middle of Piccadilly Circus in 1893, sculptor Alfred Gilbert thought the playful maritime-themed sculptures on its base would be celebrated. Audiences, however, have minds of their own: They responded instead to the archer god on top. But they got even that bit of admiration wrong—they thought he represented **Eros,** god of erotic love, when Gilbert had actually intended Anteros, god of requited love. Today, Piccadilly Circus isn't a roundabout anymore—it's an interchange—but the ceaseless tourist crowd photographing Gilbert's misunderstood masterpiece at least puts the circus back into Piccadilly. Gilbert's fabulous fountain is now dry and full of McDonald's wrappers, but his misidentified god blesses the city as an icon. (Tube: Piccadilly Circus)

The original Cleopatra's Needles obelisks—which Cleopatra had nothing to do with—were erected in Heliopolis, Egypt, around 1450 B.C., and inscriptions were added 200 years later. The Romans moved the granite spires to Alexandria, where they toppled and were buried in the sand, which preserved them until the early 1800s. After a perilous delivery, London's 224-ton **Cleopatra's Needle** was erected here on the river in 1878 (New York City got one in 1881, and a third went to Paris). Two sphinxes were installed to guard it (some say backward, since they face the sculpture, not away from it). Just 140 years here wrecked what 20 Saharan centuries didn't: Pollution has rendered the hieroglyphs illegible. In 1917, German bombs scarred the western sphinx. The cast iron benches in the area were installed in preparation of its arrival in the 1870s. Look closely; you'll find sphinxes and camels hidden in the armrests. (Tube: Embankment or Temple) classical art as a way of stocking up on a sense of righteousness—but that doesn't mean it's not wondrous.

12 Lincoln's Inn Fields, WC2. www.soane.org. © **020/7405-2107.** Free admission. Tues–Sat 10am–5pm, last entry 4:30pm; candlelit nights 1st Tues of month 6–9pm (be in line by 5:30pm). Tube: Holborn.

Other West End Attractions

The Benjamin Franklin House ★ HISTORIC HOME The only surviving residence of the portly politico is a sort of architectural preserve. Shocker: Franklin lived in this boarding house by the Thames without his wife for nearly 16 years—he was here for the Boston Tea Party, the enactment of the Stamp Act, and his invention of the armonica—and it was only the Revolution (and scandal) that forced him from his adopted home back to the Colonies. For much of his life Franklin was a fervent Loyalist who, even as late as 1775, felt the differences between Britain and the Colonies could be settled in "half an hour." Tours are conducted by a young actress playing the landlady's daughter, Polly Hewson, who became such a dear friend that she moved to Philadelphia and was with him when he died. In empty rooms, Polly tells wistful tales as recordings chime in with voices from her memory. (Mon are for architectural tours without the actress.) Rewards are mixed. Exhibits are sparse (one exception is the ghoulish deposit of human bones in the backyard, likely left over from dissections by Franklin's doctor neighbor), and there are few kids' activities. But on the other hand, it's rare for a famous home of this age to have survived into our lifetime. It's also humbling to see how this giant man made do with such small quarters. The worn wooden staircase, on which he got his exercise when French trollops weren't available, is so well preserved it feels ghostly.

36 Craven St., WC2. www.benjaminfranklinhouse.org. © **020/7925-1405.** Admission and tour (required) £8 adults, £6 seniors and students, free for children 15 and under. 5 timed tours daily, Mon (architectural tour) and Wed–Sun (historical tour) noon–4:15pm. Tube: Embankment or Charing Cross.

WESTMINSTER & ST JAMES'S

For information on the **Changing the Guard** ceremony, please see p. 187.

Buckingham Palace ★★ PALACE If you were to fall asleep tonight and wake up inside one of the **State Rooms,** you'd never guess where you were. Is it opulent? No question. But if gilding, teardrop chandeliers, 18th-century portraits, and ceremonial halls could ever be considered standard-issue, Buckingham Palace is your basic palace. Queen Elizabeth's mild taste—call it "respectable decadence" of yellows and creams and pleasant floral arrangements, thank you very much—is partly the reason. Remember, too, that much of this palace was built or remodeled in the 1800s—not so long ago in the scheme of things—and that the queen considers Windsor to be her real home. That's right: Buckingham Palace is a mere *pied-à-terre.*

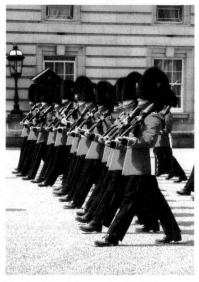

The changing of the guard at Buckingham Palace is a must-see.

All tickets are timed and include an audio tour that rushes you around too quickly. (If you want to see highlights of the formal gardens, that's another £9.) The route threads through the public and ceremonial rooms at the back of the Palace—nowhere the Royal Family spends personal time (and besides, tours are held only when they're in Scotland, 2 months a year). Highlights include the 50m-long (164-ft.) **Picture Gallery** filled mostly with works amassed by George IV, an obsessive collector; the 14m-high (46-ft.) **Ballroom,** where the queen confers knighthoods; the parquet-floored **Music Room,** unaltered since John Nash decorated it in 1831, where the queen's three eldest children were baptized in water brought from the River Jordan; and a stroll through the thick **Garden** in the back yard. It's definitely worth seeing—how often can you toddle around the spare rooms in a queen's house, inspecting artwork given as gifts by some of history's most prominent names? But it's no Versailles. If you're in London any time other than August or September and spot her standard of red, gold, and blue flying above, you'll at least know the queen is home. If it's the Union Jack, she's gone.

Buckingham Palace Rd., SW1. www.royalcollection.org.uk.© **020/7766-7300.** Admission £23 adults, £21 seniors and students, £13 children 5–16. Generally open late July to late Aug daily 9:30am–7:30pm; Sept daily 9:30am–6:30pm; last admission 2¼ hr before closing. Tube: Victoria or Green Park.

Churchill War Rooms ★★★ MUSEUM/HISTORIC SITE   One of London's most fascinating museums is the secret command center used by Winston Churchill and his staff during the most harrowing moments of World War II, when it looked like England might become German. We regard the period with nostalgia, but a staggering 30,000 civilians were killed by some 18,000 tons of bombs in London alone and more than 65,000 innocent people were killed in Britain as a whole. Here, in the cellar of the Treasury building, practically next door to 10 Downing St., the core of the British government hunkered down where one errant bomb could have incinerated the lot of them.

When the War ended, the bunker was abandoned, but everything was left just as it was in August 1945. When it came time to make it a museum, everything was intact—from pushpins tracing convoy movements on yellowed world maps to rationed sugar cubes hidden in the back of a clerk's desk drawer. Although the hideout functioned like a small town for 526 people,

5

EXPLORING LONDON | Westminster & St James's

with sleeping quarters, kitchens, radio rooms, and other facilities that would enable leaders to live undetected for months on end, it feels a lot more like your old elementary school, with its painted brick, linoleum walls, and round clocks.

Midway through, you disappear into the **Churchill Museum,** surely the most cutting-edge biographical museum open at this moment. Exhaustively displaying every conceivable facet of his life (his bowtie, his bowler hat, and even the original front door to 10 Downing St.), it covers the exalted states-man's life from entitled birth through his antics as a journalist in South Africa (where he escaped a kidnapping and became a national hero) to his stints as prime minister. You even learn his favorite cigar (Romeo y Julieta) and brandy (Hine). The entire museum is atwitter with multimedia displays, movies, and archival sounds, but the centerpiece will blow you away: a 15m-long (50-ft.) Lifeline Interactive table, like a long file cabinet illuminated by projections, that covers every month of Churchill's life. Touch a date, and the file "opens" with 4,600 pages of rare documents, photos, or, for critical dates in history, animated Easter eggs that temporarily consume the entire table (select the original Armistice Day or the *Titanic* sinking to see what I mean). You could play for hours, dipping into his life day by day.

Clive Steps, King Charles St., SW1. www.iwm.org.uk. © **020/7930-6961.** Admission £17 adults, £14 seniors and students, £8.60 children 5–15 (higher posted prices include a "voluntary donation"). Daily 9:30am–6pm; last admission 5pm. Tube: Westminster or St James's Park.

Houses of Parliament ★★ LANDMARK   In olden days, England's rich overlords got together at the king's house, Westminster Palace, to figure out how to manage their peasants. Over time, the king was forced out of the proceedings and most of the Palace burned down. What remains is con-structed to express the might of Empire riches and the lofty aesthetics of Gothic-revival architecture. Luckily, the nation allows you to tour a dozen stately halls and even to wander through its vaunted House of Lords and House of Commons when they're not in session. There are now two ways to see it: Choose a 100-minute guided group tour, which presents the usual issues of audibility and pace, or take it easy with the new 2-hour audio guide (and eavesdrop on groups whenever you want).

The historical highlight is massive **Westminster Hall,** one of the world's most precious spaces and a UNESCO World Heritage Site, built in 1097 by William Rufus, son of William the Conqueror. Richard II commissioned its cherished oak hammer-beam ceiling before he was deposed in the 1390s. Charles I, William Wallace, Sir Thomas More, and Guy Fawkes were all con-demned in it, monarchs lie in state in it—and your role in it is to pick up your audio tour. The rest of the Palace is roughly divided into three areas: those for the **House of Lords** (whose members inherit seats upholstered in rose with an unbelievable gilt sitting area where Queen Victoria would preside on desig-nated occasions); the **House of Commons** (by far the more powerful, elected by the people, but plainer, with seats of blue-green under a hanging forest of microphones); and some flabbergasting lobbies, sitting rooms, and the

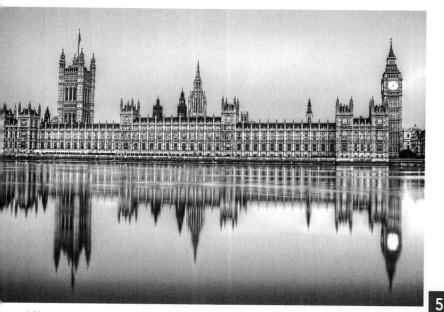
You can tour portions of the Houses of Parliament.

Robing Room (golds, browns, burgundies), which the Sovereign flits through when she shows up once a year to kick off sessions. You walk right onto the floor of both Houses. Many delicious details are elucidated, from the knock-marks on the Commons door made by the Crown's emissary, the Black Rod, to the line in the carpet members may not cross when in the throes of vigorous debates. Booking ahead is advisable; otherwise, try your luck for openings at the ticket office next to the Jewel Tower, across the street.

Overseas visitors are permitted to observe some debates, but the wait can be as long as 2 hours (line up outside the Cromwell Green visitor entrance). Check ahead, since security concerns may cause the government to review public access. The website also posts times of lower-level "Westminster Hall debates" in a committee room, where anyone can come on a first-come, first-served basis. Question Time is only allowed for U.K. residents by previous arrangement with their MP or a Member of the House of Lords.

The Palace runs an afternoon tea service (p. 90) overlooking the river (not the most posh, but a cool place). Sorry, but Elizabeth Tower (1859) beside the Houses—it contains the 13½-ton bell known as Big Ben plus four smaller bells—is only open to U.K. residents. If the green Ayrton Light atop it burns, Parliament is sitting after dark.

Bridge St. and Parliament Sq., SW1. www.parliament.uk/visit. ℂ **020/7219-4114.** Admission £26 adults, £21 seniors and students, £11 children 5–15, free for children 4 and under, add £2 if booked the same day. Tours: Sat and most weekdays during Parliamentary recesses; times vary; always check ahead. Reservations recommended. Tube: Westminster.

Spencer House ★★ HISTORIC HOME   Currently owned by Roths-childs banking company, which hosts diplomatic and corporate events here, this lush home is the only surviving London mansion with an intact 18th-century interior; tours let you see the ground floor and a portion of the first floor. The house was begun in 1756 as a love nest by Diana Spencer's ances-tors (and, by extension, the future king's); its lavish gilt and carved decor repeatedly invoke the symbols of fidelity and virility. Great War damage spooked the Spencer clan, who moved out in the 1920s, and since then, they've gradually transferred the most precious elements to their estate at Althorp, 193km (120 miles) north of the city, and replaced them with equally fantastic facsimiles—the library fireplace, for instance, took 4,000 hours to carve. The original Painted Room suite was once at the V&A. Groups are limited to 20, so arrive early to secure a spot.

27 St James's Place, SW1. www.spencerhouse.co.uk. ⓒ **020/7514-1958.** Tours £13 adults; £11 students, seniors, and children 15 and under. Sun 10:30am–4:30pm; closed Jan and Aug. Tube: Green Park.

Tate Britain ★ MUSEUM   Tourists often wonder about the difference between the Tate Modern and this, its sister upstream on the Thames. Well, the Modern is for contemporary art of any origin, and the Britain, besides its calmer and more civilized affect, is mostly for British-made art made after 1500. Its art is far more approachable than the esoteric stuff at Bankside, and

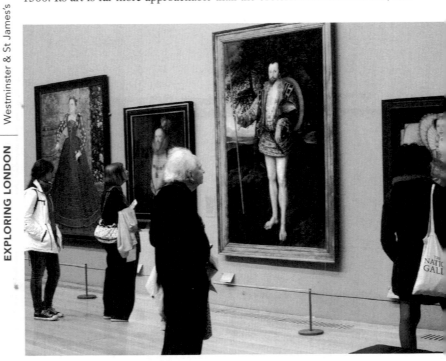

The Tate Britain museum is for British-made art made after 1500.

you'll see plenty of grade-A work, though not many recognizable masterpieces. Britain has a historic knack for collecting masterpieces, not so much for creating them, so a lot of the work is rich with relevance but highly imitative of classical or Renaissance styles—it's hard to shake the feeling that, artistically speaking, Britain was playing catch-up with the rest of Europe. The oldest portion of the collection, full of documentary or moralist works by William Hogarth, William Blake, and Joshua Reynolds, dips into British life from centuries ago, but it's not until the galleries progress chronologically into the modern era that you find works by visionaries such as Francis Bacon, John Singer Sargent, and James Abbott McNeill Whistler (those last two, granted, were not English but Americans in England) that reveal ebullient colors latent in the national mind.

Descriptions are pedantic ("this picture bridges the historical and the sublime") and paintings are hung salon-style, many at such altitude that lighting glare makes them inscrutable. But the 1-hour tours (at 11am, noon, 2pm, and 3pm) help get around such shortcomings. The last tour of the day focuses on paintings by J. M. W. Turner, a highlight of the collection (see below).

Beloved paintings are constantly being rotated into storage, a frustrating habit with Tate, but some masterpieces can be relied upon. Turner's trenchant *The Field of Waterloo* (room 1810) was painted in 1818, 3 years after the battle; its shadowy piles of corpses, and of bereaved family members searching them, is still considered a daring exposure of the true price of war. The oil-on-canvas *Carnation, Lily, Lily, Rose* (1840) by John Singer Sargent depicts children holding paper lanterns so luminous that when it was first exhibited in 1887, its worth was instantly recognized and it was purchased for the nation. John Everett Millais' depiction of a drowning *Ophelia* (1840) is also considered a treasure for its phenomenally tricky depiction of water; the artist painted the plants in the summer so he'd get them right and waited until winter to paint his model, a hat-shop girl, in a tub of water. Naturally, she caught a severe cold (he paid for her doctor's bill after her father threatened to sue). Kids love the double vision of *The Cholmondeley Ladies* (room 1540), two new mothers "born the same day, Married the same day, And brought to Bed the same day"; look closely and you'll realize they're not identical. Check out the sculptures, too, including forms by **Henry Moore,** who gets two rooms, and Barbara Hepworth. But the crowning attraction here is the **Turner Galleries,** with their expansive collection of J. M. W. Turners. Turner (1775–1851), the son of a Covent Garden barber, was a master of landscapes lit by gauzy, perpetual sunrise, and the dozens of paintings testify to both his undying popularity and his doggedly British tendency to convey information mostly by implication. Turner's work is lovely, if sleepy, but it's best appreciated if you understand its influence on subsequent artists. The free Tate App supplies some additional descriptions of major works. Maps are £1. There are two places to eat: a casual underground café and the **Rex Whistler** (p. 91), which in 1927 kicked off the trend of high museum dining.

Millbank, SW1. www.tate.org.uk/britain. ✆ **020/7887-8888.** Free admission. Daily 10am–6pm; closes 10pm 1 Fri/month. Tube: Pimlico.

Westminster Abbey ★★★ HISTORIC SITE/CHURCH   If you have to pick just one church to see in London—nay, one church in the entire *world*—this is the one. The echoes of history are mind-blowing: The current building dates from the 1200s, but it was part of a monastery dating to at least 960. Every English monarch since 1066 has been crowned here (with three minor exceptions: Edward V, Edward VIII, and possibly Mary I). There are 17 monarchs interred here (deaths dating from 1066 to 1760—the crypts here are overstuffed, so now they go to Windsor), as are dozens of great writers and artists. Even if England's tumultuous history and the thought of bodies lying underfoot don't stir your imagination, the interior—in places, as intricate as

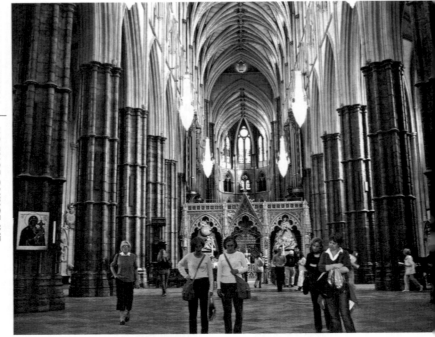

Westminster Abbey is the one church you must see.

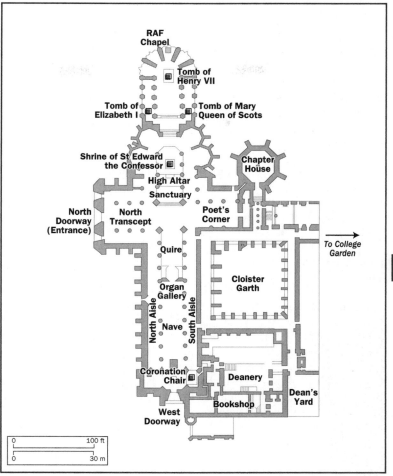

RAF
Chapel

Tomb of
Henry VII

Tomb of
Elizabeth I

Tomb of Mary
Queen of Scots

Shrine of St Edward
the Confessor

Chapter
House

High Altar

Sanctuary

North
Doorway
(Entrance)

North
Transcept

Poet's
Corner

To College
Garden

Quire

Cloister
Garth

Organ
Gallery

North Aisle

South Aisle

Nave

Coronation
Chair

Deanery

Dean's
Yard

Bookshop

West
Doorway

| 0 | 100 ft |
| 0 | 30 m |

lace—will earn your appreciation. A visit should take about 3 hours and should begin early, since entry lines can be excruciating.

Unlike St Paul's Cathedral (p. 161), which has an airy, stately beauty, the much smaller Westminster is more like time's attic, packed with artifacts, memorials, tombs, and virtuosic shrines—a confluence of God, art, and dense history. It's easy to feel overloaded after just a few minutes. Take your time and don't get swept along in the current of visitors. Let them pass. There are stories to be told in every square meter of this place—name another building where there is such a staggering continuity of a nation's heritage.

A visit is likely to start with a welcome from a volunteer; the Abbey follows the Benedictine tradition, which dictates a warm reception for everyone. It's also still a functioning spiritual center, so there may be calls for prayer or moments of silence as you tour. You'll be in the Nave, passing Darwin's resting place (just after the first blue gate), and it only accelerates from there. Bombastic tombs abound; take your time absorbing their colonialist self-importance. Google one and you'll unravel a tale, such as the one Thomas Banks sculpted (1789) for Sir Eyre Coote, commander of the British Forces in India—"death interrupted his career of glory." Although his battles of conquest slaughtered thousands of Indians, he is attended by a weeping naked savage. All that ponderous stone, yet he (like many others memorialized in the Abbey) is not even buried here—he's in Hampshire.

The royal tombs are clustered in the region of the High Altar, where coronations and funerals are conducted. The most famous rulers of all time are truly *here*—not in story, but in body, a few inches behind marble slabs. Some are stashed in cozy side chapels (which once held medieval shrines before Cromwellians bashed them to pieces during the Reformation; some vandalism is still visible), but the oldest are on the sanctuary side of the ambulatory (aisle). The executed **Mary Queen of Scots** was belatedly given a crypt of equal stature to her rival, **Elizabeth I,** by Mary's son **James I,** who gave himself only a marker for his own tomb beneath **Henry VII**'s elaborate resting place. Some **Stuart and Hanoverian monarchs** are also here (Charles II, Queen Anne, William and Mary) but don't have elaborate tombs. James I's infant daughter Sophia, who died aged 3 days, was given a creepy bassinet sarcophagus in the Lady Chapel (peer into it using a mirror).

The audio tour only picks up highlights, and that pushes you along too quickly if you're truly interested. The *Treasures of Westminster Abbey* book in the gift shop is useful for identifying oddities and learning about people buried under them, but it's £15. If you have questions, approach anyone in a red robe; they're "vergers," or officers who attend to the church. They lead 90-minute tours (usually at 10am, but up to five times daily, for £5) and if you stump them, you may win an invitation to the atmospheric Library, a creaking loft that smells of medieval vellum and dust, where an archivist can answer you.

The South Transept is **Poet's Corner,** where Britain's great writers are honored. You'll see many plaques, but 60% (Shakespeare, Austen, Carroll, Wilde, the Brontës) are merely memorials. The biggest names who truly lie underfoot are Robert Browning, Geoffrey Chaucer (he was placed here first, starting the trend), Charles Dickens, Thomas Hardy (without his heart, which was buried in Dorset), John Gay, Rudyard Kipling, George Frideric Handel (who popularized the use of the Abbey as a concert venue), Dr. Samuel Johnson, Laurence Olivier, Edmund Spenser, and Alfred Lord Tennyson. Ben Jonson is commemorated here, but is actually buried in the Nave near Isaac Newton and Charles Darwin. Also in the Nave, in the northwest corner, look out for a batch of prime ministers underfoot.

Now for a few Abbey secrets:

o That oak seat in the last niche before your exit is the **Coronation Chair.** Unbelievably, nearly every English monarch since 1308 has been crowned on this excruciating-looking throne. The slot under the seat is for the 152kg (336-lb.) Stone of Scone, said to be used as a pillow by the Bible's Jacob, and a central part of Irish, Scottish, and English coronations since at least 700 B.C. After spending 7 centuries in the Abbey (except for when Scottish nationalists stole it for 4 months in late 1950), the Stone was returned to Scotland in 1996, where it's on view at Edinburgh Castle. It will return for every future coronation.

o **Oliver Cromwell,** who overthrew the monarchy and ran England as a republic, was buried with honors behind the High Altar in 1658. Three years later, after the monarchy was restored, his corpse was dug up, dragged to Tyburn (by the Marble Arch), hanged, decapitated, the body tossed into a common grave, and its head put on display outside the Abbey. (Didn't they realize he was already dead?) Today his much-abused cranium is at Sidney Sussex College in Cambridge. Cromwell's daughter, who died young, was mercifully allowed to remain buried in the Abbey. In the window above the grave, look for a hole that was left after a 1940 Blitz bombing.

o The **High Altar,** with a mosaic floor laid in the year 1268, is where coronations take place. The actual event sounds glamorous, but it's actually excruciating for everyone involved: Some 8,500 spectators are packed into this small space and the monarch's crown weighs a brutal 5.5 pounds.

o The **Quire** is where the choir sings; it comprises about 12 men and 30 or so boys who are educated at the adjoining Westminster Choir School, the last of its type in the U.K. The wooden stalls, in the Gothic style, are Victorian, and are so delicate they're dusted using vacuum cleaners.

2018 is a big year for the Abbey, because for the first time in 700 years it will open the 13th-century **Triforium,** a sort of attic 70 feet above the sanctuary floor, as a sensational new exhibition and public viewing area—a lift was grafted to the venerable building just for it. Look also for the panel concealing the **Chapter House,** which was made between 924 and 1030 and is Britain's oldest door. Time seems suspended in the **Cloister,** or courtyard. Even better gardens are hidden away: Look for the fragrant and fountained **Little Cloister Garden,** blackened by 19th-century coal dust, and beyond that to the right, the wide **College Garden** (open Tues–Thurs), a tempting courtyard with daffodil beds, green lawns, and five plane trees dating to 1850. The garden is thought to be Britain's longest-established one, having been cultivated for nearly a millennium. **Westminster School,** started by the abbey's monks in the 1300s, stands nearby. (Incidentally, there haven't been monks in this complex for 550 years, yet Londoners persist in calling it an "Abbey.")

Get a real sense of the majesty of the space at a service. Evening prayer services with choirs from around the world are at 5pm weekdays; sung Eucharist is on Sundays at 11am, plus a Sunday organ recital at 5:45pm and evening service with simple hymns at 6:30pm (but check ahead, since services are sometimes shuffled to smaller, but equally historic, chapels). Holy Communion is daily at 8am, Matins are at 10am, and Evensong is Saturdays at 3pm. There's also a daily Eucharist at 12:30pm in the Nave. Next door, pop into **St**

Margaret's Chapel (free), which the monks built in 1523 so they'd be left alone in peace. The Germans didn't comply: Some southern windows were destroyed by a bomb and were replaced by plain glass, and in addition to damage to the north wall, Pew 3 remains charred.

Broad Sanctuary, SW1. www.westminster-abbey.org. ℭ **020/7222-5152.** Admission £20 adults, £17 seniors and students, £9 children 6–16, free for children 5 and under. Generally Mon–Tues and Thurs–Fri 9:30am–3:30pm; Wed 9:30am–6pm; Sat 9:30am–1:30pm; last admission 1 hr before closing. Closed Sun for worship. Check ahead for closures. Tube: Westminster.

Other Westminster & St James' Attractions

The Banqueting House ★ HISTORIC SITE The storied palace of Whitehall was home to some of England's flashiest characters, including Henry VIII. In a wrenching loss for art and architecture—to say nothing of bowling heritage, since Henry had an alley installed—it burned down in 1698. But if you had to pick just one room to survive, it would have been the one that did, designed with Italianate Renaissance assurance by Inigo Jones and completed in 1622. Henry never set foot in it, but another fateful king set his *last* foot in it: In 1649, Charles I walked onto the scaffold from a window that stood in the present-day staircase, and met his doom under an axe wielded by Cromwell's republicans, many of whom (shades of modern fundamentalism here) thought that by executing the king of Divine Right, they were heralding the return of Christ himself. The reason to come here is to gape at the nine grandiose ceiling murals by Peter Paul Rubens in which the king is portrayed as a god. They give you a bold clue as to why the rabble would want to see His Highness brought low. Thoughtfully, mirrored tables help you inspect the ceiling without craning your head to behold why Charles lost his.

Whitehall at Horseguards Ave., SW1. www.hrp.org.uk. ℭ **084/4482-7777.** Admission £6.50 adults, £5.50 seniors and students (including audio tour), free for children 15 and under (posted rates are higher and include a "voluntary donation"). £1 cheaper if bought online. Daily 10am–5pm; last admission 30 min before closing. Tube: Charing Cross or Westminster.

Clarence House ★ HISTORIC HOME The queen dictates who lives at which palace, and she herself lived at this four-story mansion, a part of St James's Palace, before she took the throne. Her mother dwelled here for nearly half a century until her 2002 death at age 101, and now it's chez Charles and Camilla. Charles, having a keener sense of public relations than any royal before him, decided to open the house, where royals have lived since 1827, during the summer when the family is away. You won't get to poke around the Prince's medicine cabinet, though; you can only see the ground floor. Clarence is more like a grand town house than a king's mansion, and that reflects the Windsors' homey, cluttered style, heavy on horse paintings and light on gilding and glitter.

Stableyard Rd., SW1. www.royalcollection.org.uk. ℭ **020/7766-7303.** Admission £10 adults, seniors, and students, £6 children 5–16. Aug Mon–Fri 10am–4:30pm; Sat–Sun 10am–5:30pm; last admission 1 hr before closing. Tube: Green Park.

Jewel Tower ★ HISTORIC SITE   Built around 1365, it's one of only two remnants left from the 1834 fire that ravaged the Royal Palace of Westminster. Quiet and easily overlooked, this three-level stone tower, once a moatside storehouse for Edward III's treasures, has walls so thick it was later considered an ideal setting for taking accurate measurements. So you'll see some explanation of weights-and-measures standards and some relics dug up from the moat (including a 1,200-year-old sword, and a bulbous bottle from the Sun, a 17th-c. tavern where Samuel Pepys drank).

Abingdon St., SW1. www.english-heritage.org.uk. ⓒ **020/7222-2219.** Admission £5 adults, £4.50 seniors and students, £3 children 5–15. Apr–Sept daily 10am–6pm; Oct–Nov 2 daily 10am–5pm; Nov 3–Mar Sat–Sun 10am–4pm. Tube: Westminster.

The Queen's Gallery ★ MUSEUM   The queen inherited the mother of all art collections—7,000 paintings, 30,000 watercolors, and half a million prints, to say nothing of sculpture, furniture, and jewelry—but she shows only a tiny fraction. The few works (budget 1 hr.) are undoubtedly exceptional (one of the world's few Vermeers, a Rubens' self-portrait given to Charles I, glittering ephemera by Fabergé), but depending on what temporary exhibition supplements them, they may not be the cream of what she owns, and it may bore kids. The Gallery and the Royal Mews can be seen on a joint ticket (£19 adults, £17 seniors and students, £10 children 5–16).

Buckingham Palace Rd., SW1. www.royalcollection.org.uk. ⓒ **020/7766-7301.** Admission £11 adults, £10 seniors and students. £5.50 children 5–16. Sept–July daily 10am–5:30pm; Aug–Sept daily 9:30am–5:30pm; last admission 4:30pm. Tube: Victoria.

The Royal Mews ★ MUSEUM   Most visitors pop in to what amounts to the queen's garage in about 15 minutes. You'll see stables fit for a you-know-who (they barely smell at all) and Her Majesty's Rolls-Royces (many of which, at Prince Charles's behest, run on green fuels). You'll also overdose on learning about regulations for when this set of harnesses may be used and when that leather must be polished. The Queen's Gallery and the Mews can be seen on a joint ticket (£19 adults, £17 seniors and students, £10 children 5–16).

Buckingham Palace Rd., SW1. www.royalcollection.org.uk. ⓒ **020/7766-7302.** Admission £10 adults, £9.20 seniors and students, £5.80 children 5–17. Apr–Oct 10am–5pm; Nov–March 10am–4pm; last admission 45 min before closing. Tube: Victoria.

MARYLEBONE & MAYFAIR

Apsley House ★★ HISTORIC HOME   This is how you'd be rewarded if you became a colonial war hero: You'd get Hyde Park as a backyard. In 1815, Arthur Wellesley defeated Napoleon and became the Duke of Wellington, and later prime minister. The mansion, still in the family (they maintain private rooms), was filled with splendid thank-you gifts showered upon him by grateful nations, including a thousand-piece silver set from the Portuguese court. Still, he never seemed to get his nemesis off his mind: Under the grand staircase stands a colossal nude statue of Napoleon that the little emperor despised; the Duke cherished it as a token of victory. Apsley's supreme art stash, which was largely looted by the French from the Spanish royal family and never went home, includes a few Jan Bruegel the Elders, Diego Velasquez's virtuosic *The Waterseller of Seville* (you can understand why it was the artist's favorite work—just looking at it makes you thirsty); and Correggio's *The Agony in the Garden,* in a case fitted with a keyhole so the Duke could open it and polish it with a silk hankie. The Duke and his best friend lived here together after their wives died, and the whiff of faded masculine glory pervades the place like cigar smoke. In other circumstances, the Duke and Napoleon, who both liked fancy finery and fancier egos, would have been buddies. If you're also visiting Wellington Arch (p. 142), a joint ticket will save a couple of pounds.

149 Piccadilly. www.english-heritage.org.uk. ⓒ **0870/333-1181.** Admission £9.30 adults, £8.40 seniors and students (including audio tour), £5.60 children 18 and under. Apr–Oct Wed–Sun 11am–5pm; Nov–Mar Sat–Sun 11am–5pm. Check ahead for closures. Tube: Hyde Park Corner.

Handel & Hendrix Museum ★ HISTORIC HOME   Here's a pleasant *Messiah* complex. This Mayfair building, the German-born composer's home from 1723 (he was its first tenant) to his death in 1759, has lived many lives—before the museum's 2001 opening, conservators chipped 28 layers of paint off the interior walls to uncover the original grey color. In its day, it was a factory for his celebrity: Handel would compose in one room, debut his work in another (there are still frequent performances; check the website), sleep in a third, and sell scores and tickets to the public from a ground-floor shop. None of the furniture was his, but Handel fans should investigate the composer's collection at the Foundling Museum (p. 117), where he was a crucial patron. In 2016, the museum expanded to encompass the top floors of a neighboring building, where legendary guitarist Jimi Hendrix lived in 1968 and 1969. Here, in a cozy flat, his girlfriend Kathy Etchingham tried to give him his first stable home; here he made music and love, entertained, filmed interviews (which gave curators images to reconstruct it down to the last detail)—and played Handel records to absorb the genius of his neighbor across the centuries. But Etchingham's nurturing efforts were to no avail; soon after they broke up, he died at age 27 in Notting Hill.

25 Brook St., W1. www.handelhendrix.org. ⓒ **020/7495-1685.** Admission £10 adults, £5 children 5–16 (Handel House only: £7.50 adult, £3 child). Mon–Sat 11am–6pm, last admission 5pm. Tube: Bond St.

Royal Academy of Arts ★ MUSEUM   Britain's first art school, founded in 1768, relocated here to Burlington House, a Palladian-style mansion that now has a splendid courtyard in which to enjoy a coffee away from Piccadilly's fumes (plus an exclusive restaurant, the Keeper's House). The main reason to come is whatever crowd-pleasing paid exhibition is on, so you're always at risk of not having much fun. A few permanently available

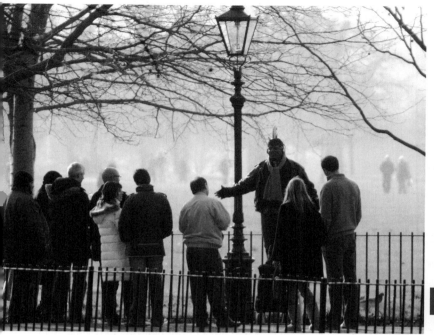

Speaker's Corner in Hyde Park is an authorized place of free speech.

objects on the third floor include Michelangelo's only marble sculpture in Britain, an unfinished circular relief of Mary with the babies Jesus and John. The biggest event, and always worth it, is the annual **Summer Exhibition,** which since the late 1700s has displayed the best works from anonymous submissions; careers are made by it. Charles Darwin's *Origin of the Species* papers were delivered for the first time on July 1, 1858, in the Reynolds Room, now part of the John Madejski Fine Rooms. Don't miss the wooden red "Phone Box No. 1" tucked behind the stone front gate—it was the 1924 prototype for what we now recognize as an international icon.

Burlington House, Piccadilly, W1. www.royalacademy.org.uk. ⓒ **020/7300-8000.** Free admission. Daily 10am–6pm (Fri until 10pm); last admission 30 min before closing. John Madejski Fine Rooms by free tour only: Tues 1pm, Wed–Fri 1pm and 3pm; Sat 11:30am. Tube: Piccadilly Circus or Green Park.

Speakers' Corner ★ LANDMARK

Near the northeast corner of Hyde Park, where Edgware Road meets Bayswater Road, Londoners of yore congregated for public executions. By the early 1800s, the gathered crowds were jeering at hangings instead of cheering them, and the locale's reputation for public outcry became entrenched. An Act of Parliament in 1872 finally legitimized it as a place of free speech, and its tradition of well-intentioned protest has evolved into a quirky weekend attraction. Laborers and suffragettes fomented social change here, but these days, you're more likely to encounter a rogues' gallery of idealists and religious nutters. Anyone can show up, always on Sunday mornings after 7am, with a soapbox (or, these days, a stepladder), plus an axe to grind, and orate about anything from Muslim relations to the superiority of 1970s disco—but if they don't have the wit to appease the crowd, they stand a good chance of being jibed, or at the very least vigorously challenged. In true British style, most speakers refrain from profanity. Even the heckling is usually polite. ("Communists, violent racists, vegetarians," reported Arthur Frommer in 1957. "They undergo the finest heckling in the world, a vicious repartee. . . .")

Tube: Marble Arch, exits 4, 5, 8, or 9.

The Wallace Collection ★★★ MUSEUM   A little bit V&A (decorative arts and furniture), a little bit National Gallery (paintings and portraits), but with a boutique French flair, the Wallace celebrates fine living in an extravagant 19th-century city mansion, the former Hertford House. Rooms drip with chandeliers, clocks, suits of armor, and furniture, usually of royal provenance, and there's not a clunker among the paintings. While other museums were stocking up on Renaissance works, the Wallaces, visionaries of sorts, were buying 17th- and 18th-century artists for cheap, and now its collection shines. You might recognize Jean-Honoré Fragonard's *The Swing* (Oval Drawing Room), showing a maiden kicking her slipper to her suitor below. Peter Paul Rubens' *The Rainbow Landscape* is also here (East Drawing Room), as is the world's most complete room of furniture belonging to Marie-Antoinette (Study; look for her initials hidden around a keyhole on one cabinet). Thomas Gainsborough's *Mrs. Mary Robinson "Perdita"* (West Room) depicts the sloe-eyed actress in mid-affair with the Prince of Wales; she holds a token of his love, a miniature portrait, in her right hand. If she exudes suspicion, it's for good reason—the Prince dumped her before the paint was dry. Don't miss the recently restored Great Gallery, a stupendous tour de force of world-class old master paintings. Red folders contain descriptions of pictures, and gold ones are for furniture—the information even tells who owned them before they got here. Be in the Ground Floor State Rooms at the top of the hour, when a chorus of golden musical clocks announce midday direct from the 1700s. Kids should grab a free trail map, which leads them to the most attention-holding works, but adults should get the audio guide which highlights 80 of the best items for £4. The Wallace Restaurant, in the covered courtyard, has an exemplary atmosphere but stupidly high prices, although its French-styled afternoon tea is under £19 or just £7 if you only want tea and scones.

Hertford House, Manchester Sq., W1. www.wallacecollection.org. ✆ **020/7563-9500.** Free admission. Daily 10am–5pm. Tube: Bond St.

Wellington Arch ★ LANDMARK   When it was finished in 1830, it was intended as a triumphal entry to central London (Marble Arch, at Hyde Park's northern corner, was originally Queen Victoria's triumphal entry to

DEATH TAKES A holiday

If you're a major musical star, stay away from London! It seems a disproportionate number of singers have met untimely ends here (especially in the summer). These houses aren't open to the public, but their grim pasts make them music landmarks:

o **June 22, 1969, 4 Cadogan Lane, Belgravia** (Sloane Square tube): **Judy Garland** overdosed on barbiturates (Seconal) and expired in the bathroom of the two-room flat owned by her fifth husband of three months, Mickey Deans. The public outpouring of grief, and its suppression by police in New York City, is credited with starting, or at least fueling, the gay rights movement as we know it today.

o **September 18, 1970, 22 Lansdowne Crescent, Notting Hill** (Notting Hill Gate tube): In a basement flat of the Samarkand Hotel, **Jimi Hendrix** washed down nine Vesperax sleeping pills with alcohol. An ambulance was summoned, but arrived too late. The plot thickened 26 years later, when the last person to see him alive, girlfriend Monika Dannemann, was found asphyxiated in a car in Seaford, East Sussex, not long after being accused in court of keeping secrets about Hendrix's final moments.

o **July 29, 1974 and September 7, 1978, Flat 12, 12 Curzon Place, Mayfair** (Hyde Park Corner tube): **"Mama" Cass Elliot** of The Mamas and the Papas was found dead in between solo performances at the London Palladium in a flat owned by songwriter Harry Nilsson, who wasn't home. Contrary to lore, she didn't die by choking on a ham sandwich but from a heart attack in her sleep brought on by morbid obesity (she was 165cm/5'5" and weighed 108kg/238 lb.). Four years after Elliot's death, **Keith Moon**, drummer of The Who, died in the same flat. His undoing: chlormethiazole edisylate, a prescribed anti-alcohol drug. Horrified that two of his friends should die while borrowing his apartment, Nilsson quickly sold it to Moon's bandmate Pete Townshend.

o **July 23, 2011, 30 Camden Square, Camden** (Camden Town tube): After a period of abstinence, **Amy Winehouse** binged on vodka and succumbed to alcohol poisoning in her bedroom in this 2,500-square-foot townhouse, where she'd lived only a few months. Security guards were there but thought she was only sleeping. For years afterward, fans would leave bottles and cans of booze outside as a macabre tribute.

Buckingham Palace). Now it's the equivalent of a shrug. Minor anecdotes of its relocation and the switch from Wellington's original statue on top to a smaller statue (*Peace Descending upon War,* the largest bronze sculpture in Europe) are all this handsome landmark can muster in its little museum, which also discusses the period when the Arch served as a police station. If you buy a joint ticket with the Apsley House, across Piccadilly (p. 139), you'll save a couple of pounds; you can take an elevator up with the admission price.

Hyde Park Corner, Apsley Way, W1. www.english-heritage.org.uk. © **020/7930-2726.** Admission £5 adults, £4.50 seniors and students, £3 children 5–15. Apr–Sept daily 10am–6pm; Oct daily 10am–5pm; Nov–Mar daily 10am–4pm. Tube: Hyde Park Corner.

KENSINGTON & KNIGHTSBRIDGE

Diana Memorial Fountain ★ LANDMARK   In July 2004, the queen came to Hyde Park, probably grudgingly, to open an unusual gated fountain designed to conjure the memory of the mother of her grandchildren and a longtime thorn in her side, Princess Diana. As designed by American architect Kathryn Gustafson, this graceful, O-shaped fountain undulates down a gentle slope, sending two flumes of water gurgling into a collecting pool. At three points, bridges carry you to the center. Rather than putting you in a state of remembrance, it may put you into a state of wanting to ride it on an inner tube. Reach it from the Alexandra Gate at Kensington Gore, Knightsbridge, up Exhibition Road, and don't confuse it for the Diana, Princess of Wales Playground in Kensington Gardens or the 17th-century Diana Fountain.

Between West Carriage Dr., Rotten Row, and The Serpentine, Hyde Park. www.royal parks.org.uk. *©* **030/0061-2350.** Free admission. Apr–Aug daily 10am–8pm; Sept daily 10am–7pm; Mar and Oct daily 10am–6pm; Nov–Feb daily 10am–4pm. Check website for maintenance closures. Tube: South Kensington.

Kensington Palace ★ PALACE   Most people know it as the place where Lady Diana raised Princes William and Harry with Prince Charles from 1984 to 1996, but now it's where Prince William, Kate, George, and Charlotte live when they're in town. (No, you won't run into them in the bathroom.) It has

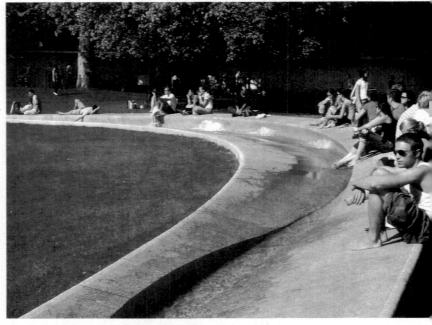

Enjoying a summer day at the Princess Diana Memorial Fountain.

been a royal domicile since 1689, when William and Mary took control of an existing home (then in the country, far from town, to ease William's asthma) and made it theirs. Handsome and haughty, with none of the symmetry that defined later English tastes, the redbrick palace is not as ostentatious as you might expect. At least from the outside. A 2013 "transformation" ruined the experience within. Historic Royal Palaces, grasping for currency, installed junky art installations (voices whispering from gramophones, graffiti-like quotations scrawled across carpets and walls) based on scandals that happened here. The venerable palace was stripped of most of its context and now it's a spook house for art snobs. The newly reopened King's Apartments, pegged to King George III and Queen Caroline, is explained to visitors not with a thoughtful historical dossier but with a scratch-and-sniff guide to odors that might have filled the palace once. Kids may appreciate the costumed characters wandering about, but anyone who can reach the pedals knows it's all style over substance. Queen Victoria has her own section, but she's given the trashy treatment, too—rather than teaching visitors what enabled a girl of 18 to rise to master the most powerful empire in the world, it shows her, misogynistically, in terms of gender roles: as a good girl, a loving wife, and a grieving widow. It's also misleading: One room draped in black leads you to believe Prince Albert died here, but no, he died at Windsor.

Thankfully, the walk-through still includes the magnificent King's Staircase, lined with delicate canvas panels whose perimeters are rigged with tissue paper slivers that will tear as a warning of shifting or swelling. The staircase is considered so precious that it wasn't opened to the public until 2004, 105 years after the rest of the palace first accepted sightseers. In the Gallery there's a working Anemoscope, which has told the outside wind direction since 1694, and a map of the world as known in that year; you'll also see gowns worn by HM the Queen, Diana, and Princess Margaret, who lived here as well. Overall, though, if you're short on time, this pandering Palace is no longer a must-see.

Kensington Gardens, W8. www.hrp.org.uk. ⓒ 084/4482-7777. Admission £17 adults, £14 seniors and students (including audio tour), free for children 15 and under (higher posted prices include a "voluntary donation"). Mar–Oct daily 10am–6pm; Nov–Feb daily 10am–5pm; last admission 1 hr before closing. Tube: High Street Kensington or Queensway.

THE SECRET tube line

New for 2018, the **Postal Museum & Mail Rail** is two attractions in one. The first holds exhibits about the social history of mail delivery in the capital, or "centuries of inspiring and surprising British history through the colourful lens of the postal service." But the most anticipated aspect of a visit will be the Mail Rail, a little-seen 22-mile underground line that from 1927 to 2003 was used for postal delivery, but a short portion now carries curious tourists on a one-mile looping journey 70 feet below the streets on its diminutive carriages. *Phoenix Place, WC1. www.postalmuseum.org. Daily 10am–5pm, last admission 4:15pm. Admission £9 plus Mail Rail ride £5.50. Tube: Chancery Lane or Russell Square.*

Natural History Museum ★★ MUSEUM   The commodious NHM, which attracts 5.5 million visitors a year (mostly families, and by far the most of the three big South Ken museums), is a true blockbuster and it's good for several hours' wander, but you'll have plenty of company. In all ways, it's a zoo. You get a hall of dinosaur bones, a taxidermist's menagerie, and case after case of stuffed goners. Mostly, you'll encounter the wildest creatures of all: lurching, wailing, scampering children in all their varieties. On weekends and school holidays, the outdoor queue can be an hour long, so go at opening and enter through Exhibition Road for lighter crowds. The trove is rich: At the top of the stairs, the **Treasures** gallery holds such historically meaningful stuff as a dodo skeleton and Britain's only moon rock. The pretend kitchen full of hiding places for insects and **Creepy Crawlies** (the **Green Zone**) are longtime visitor favorites, as is the **Red Zone** (the Earth Galleries), anchored by a toned-down, ride-along mock-up of a Japanese supermarket jolted by the 1995 Kobe earthquake. Even the dinosaurs (in the **Blue Zone**) are supplemented by scary robotic estimations of how they sounded and moved. The **Darwin Centre**'s Cocoon looks like a seven-story egg laid in the back atrium; hidden inside are some 20 million bottled specimens (including those that came back on the *Beagle*) on 27km/17 miles of shelves, which you will not see. Most of the discussion here, and throughout the museum, is aimed at a child's mind, with signs answering such unasked questions such as why we study nature, but now and then you'll see an expert through a window into the stacks of the Centre who can use a microphone to respond to more intelligent concerns.

Even if you don't give a hooey about remedial ecology, the cathedral-like 1880 Victorian building is unforgettable. Columns crawl with carved monkeys whimsically clinging to the terra-cotta and plants creeping across ceiling panels. Daily Nature Live talks are given at 2:30pm on a huge range of topics; they're put online, too. The Museum's brainiacs even cultivate a garden and pond (the **Orange Zone;** open Apr–Oct) that attracts a range of English creatures and flowers. Kids under 7 can borrow free Explorer backpacks with pith helmets, binoculars, and activities themed to Monsters, Birds, Oceans, or Mammals (they tend to run out early on weekends); and those 7 to 14 should look for the hands-on **Investigate** lab in the basement

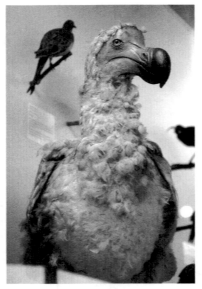

The Dodo bird, now extinct, lives on at the Natural History Museum.

(afternoons are less crowded). All that and the requisite ceiling whale.

Cromwell Rd., SW7. www.nhm.ac.uk. ⓒ **020/7942-5000.** Free admission. Daily 10am–5:50pm. Tube: South Kensington.

Royal Albert Hall ★★ CONCERT HALL   In addition to being a great concert venue, the Royal Albert is also one of London's great landmarks, and you don't need a seat to enjoy it. Conceived by Queen Victoria's husband Albert, it opened in 1871, a decade after his death from typhoid (Vicky was so distraught that she didn't speak at the opening ceremonies). If you don't mind stairs, you can take a 1-hour tour. The hall contains such oddities as Britain's longest single-weave carpet (in the corridors), the Queen's Box (still leased to the monarchy), and a spectacular glass dome (41m/135 ft. high and supported only at its rim). Only groups can go backstage, however: Some 320 performances a year are presented, many with less than 24 hours' set-up time, and a flow of sightseers would be in the way.

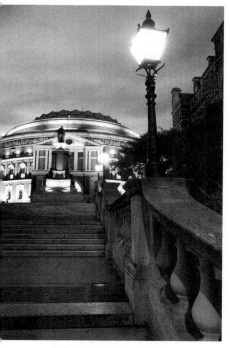

Royal Albert Hall is one of London's great landmarks.

Kensington Gore, SW7. www.royalalberthall.com. ⓒ **020/7589-8212.** Free admission to lobby, tours £13 adults, £11 seniors and students, £6 children 18 and under. Tours available most days; times vary, generally 9:30am–4:30pm. Tube: South Kensington.

Science Museum ★★ MUSEUM   It's really two museums, one old-fashioned and one progressive, that have been grafted together and embellished with a few tacky gimmicks and blatant corporate propaganda, but it's a firm family favorite, attracting 3.4 million visits in 2015. So many interesting exhibitions are on display here that you'll probably run out of time. The old-school section, which began collecting in 1857 and is split over six levels, is an embarrassment of riches from the artifact archives of science and technology: 1969's *Apollo 10* command module; "Puffing Billy," the world's oldest surviving steam engine; and the first Daguerreotype camera from 1839. In 2015, the rare clocks and watches of London's prestigious Clockmakers' Museum, most dating from 1600 to 1850, moved here from their overlooked space in Guildhall (p. 163). Upper floors are full of model ships and 1950s computers (second floor, where a £16.5-million hall about the Information Age has been installed), veterinary medicine (fifth floor), and in the hangarlike third floor, aviation. Highlights there: a complete De Havilland Comet, which was the first jetliner (1952), a slice of a jumbo jet, and a modified Vickers Vimy bomber, the first plane to cross the Atlantic without stopping. It was flown by Arthur Whitten Brown, who promptly became the first person to report jet lag. He called it something less catchy: the "difficulty of adjustment to the sudden change in time." New is the Mathematics gallery (second floor), one of the last projects overseen by the late architect Zaha Hadid, full of lovely swooping forms inspired by the aerodynamic flow around its central object: an experimental Handley Page aircraft from 1929 that was only made possible by math (or as the English call it, "maths").

The high-concept wing buried in the back of the ground floor is easy to miss, but seek it out. A cobalt-blue cavern for interactive games and displays, it bears little relation to the mothballed museum you just crossed through. The Antenna exhibition (ground floor) is exceptionally cutting-edge, and updated regularly with the latest breakthroughs; past topics have included biodegradable cell phones implanted with seeds and building bricks grown from bacteria. The interactive exhibits of Launchpad (third floor; heat-seeking cameras, dry ice, and the like) enchant kids. But not everything in the museum is enchanting. The gift shop (mostly mall-style toys) and guidebook disappoint. And when you've got the actual Model T, why charge an extra £11 for a gimmicky IMAX 3D cinema or £6 on motion simulator rides? Fortunately, the merits override the patronization.

Exhibition Rd., SW7. www.sciencemuseum. org.uk. © **087/0870-4868.** Free admission. Daily 10am–6pm. Tube: South Kensington.

V&A ★★★ MUSEUM   If it was pretty, well-made, or valuable, the British Empire wanted to possess it. As a decorative arts repository, the Victoria & Albert, occupying a haughty High Victorian edifice (it was endowed by the proceeds from the first world's fair, the Great Exhibition of 1851), is about the eye candy of objects—not so much for paintings—and if you're paying attention, it tells the story of mankind through the development of style and technique.

As for how to tour it, the ground floor, a jumbled grid of rooms, has

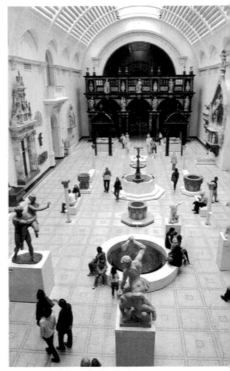

The interior of the V&A Museum is all about eye candy.

lots of good stuff, but lots more bric-a-brac (Korean pots, 1,000-year-old rock crystal jugs from Egypt) that you'll probably walk past with polite but hasty appreciation. The second, third, and fourth levels have less space and therefore are more manageable. Look for the **Theatre & Performance** collection (103–106b), which was rescued from the bygone Theatre Museum in Covent Garden and adds the spark of modern familiarity to the proceedings; you can see, for example, Vivien Leigh's Tony Award and costumes from *The Lion King.*

Rooms are arranged by country of origin or by medium (ironwork, tapestries, and the like) but you'll want to see the **20th Century** (rooms 74, 76; level 3), which surprises by including objects you may have once kept in your home (a Dyson vacuum cleaner, mobile phones); the U.K.'s only permanent **Architecture** gallery (rooms 127–128a, level 4), for a nautilus-like preconstruction model of the Sydney Opera House; and endless slices of **medieval stained glass** (rooms 83–84, level 3). Wherever you go, if you see a drawer beneath a display case, open it, because many treasures are stored out of the light. More not to miss:

o The **Europe 1600–1815 galleries,** to the left as you enter, were recently renovated to be bright, rich, and instructive. They're crammed with 1,100 precious objects including 300-year-old furniture, 18th-century court clothing that looks like it was made yesterday, and even an entire bedchamber from the 1600s. Stream the audio guide from vam.ac.uk/europeaudio (there's free Wi-Fi).

o The seven **Raphael Cartoons** (room 48a), 500 years old in 2015, are probably the most priceless items. These giant paper paintings—yes, paper—were created by the hand of Raphael as templates for the weavers of his 10 tapestries for the Sistine Chapel. Before Queen Victoria moved them here, they hung for around 175 years in the purpose-built Cartoon Gallery at Hampton Court Palace (p. 179). The colors are fugitive, meaning they're fading: Christ's red robe, painted with plant-based madder lake, has turned white—his reflection in the water, painted with a different pigment, is still red. Yet the queen recently decided people could take flash photos of it.

o None of the sculptures in the sky-lit **Cast Court** (rooms 46 and 46a) are original. They're casts of the greatest hits in Renaissance art, and they crowd the room like a yard sale. They were put here in 1873 for the poor, who could never hope to see the real articles for themselves. Find Ghiberti's doors to the baptistery at Florence's San Giovanni, whose design kicked off the artistic frenzy of the Renaissance, and Michelangelo's *David,* floppy puppy feet and all; he was fitted with a fig leaf for royal visits. Depressingly, many of these replicas are now in better shape than the originals.

o Tipu Sultan of India hated imperialists. So, in the 1790s he commissioned an automaton of a tiger devouring one. A crank on **Tippoo's Tiger** (room 41) activates a clockwork that makes an Englishman's hand flail and an organ makes his gaping mouth moan. In the end, Tipu was killed by

Kensington & Knightsbridge

Europeans and the English got his Tiger after all. It has been a crowd favorite since 1808, when it was part of the East India Company's trophy museum.

o The **Great Bed of Ware** (room 57), a 10-by-11-foot four-poster of carved oak that dates to about 1590, was once a tourist attraction at a country inn, renowned enough for Shakespeare to mention it in *Twelfth Night:* "big enough for the bed of Ware." As you admire it, consider that in those days, bed canopies were installed to protect sleepers from insects that might tumble out of their thatched roofs and into their mouths. Canopied beds, a mark of luxury today, were a sign of a humbler home. Nearby is James II's silver-embroidered wedding suit (1673, room 56).

o The **Ardabil carpet** (room 42), the world's oldest dated carpet (copies lay on the floors of 10 Downing St. and Hitler's Berlin office alike), is from 1539. To preserve its dyes, it's lit 10 minutes at a time on every half-hour.

o The **Hereford Screen** (1862, Ironworks balcony) is a liturgical riot by Gilbert Scott, the architect of the "Eros" (p. 127) and the St Pancras Renaissance (p. 36). It took 38 conservators 13 months to restore the 8-ton choir screen to its full golden, brassy, painted Gothic Revival glory.

o The **Gilbert Collection** (rooms 70–73) of impossibly fine jewel boxes, cameos, silver, and mosaics was amassed by a rich enthusiast who originally gave them to LACMA in California, where he made his fortune. But in a museum-world scandal, he stripped them from it for not showing the whole collection at once. Despite that slap in the face, the V&A still displays only highlights and the galleries may be closed.

Questions about what you're seeing will be referred to the Info Desk, which in turn may be referred to a search on a computer screen, possibly your own. Such is the sad reality of today's heavily touristed museum. That's why planning pays off: Download a map and you'll save £1, and download its free app to see what hot-ticket exhibitions are coming, many of them on topics that pander to a wide paying audience (David Bowie, Pink Floyd) or are blatantly influenced by sponsors (historic underwear). The big one in 2017 was about the late 1960s; it cost £16, a typical upcharge for an exhibition here. Free 1-hour introductory tours are given at 10:30am, 12:30pm, 1:30pm, and 3:30pm, with one for the Medieval and Renaissance galleries at 11:30am and another for the British galleries at 2:30pm. Kids can borrow delightful "Back-Packs" at a dedicated Families Desk in the Learning Centre, which contain activity sets that engage them in some of the museum's most eye-catching holdings. More goodies for kids are listed at www.vam.ac.uk/families and exhibited at the Museum of Childhood (p. 172). Even the cafe (the world's first museum restaurant) is gorgeous; have a coffee in the extraordinary Gamble Room (1865–1878), a visual feast in ceramic tile and enameled iron. Also visit the V&A's western exterior; scarred during the Blitz, the stonework was left unrepaired as a memorial.

Cromwell Rd., SW7. www.vam.ac.uk. ℂ **020/7942-2000.** Free admission. Daily 10am–5:45pm (Fri until 10pm). Tube: South Kensington.

Other Kensington & Knightsbridge Attractions

Albert Memorial ★ LANDMARK Albert, Queen Victoria's German-born husband (and, um, first cousin), was a passionate supporter of the arts who piloted Britain from one dazzling creative triumph to another. But when he died suddenly of typhoid (some say Crohn's disease) in 1861 at age 42, the devastated queen abruptly withdrew from the gaiety and remained in mourning until her death in 1901, shaping the Victorian mentality. She arranged for this astounding spire—part bombast, part elegy—to be erected in 1872 opposite the concert hall Albert spearheaded. Some of its nearly 200 figures represent the continents and the sciences, and some, higher up, represent angels and virtues. It's Victorian high-mindedness in stone. At the center, as if on an altar, is Albert himself, gleaming in gold. Guided explanations happen at 2 and 3pm on the first Sunday of each month, March to December (© **020/8969-0104;** no reservations required; 45 minutes; £8).

Kensington Gardens. www.royalparks.org.uk. Tube: South Kensington.

The Design Museum ★ MUSEUM Newly relocated to a cavernous landmark modernist building in Kensington, The Design Museum is where you'll find the cool kids of current style and architecture waxing esoteric about their thought processes in themed exhibitions. The top floor balcony celebrates everyday objects (typeface, laptops) that have been designed well. In point of fact, it's more of a gallery than a museum, appealing more to designers than to scholars. Everything is imbued with an awareness of how design can improve the lives of the less fortunate, a notion that's at best Victorian and at worst condescending, and the curators occasionally appear to sell out to sponsors (a recent show rhapsodized about Cartier wristwatches), but the rewards may be richer if there's a good temporary exhibition on. The shop has some interesting finds, as you might suspect.

224–238 Kensington High St., W8. www.designmuseum.org. © **020/3862-5900.** Permanent collection free, exhibitions charge £10–16. Daily 10am–6pm; last admission 5pm. Tube: High Street Kensington.

THE SOUTH BANK, SOUTHWARK & BOROUGH

Florence Nightingale Museum ★ MUSEUM You probably don't know much about her now, but spend 45 minutes in this small and well-designed biographical museum (on the grounds of the hospital with which she worked) and you'll brim with newfound respect for this consequential person—as a founder of sensible nursing practices, as a leader who took no guff, and ultimately, as an all-around hard-core badass. It's broken into three sections, attractively presented and with kid-friendly elements: her headstrong youth, her fame-making work whipping the troop hospitals of the Crimean

War into shape, and her subsequent years of cranky reclusiveness and ceaseless writing.

2 Lambeth Palace Rd., SE1. www.florence-nightingale.co.uk. ℭ **020/7620-0374.** Admission £7.50 adults, £4.80 seniors and students, £3.80 children 15 and under. Daily 10am–5pm. Tube: Westminster, Waterloo, or Lambeth North.

Garden Museum ★ MUSEUM Ordinarily, I'd say that given the niche subject matter of British gardening, you could skip this one—but in 2017, it revealed a macabre secret about what was *really* planted here: a tomb heaped with 30 crumbling lead coffins, containing among them as many as five Archbishops. In 1977, the museum had been set up as a way to preserve this site, the abandoned church of St Mary's, but—garden museum irony alert—no one had thought to dig down until 2017, when they had to even out some paving stones. Workers found a hole leading into a chamber, put a smartphone on a selfie stick, and nearly died of heart attacks when they captured a collapsing pile of blackened and rotten coffins, topped with a gilded tin mitre hat—like your nightmare's nightmare. You can peer into the chamber, too, through a glass panel, but you're not allowed to go into the resting place because of the risk of viscous black "coffin liquor" spraying all over you. There are other graves you can see: Captain Bligh of *Bounty* fame is buried in the yard. Oh, yeah, and there's gardening stuff, too—an assortment of antique gardening implements and a collection of gardening-related art. Fun fact: The roundabout to the south, at Lambeth Bridge, is where, in *National Lampoon's European Vacation*, Clark Griswold told his kids, "Big Ben! Parliament!"

5 Lambeth Palace Rd., SE1. www.gardenmuseum.co.uk. ℭ **020/7401-8865.** Admission £10 adults, £8.50 seniors, £5 students, children under 6 free. Church tower another £3. Sun-Fri 10:30am–5pm, Sat 10:30am–6pm (but check ahead). Closed first Mon of month. Tube: Westminster, Waterloo, or Lambeth North.

Imperial War Museum London ★★ MUSEUM One of London's unexpectedly gripping museums has a deceptive name. It's not just for military buffs, and it's no gun-fondling armory, even if there is a Spitfire hanging from the rafters. Instead of merely showcasing heavy implements of death, which it does, this museum—the latest tenant of the commodious former mental hospital known as Bedlam—takes care to convey the sensations, feelings, and motivations of soldiers and civilians caught in past conflicts. It is ultimately not about weapons but a museum about *people* at war. In addition to easy-to-grasp background on major conflicts, the museum intelligently balances tanks and planes with storytelling that unravels propaganda. In 2014, the IWM was expensively renovated from a brick storehouse into a gleaming facility—while some exhibits were perhaps oversimplified, the First World War Galleries (reserve ahead in peak season) are the most advanced, best-stocked, most comprehensible, and most moving you'll ever see on the topic, followed by the segment on the Holocaust.

Lambeth Rd., SE1. www.iwm.org.uk. ℭ **020/7416-5000.** Free admission. Daily 10am–6pm, last admission 5:30pm. Tube: Lambeth North or Elephant & Castle.

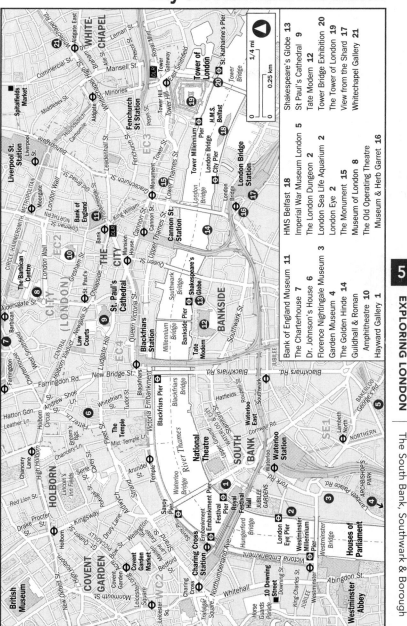

Bank of England Museum **11**
The Charterhouse **7**
Dr. Johnson's House **7**
Florence Nightingale Museum **3**
Garden Museum **4**
The Golden Hinde **14**
Guildhall & Roman
Amphitheatre **10**
Hayward Gallery **1**

HMS Belfast **18**
Imperial War Museum London **5**
The London Dungeon **2**
London Sea Life Aquarium **2**
London Eye **2**
The Monument **15**
Museum of London **8**
The Old Operating Theatre
Museum & Herb Garret **16**

Shakespeare's Globe **13**
St Paul's Cathedral **9**
Tate Modern **12**
Tower Bridge Exhibition **20**
The Tower of London **19**
View from the Shard **17**
Whitechapel Gallery **21**

5

EXPLORING LONDON | The South Bank, Southwark & Borough

London Eye ★★★ OBSERVATIONAL WHEEL   The Eye was erected in 1999 as the Millennium Wheel, and like many temporary vantage points, it became such a sensation—and a money-spinner—that it was made permanent. It rises above everything in this part of the city—at 135m/443 ft. high, it's 1½ times taller than the Statue of Liberty. The 30-minute ride above the Thames affords an unmatched and unobstructed perspective on the prime tourist territory; there's no narration, but six tablets elucidate what's before you. On a clear day, you can see to Windsor, but even on an average day, the entire West End bows down before you. That's why you should either go as soon as you arrive in the city, to orient yourself, or on your last day in town (my choice), when you can appreciate what you've seen. The whirl is adulterated by a lame "4D Experience" movie (a camera flies over London while a fan and bubbles blow in your face—it's Orlando-fied twaddle) but it's included in the price and you can skip that if you want. Each of the 32 enclosed capsules, which accommodate up to 28 people, is climate-controlled and rotates so gradually that it's easy to forget you're moving—which means this ride will upset only the desperately height-averse. By the time you summit, you'll have true 360-degree views unobstructed by the support frame. The ticket queue often looks positively wicked (book ahead if possible), but it moves quickly, chewing through 15,000 riders a day, 800 per revolution. The Shard (p. 157) is much taller (and costs much more), which is why you have a much better chance of appreciating what you're seeing aboard the Eye. *Tip:* Booking online saves waiting in the first queue, but you will be bewildered by the ticket options. Basically, a Standard timed ticket will do, although you can pay up to £30 to go anytime you want ("Flexi") rather than stick to a reservation or to wait in a shorter line ("Fast Track").

Riverside Building, County Hall, SE1. www.londoneye.com. ⓒ **0871/781-3000.** Advance purchase prices for standard ticket: £23 adults, £19 children 4–15, free for children 3 and under. Walk-up prices 10% higher. Apr–June 10am–9pm; July–August 10am–9:30pm; Jan–Mar and Sept–Dec 10am–8:30pm. Tube: Waterloo or Westminster.

The Old Operating Theatre Museum & Herb Garret ★★ MUSEUM

In the mid-1800s, before general anesthesia, St Thomas' Hospital used the attic of a neighboring church as a space where surgeries, mostly amputations and other quick-hit procedures, could be conducted where students could watch but other patients couldn't hear the agonized screams. When the hospital moved in 1862, it was abandoned, sealed away, and forgotten. It was considered lost until 1956, when an enterprising historian thought to look in the attic, and found the secret surgical stadium behind a wall. Creep up a tight wooden spiral staircase once used by the bell ringer and you'll find the theater, now the centerpiece of a ghoulish, but carefully educational, museum delving into medical methods of the early 1800s, from herbal remedies to leeches. On a recent visit, a 7-year-old boy in a visiting school group nearly passed out during a mock bloodletting show-and-tell; the staff, accustomed to fainters, casually produced a pillow and a glass of water without halting the demonstration, proving that in the old days, medicine was less about science and more about soldiering on.

9a St Thomas St., SE1. www.oldoperatingtheatre.com. ✆ **020/7188-2679.** Admission £7 adults, £5 seniors and students, £4 children 15 and under. Daily 10:30am–5pm. Closed late Dec–early Jan. Tube: London Bridge.

Shakespeare's Globe ★ LANDMARK   A painstaking re-creation of an outdoor Elizabethan theater, it tends to bewitch fans of history and theater, but it can put all others to sleep. Arrive early since the timed 40-minute tours fill up. Get a bad time, and you'll be stuck waiting for far too long in the Under-Globe, a well-crafted but exhaustible exhibition about Elizabethan theater. Also avoid matinee days, since tours don't run during performances. Opened in 1997, the open-air theater was made using only Elizabethan technology such as saws, pillars made from solid oak trees, 17,000 bundles of Norfolk water reed, and plaster panels mixed with goat's hair (the original recipe called for cow's hair, but the breed they needed is now extinct). The first Globe burned down, aged just 14, when a cannon fired during a performance caused its thatched roof to catch fire; it took a special act of Parliament, plus plenty of hidden sprinkler systems, to permit the construction of this, the first thatched roof in London since the Great Fire. The original theater was the same size (and stood 180m/591 ft. to the southeast), but it crammed in 3,000 luckless souls. Today, just 1,600 are admitted for performances. If you'd like to see the location of the **Rose Theatre,** a true Shakespeare original, go around the corner to 56 Park St., where its foundations, discovered in 1989 and now squatted over by a modern office building, are open for visitors on Saturdays from 10am to 5pm. There's a video on how it was discovered and it also hosts regular performances (www.rosetheatre.org.uk; ✆ **020/7261-9565;** free admission).

21 New Globe Walk, SE1. www.shakespearesglobe.com. ✆ **020/7401-9919.** Exhibition admission £16 adults, £15 seniors, £13 students, £9 children 5–15. Exhibition: daily 9am–5pm. Theater tours: daily 9:30am–5pm; check ahead for schedule changes. Tube: London Bridge.

Tate Modern ★★★ MUSEUM   In 2000, Bankside's most reviled eyesore, a goliath power station—steely and cavernous, a cathedral to the soulless machinery of industry—was ingeniously converted into the national contemporary art collection of pieces made since 1900. Now it's a temple to the machinery of the art world. It's as integral to London as the Quire of Westminster Abbey or the Dome of St Paul's, attracting 4.7 million annual visitors. The mammoth Turbine Hall, cleared of machinery to form a meadowlike expanse of concrete, often hosts works created by major-league artists for its periodic Hyundai Commission. People of every background frolic there as if it were a park.

In 2016, behind schedule and over budget, the Tate took on declining attendance by expanding its exhibition spaces by 60% with a newly built expansion in back. Now the Turbine Hall connects the original post-industrial, three-level galleries (the riverfront Boiler House) with a twisting 10-story custom-built tower behind them (Switch House) that's topped with a terrace for views of St Paul's' dome. Beneath the new tower, in the power station's former oil

MUSEUMS: after hours

Many attractions offer extended opening times for evening viewing. Often, extra inducements are tossed in, such as wine and sketch classes at the National Portrait Gallery or DJs at the V&A. These are the major "Lates" events that can really free up your daytime touring to include more sights:

ATTRACTION	LATE OPENING
British Museum (p. 113)	Friday to 8:30pm
British Library (p. 109)	Tuesday–Thursday to 8pm
Design Museum (p. 151)	Friday to 8pm (first of month)
Handel House Museum (p. 140)	Frequent evening concerts
London Canal Museum (p. 191)	Thursday to 7:30pm (first of month)
London Zoo (p. 186)	Friday to 10pm (selected nights)
National Gallery (p. 122)	Friday to 9pm
National Portrait Gallery (p. 124)	Thursday–Friday to 9pm
Natural History Museum (p. 146)	Friday to 10:30pm (last of month)
Royal Academy (p. 140)	Friday to 10pm
Science Museum (p. 147)	Wednesday to 10pm (last of month)
Sir John Soane's Museum (p. 126)	Tuesday to 9pm (first of month)
Tate Britain (p. 132)	Friday to 10pm (once bi-monthly)
Tate Modern (p. 155)	Friday–Saturday to 10pm
Victoria & Albert Museum (p. 148)	Friday to 10pm
Wellcome Collection (p. 119)	Friday to 10pm (first of month except Jan & Aug)
Whitechapel Gallery (p. 168)	Thursday to 9pm

tanks, new performance spaces try to engage visitors (check online ahead of time for what's on).

The addition is impressive but it doesn't solve some of the core problems with the Tate: Great works are too often rotated into storage, so there's no guarantee of what you'll find, and the pieces that are on display annoy many visitors as joyless or overly esoteric. The commissions in the Turbine Hall are so massive they take weeks to assemble, so there's a good chance you won't be able to enjoy that part of the facility when you visit. And descriptions dwell on pretentious doubletalk and the incestuous art world culture—"works gathered in this wing capture making as gesture, the trace of an action," whatever that means—something you may ameliorate with the "Modern Art Terms" glossary smartphone app ($3), one of many apps the museum puts out to explain what its signs won't (warning: The free Wi-Fi is inadequate on busy days). On the second floor, rent a multimedia guide of the highlights (£4.25, one version for adults, another for kids, and you can swap between them) on a video device that embellishes on the works' meaning and context. Maps cost £1, so consider going online ahead of time to print floor plans for free. Also see what temporary exhibitions are on—in early 2018, the blockbuster is an examination of Pablo Picasso in 1932, a pivotal year of his life—which can make or break your visit.

The formidable permanent collection, one of the world's best for breadth, is always shifting, not just because the museum owns more than it can display (even with the new tower), but also because works vanish on short-term loans. Some heavy hitters never leave, though. My favorite: Seven of the nine monotonal series created by Mark Rothko for New York City's Four Seasons restaurant, which never fail to put visitors in a meditative mood (one of them, *Black on Maroon,* was restored after a 2012 vandalism incident). There are four free daily guided tours, usually at 11am, noon, 2pm, and 3pm; ask at the ground-floor desk to find out where to join them. At the family desk, open on weekends and busy days, kids pick up free drawing kits or tours based on sounds. One thing not to miss is the shop on the bottom floor. Also carve out refreshment time: The restaurant on Level 6 can be inhospitable due to crowds—but when I'm here, I beeline for the 30 first-come bar stools facing floor-to-ceiling glass over St Paul's and the Thames. Afternoon tea is just £15 (Fri–Sun), and the fish and chips platter with mushy peas has my approval for flavor if not price (£18).

Bankside, SE1. www.tate.org.uk/modern. © **020/7887-8888.** Free admission. Sun–Thurs 10am–6pm; Fri–Sat 10am–10pm. Tube: Southwark.

View from the Shard ★ OBSERVATION DECK In 2013 the Shard, the tallest building in Europe (but not even in the top 50 worldwide), added an extremely expensive observation deck with timed tickets—sunset sells out ahead of time, but if you come during the day, you can come back after dark on the same ticket. Jude Law called it "about the most unfortunate name for a building in the world," and the jagged 306m/1,016 ft.-tall tower doesn't exactly fit in with its neighbors. Even its prices are outsized: green-screen souvenir photos, which staff members desperately hustle you to purchase, start at £22, and a glass of champagne will be £10 to £12. After airport-style security and two ear-popping fast elevator rides, you emerge 244m/800 feet up to some weird angel-like choir music and vertiginous floor-to-ceiling windows far, far over the city—so far that, after the initial impression, casual visitors aren't likely to discern most of what they're seeing. A few levels up (hoist yourself upstairs for the last three floors), there's a second patio level shielded at body-level from the elements. You can stay as long as you want, but there's no seating and no washrooms up there, so take care of business on Earth. There is one novel addition: Point a digital "TellScope" in the distance, and its screen reveals the same view at different times of day. The unblinking truth? The London Eye is more memorable and a better experience than a £31 elevator ride.

Joiner St., SE1. www.theviewfromtheshard.com. © **0844/499-7111.** Admission £31 adults, £26 student, £25 children 4–15, £5 discount if booked 24 hr ahead. Apr–Oct daily 10am–10pm; Nov–Mar Sun–Wed 10am–7pm and Thurs–Sat 10am–10pm. Tube: London Bridge.

Other Bankside/Southwark Attractions

Brunel Museum ★ MUSEUM/HISTORIC SITE Although the engineering contributions of Marc Brunel and his son Isambard Kingdom Brunel are commonly taken for granted, here they're given their due. With the help of a shield system they invented, these pioneers executed the first tunnel to be built under a navigable river. London's soft earth didn't make it easy, though—it took from 1825 to 1843. This red brick building marked by a chimney was where steam engines pumped the seeping water out as diggers toiled. The tunnel, lined with arches and Doric capitals, was a commercial flop that deteriorated into a subterranean red-light district. It later found new purpose, however, as a part of the Overground Line, and it has gained new respect through this museum, which often creates special events to bring guests into the tunnel. Maximize immersion by combining it with a London Walks tour from Bermondsey Station to the museum door (current times are listed on the website; no reservations needed).

Railway Ave., SE16. www.brunel-museum.org.uk. © **020/7231-3840.** Admission £6 adults, £4 seniors, students, and children. Daily 10am–5pm. Tube: Rotherhithe.

The Golden Hinde ★ HISTORIC SHIP Tucked into one of the few remaining slips that enabled ships to unload in Southwark (another is Hay's Galleria, downstream by the HMS *Belfast* [see below], now a boutique shopping area), is a 1:1 replica of Sir Francis Drake's square-rigged Tudor galleon, which circumnavigated the world from 1577 to 1580. This 1973 version, which is so tiny you will forever feel pity for those old explorers, made its own circumnavigation in 1980. Self-guided and hour-long guided tours are available daily (usually at 1pm), but check the schedule for regular Pirate Fun Days, Battle Experience events, and Tudor Fun Days for kids, as well as sleepovers (Mar–Oct) during which the little ones can dress in period clothes, hear tales from costumed actors, and help with shipboard tasks on an imaginary voyage.

Pickfords Wharf, Clink St., SE1. www.goldenhinde.com. © **020/7403-0123.** Adults £6, £4.50 seniors and students and children 4–16.

HMS *Belfast* ★ HISTORIC SHIP It's as if the powerful 1938 warship, upon being retired from service in 1965, was motored straight to this dock and opened to visitors the next day. Nearly everything, down to the checked flooring and decaying cables, is exactly as it was, making the boat a fascinating snapshot of midcentury maritime technology, and smart exhibits do a lot to make it come alive again. Authenticity also makes it a devil to navigate, especially if you have any bags with you—sorry, no cloakrooms, sailor. Getting around its labyrinth of decks, engine rooms, ladders, and hatches requires dexterity and a well-calibrated inner compass—it seems the Health and Safety rules that bedevil every aspect of British life do not apply here. You can roam as you wish, visiting every cubby of the ship from kitchen to bridge, touching nearly anything you want, while being thankful that it wasn't you who was

The South Bank, Southwark & Borough

EXPLORING LONDON

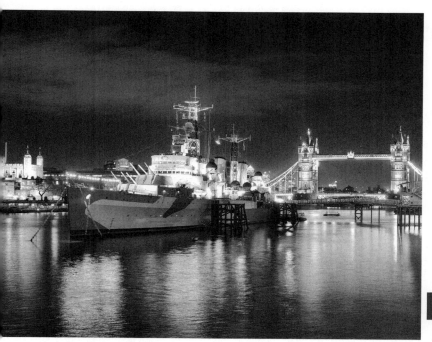

HMS *Belfast* and Tower Bridge.

chasing German cruisers (the *Belfast* sank the *Scharnhorst*) and backing up the D-Day invasion in this tough tin can. Admission includes an excellent audio guide, but privately, crew members tell me that they wish visitors would pause and ask them questions in person—there's so much more to point out to you. The price is too high for those with a lukewarm interest, but the Tom's Kitchen bar, atop the visitor center (a wine bar overlooking a warship—appropriate?), has stellar views of the Tower of London and Tower Bridge—and an afternoon champagne tea that's just £15. Thanks, World War II!

Morgan's Lane, Tooley St., SE1. www.iwm.org.uk. © **020/7940-6300.** Admission £15 adults, £12 seniors and students, £7.25 children 5–15 (higher posted prices include a "voluntary donation"). Mar–Oct daily 10am–6pm; Nov–Feb daily 10am–5pm; last admission 1 hr before closing. Tube: London Bridge.

THE CITY

Museum of London ★★★ MUSEUM This repository's miraculous cache of rarities from everyday life would do credit to the greatest national museums of any land, and it's sure to satisfy history buffs. Displays contain so many forehead-smackingly rare or fascinating items that by the time you're two-thirds through it, you'll start to lose track. Exhibits start with local archaeological finds (including elephant vertebrae and a lion skull) before

A Poignant Pocket Park

Little-known **Postman's Park** is beloved by those lucky enough to have stumbled across it. Hemmed in between buildings, its central feature is the moving **Watts Memorial,** a collection of plaques dedicated to ordinary people who died in acts of "heroic self sacrifice." Have a seat on a bench and ponder John Clinton, 10, "who was drowned near London Bridge in trying to save a companion younger than himself" in July 1894. In 1893, William Freer Lucas tantalizingly "risked poison for himself rather than lessen any chance of saving a child's life and died." Alice Ayres saved three children from a burning house in 1885 "at the cost of her own young life." The commemorations mostly ceased in Edwardian times (poor Leigh Pitt squeaked in after saving a drowning child in 2009), making these forgotten faces obscure once again. (West side of St Martin's-Le-Grand between St Paul's Cathedral and the Barbican Centre; 8am–dusk; St Paul's or Barbican tube.)

continuing to 3,500-year-old spearheads and swords found in the muck of the Thames. Voices from the past come alive again in chronological order: There's a 1st-century oak ladder that was discovered preserved in a well, Norman chain mail, loaded gambling dice made of bone in the 1400s, a leather bucket used in vain to fight the Great Fire of 1666, a walk-in wooden prison cell from 1750, Selfridge's original bronze Art Deco elevators, and far, far more. The biggest drawback is that you need to budget a few hours, otherwise you'll end up in a mad rush through the entire lower floor covering the Great Fire to now—and it'd be such a shame to miss diver Tom Daley's teeny Stella McCartney swim trunks. You also don't want to miss the Victorian Walk, a kid-friendly re-creation of city streets, shops and all from the 1800s (grab a card at its entrance to know what you're seeing). Also seek out the Lord Mayor's state coach, carved in 1757, which garages here all year awaiting its annual airing at the Lord Mayor's Show in November, and Great Britain's petal from the Olympic flame cauldron, on display until mid-2018 alongside a re-creation of a portion of it (the original petals were given to each country they represented).

The museum, built into the Barbican complex beside a Roman wall fragment (it will move to Clerkenwell in 2022), is easy to combine with a visit to St Paul's, and it sells one of the best selections of books on city history. It also runs an excellent second museum in East London about Docklands (p. 172). Download its absorbing (and free) Streetmuseum app, which shows you archival images and historic facts that relate to wherever you're standing in London. So rich is this city in history that behind the scenes, the Museum owns the world's largest archaeological archive, which is open for tours a few times a year.

150 London Wall, EC2. www.museumoflondon.org.uk.© **020/7001-9844.** Free admission. Daily 10am–6pm, galleries close 5:40pm. Tube: Barbican or St Paul's.

St Paul's Cathedral

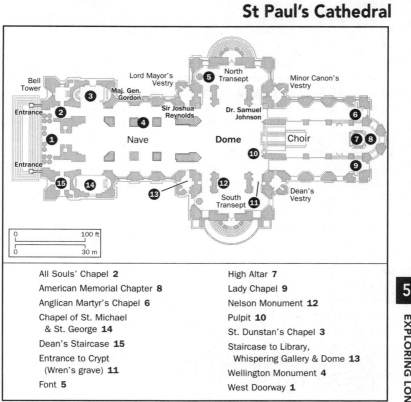

All Souls' Chapel **2**
American Memorial Chapter **8**
Anglican Martyr's Chapel **6**
Chapel of St. Michael
  & St. George **14**
Dean's Staircase **15**
Entrance to Crypt
  (Wren's grave) **11**
Font **5**

High Altar **7**
Lady Chapel **9**
Nelson Monument **12**
Pulpit **10**
St. Dunstan's Chapel **3**
Staircase to Library,
  Whispering Gallery & Dome **13**
Wellington Monument **4**
West Doorway **1**

St Paul's Cathedral ★★★ HISTORIC SITE/CHURCH The old St
Paul's, with its magnificent spire, stood on this site for 600 years before it was
claimed by 1666's Great Fire. It was so beloved that when Sir Christopher
Wren was commissioned to rebuild London's greatest house of worship, he
tried to outdo the original, devoting 40 years to the project and going one
further by crowning it with a mighty dome—highly unusual for the time. It
was also stark and plain, like the Catholics did their churches, not Gothic and
complicated like the Protestants. My, how people talked.

St Paul's cost £750,000 to build, an astronomical sum in 1697 when the first
section opened for worship, and now, it costs £3 million a year to run. Wren
overspent so badly that decoration was curtailed; the Byzantine-style mosaics
over the Quire weren't added until Queen Victoria thought the place needed
spiffing up (and some purists are still complaining). Stained glass is still

missing, but that just allows the sweep and arch of Wren's design to shine cleanly through. Many foreigners were introduced to the sanctuary during the wedding of Prince Charles and Lady Diana Spencer in 1981, but the pulpit also saw a sermon by Martin Luther King in 1964 and Churchill's funeral the next year. Frustratingly, you're not allowed to take photos on your tour.

The **Great West Doors,** largely unused unless you're important, are 27m high (90 ft.) and on their original hinges; they're so well-hung that even a weakling can swing them open. In 2005, the Cathedral completed a £10.8-million cleaning program; a stone panel beside the doors was left filthy to show just how gloomy centuries of candles had made it in here. The **High Altar** has a canopy supported by single tree trunks that were hollowed out and carved, and its 15th-century crucifix and candlesticks require two men to lift. (They're nailed down, anyway. As one docent, a half-century veteran of Cathedral tours, lamented, "You'd be surprised what people try to steal.") Behind it is the **American Memorial Chapel** to the 28,000 American soldiers who died while based in England in World War II; in a glass case, one leaf of a 500-page book containing their names is turned each day. The **organ,** with 7,000 pipes, was regularly played by Mendelssohn and Handel, and the **lectern** is original. Give special admiration to the impossibly fine limewood carvings in the Quire by Grinling Gibbons—dark wood is original and lighter wood has been replaced or restored. Nearby, there's a monument to prettyboy poet and cleric **John Donne** that still bears on its urn the scorch marks it suffered in Old St Paul's during the Great Fire (it was the only thing that survived the conflagration).

Eight central pillars support the entire weight of the wood-framed Dome; Wren filled them with loose rubble. In 1925, engineers broke them open to find the debris had settled to the bottom, and they filled them again with liquid concrete. If you're fit, you can mount the 259 steps (each just an awkward 13cm/5 in. tall, but double-wide with some spots to catch your breath) to the circular **Whispering Gallery,** 30m/98 feet above the floor. Famously, its acoustics are so fine you can turn your head and mutter something that can be understood on the opposite side, 33m/108 feet away. That's in theory; so many tourists are usually blabbing to each other that you won't hear a thing, although it is a transcendent place to listen to choir rehearsal on a mid-afternoon. Climb higher (you've gone 378 steps now, and now the stairs get tight) to the **Stone Gallery,** an outdoor terrace just beneath the Dome. Catch your breath, if you choose, for the final 152-step push to the **Golden Gallery**—you'll be scaling the inner skin of the Dome, past ancient oriel windows and along tight metal stairs. There are three domes, in fact—the inner skin with the monochrome paintings by Sir James Thornhill, the leaden outside, and in between, a brick one that holds it all together. That's what you traverse—look sharp for ancient carved graffiti by tourists who preceded you in the 1700s. It's safe, but it's not for those with vertigo or claustrophobia. The spectacular 360-degree city view from the top (85m/279 ft. up), at the base of the Ball and Lantern (you can't go up farther), is so beautiful that it defies full appreciation. For more than 250 years, this was the tallest structure in London, and therefore the top of the world.

If you miss the **Crypt,** you'll have missed a lot. In addition to memorials to the famous dead (such as Florence Nightingale and plenty of obscure war heroes), you'll find tombs, such as composer Sir Arthur Sullivan's ebullient bronze plate and the tombs of two of Britain's greatest military demigods: **Admiral Horatio Nelson** (whose body was preserved for the trip from the battlefield by soaking in brandy and wine), and **Arthur Duke of Wellington** (flanked by flags captured on the field of battle; they will hang there until they disintegrate). To the right of the OBE Chapel, in **Artists Corner,** you'll find the graves of the artists **J. M. W. Turner** and **Henry Moore,** plus, under a black slab by a window, **Christopher Wren** himself, who rests inside his masterpiece. "I build for eternity," he once said, and so far, so good: In 2010, the cathedral celebrated 300 years since its completion.

Volunteers, called "supers," lead free 90-minute tours at 10am, 11am, 1pm, and 2pm, and half-hour highlights tours six times a day between 10:30am and 3pm. Listen closely, because they are the elder statesmen; many have been here for decades. Lest you forgot it's actually a cathedral, you can also worship here outside of sightseeing hours—for free. If you're hungry, scope out the cafe, one of the cheaper options in this neighborhood. When you're done inside, head just east to the **One New Change** shopping complex, where the free rooftop terrace has some spectacular close-up views of the Dome—perfect for vacation snaps.

St Paul's Churchyard, EC4. www.stpauls.co.uk. (𝒸 **020/7246-8357.** Admission £18 adults, £16 seniors and students (up to £2 cheaper online), £8 children 6–17, free for children 5 and under. Mon–Sat 8:30am–4:30pm; Sun open for worship only. Whispering Gallery and Dome 9:30am–4pm. Tube: St Paul's.

The Forgotten Colosseum

Guildhall, a magnificent stone structure originally completed in 1440 but heavily rebuilt time and again, was once where Londoners went to pay taxes but today is used as the City's most regal events space. Partly due to World War II's wrath, the collection at its **Guildhall Art Gallery** is perhaps second-rate (for this city), although its works depicting London can be interesting. But the real reason to come is in the cellar: the foundations of the eastern entrance of **London's Roman Amphitheatre,** 2,000 years old, which were discovered when the gallery was being built in 1987. Once the largest in Britannia, the amphitheater could hold some 7,000 spectators at a time when the entire population of London was only about 25,000. Slots carved into one of the rooms suggest there was once a trap door that could release wild animals to fight in the arena. Sometimes it's hard to believe the Romans trod the same streets as you, but here in the darkness deep underground, the bones of their abandoned plaything provide an eerie reminder. (Gresham St., EC2; www.guildhall.cityoflondon.gov.uk; (𝒸 **020/7332-3803;** admission free except for exhibitions; Mon–Sat 10am–5pm, Sun noon–4pm, free 45-minute tours Tues, Fri, Sat 12:15pm, 1:15pm, 2:15pm, 3:15pm; Moorgate or St Paul's tube.)

Tower Bridge Exhibition ★★ LANDMARK   In the late 1800s, there was no bolder display of a country's technological prowess than a spectacular bridge; consider the Brooklyn Bridge or the Firth of Forth Bridge. This exhibit celebrates one such triumph, Tower Bridge. You may wonder: How did such a monument survive the Blitz when everything around it got flattened? Simple: The Luftwaffe needed its proud towers as a visual landmark. It's always free to walk across the bridge on your own, but visiting this museum is like getting two attractions in one. The first satisfies sightseers who dream of going up in the famous neo-Gothic towers and crossing the high-level observation walkways—it's a close encounter with a world icon. The second aspect delves into the steam-driven machinery that so impressed the world in 1894; those displays will hook the mechanically inclined. The original bascule-raising equipment, representing the largest use of hydraulic power at the time, remains in fine condition despite being retired in favor of electricity in 1976. The raising of the spans is now controlled by joystick from a cabin across the road from the entrance (check "Bridge Lift Times" on the website to find out when, or download the free "Raise Tower Bridge" app to watch it happen in 360-degree augmented reality). Recently, a glass floor was installed in a portion of the upper walkway so visitors can get giddy to the sight of the river 42m (138 ft.) below their feet. *Note:* Tickets are discounted if you also buy entry to the Monument (p. 169).

Tower Bridge (on the Tower of London side), SE1. www.towerbridge.org.uk. © **020/ 7403-3761.** Admission £9.80 adults, £6.80 seniors and students, £4.20 children 5–15; about £1 cheaper online. Apr–Sept daily 10am–6pm; Oct–Mar daily 9:30am–5:30pm; last admission 30 min before closing. Tube: Tower Hill or Tower Gateway DLR.

The Tower of London ★★★

MUSEUM/HISTORIC SITE   Every morning at 9am, a military guard escorts the keys to the Tower and its huge wooden doors yawn open again for outsiders. It's the most famous castle in the world, a UNESCO World Heritage Site, and a symbol of not just London, but also of a millennium of English history. Less a tower than a fortified mini-town of stone and timber, its history could fill this book. Suffice it to say that its oldest building, the four-cornered White Tower, went up in 1078, and the compound that grew around it has served as palace, prison, treasury, mint, armory, zoo, and now, a lovingly maintained tourist attraction that no visitor should neglect. Exploring its sprawl should take between 3 and 5 hours.

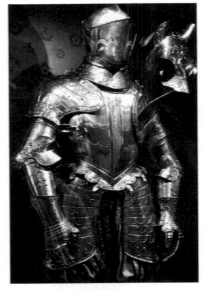

Knight's armor is on display at The Tower of London.

Tower of London

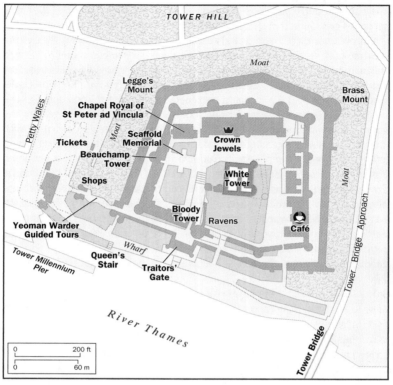

TOWER HILL

Moat

Legge's
Mount

Brass
Mount

Chapel Royal of
St Peter ad Vincula

Petty Wales

Moat

Scaffold
Memorial

Crown
Jewels

Tickets

Beauchamp
Tower

White
Tower

Shops

Moat

Bloody
Tower

Ravens

Yeoman Warder
Guided Tours

Café

Tower Bridge Approach

Tower Millennium
Pier

Wharf

Queen's
Stair

Traitors'
Gate

River Thames

0	200 ft
0	60 m

Tower Bridge

The key to touring the Tower is to arrive close to opening, since intimidating queues can form by lunchtime for the Crown Jewels, located in the Waterloo Block at the north wall (farthest from the Thames), and the White Tower, in the center. Tickets are sold outside the battlements. Hit the Welcome Centre, just past the Ticket Office, and grab a copy of the free "Daily Programme," which runs down the times and locations of all the free talks, temporary exhibitions, and mini-performances. Plenty are offered—the Tower at times feels like a theme park with 1,000 years of history behind it. As soon as you're in, between the Middle and Byward towers, note the next time of the prime excursion: the 1-hour **Yeoman Warder Tour,** led with theatrical aplomb by one of the Beefeaters who live in the Tower and preserve it. (There are about 100 Tower residents, including families, but only one of the 35 Beefeaters, Moira Cameron, is female.) The tour (don't come later than 2pm if you want one) is engaging, but juvenile—expect bellowing and histrionics, each reciting an identical script with a gleeful fetish for yarns about beheadings and torture. (In truth, you can count the people executed inside the Tower on your fingers and toes; it was considered an honor to be killed here, since it was private.) If you'd like your history delivered without vaudevillian shenanigans, head to the gift shop on the right after Middle Tower and grab an audio tour (£4) but do it early; headsets can run out. The official guidebooks (£5) here are pretty good, and they certainly help with orientation.

As you enter the **Crown Jewels** exhibition, you'll see archival film of the last time most of the jewels were officially used, at the coronation of Queen Elizabeth in 1952. After passing into a vault, visitors glide via people-movers past cases of glittering, downlit crowns, scepters, and orbs worn (awkwardly—they're 2.3kg/5 lb. each) by generations of British monarchs. Check out the legendary 105-carat Koh-I-Noor diamond, once the largest in the world, which is fixed to the temple of the **Queen Mother's Crown** (1937), along with 2,000 other diamonds; the Indian government has been begging to get the stone back. The 530-carat Cullinan I, the world's largest cut diamond, tops the Sovereign's **Sceptre with the Cross** (1661). The **Imperial State Crown**—ringed with emeralds, the 170-carat Black Prince's ruby, and diamonds aplenty—is the one used in the annual State Opening of Parliament; the solid gold **St Edward's Crown** is for coronations. After those come candlesticks that could support the roof of your house, trumpets, swords, and the inevitable traffic jam around the 1 meter-wide **Grand Punch Bowl** (1829), an elaborate riot of lions, cherubs, and unicorns that holds 144 bottles' worth and shows what it would look like if punch bowls could go insane. Because Oliver Cromwell liquidated every royal artifact he could get his hands on, everything dates to after the Restoration (the 1660s or later). Clearly, the monarchy has more than made up for the loss.

Touring the four levels of the cavernous **White Tower** requires much circuitous stair-climbing, but takes in a wide span of history, including a fine stone chapel, Norman-era fireplaces and toilets, the gleaming **Line of Kings** collection of the **Royal Armoury** (even small children can't help but notice the exaggerated codpiece of King Henry VIII's intricately etched suit from 1540), and some models depicting the Tower's evolution (it's been much altered, but the six smallest arched windows on the White Tower's south side are original to the 11th c.). Try to time your arrival on the top floor to take one of three daily tours (10:45am, 12:45pm, or 2:15pm) of the nearly 1,000-year-old **Chapel of St John.** After you're finished in here, you'll have an excellent overview of how the whole complex worked.

Once you've got those two areas under your belt, take your time exploring the rest. I suggest a stop

The Ravens, Forevermore

Ravens probably first visited the Tower in the 1200s to feast on the dripping corpses of the executed, who were taken from Tower Hill (the public execution ground, near the present-day Tube stop) and hung outside the battlements as a warning. You've probably heard the modern legend that if the ravens ever leave the Tower, England will fall—so seven of the carnivorous birds are kept in cages north of Wakefield Tower, where they are fed raw meat, blood-soaked cookies, and the occasional finger from a tourist dumb enough to get too close.

in the brick **Beauchamp Tower** (pronounced *beech*-um, built in 1280), where important political prisoners were held and where you can still glimpse graffiti testifying to their suffering. In front of it on Tower Green is the circular glass memorial designating the **Scaffold Site,** where the unlucky few (including sitting Queens Anne Boleyn and Lady Jane Grey) are said to have lost their heads. In reality, we don't know exactly where they were killed, but Queen Victoria wanted a commemorative site set, and because of the evident dangers of displeasing the monarch, this spot was chosen.

The **St Thomas's Tower,** from the 13th century, is closest to the Thames and re-creates King Edward's bedchamber with authentic materials. Beneath it, **Traitor's Gate,** once called Water Gate, originally was used to ferry prisoners in secret from the Thames. Torture was never a part of English law, but it happened here anyway, and the **Bloody Tower** was where some of the worst stuff went down. In truth, there were only 48 recorded cases of torture in the Tower, but that doesn't stop curators from devoting an entire room to a display of (mostly replica) torture devices. Don't forget to climb the ramparts for that classic photo of the Tower Bridge. Skip the Royal Fusiliers Regimental Museum, a dreary hodgepodge of military memorabilia.

Daily at 2:50pm, the guards parade outside the Waterloo Block to the Byward Tower. On Sundays, your admission ticket allows you to attend services at the **Chapel Royal of St. Peter ad Vincula,** the Tower's church with a Tudor-era Spanish chestnut ceiling, at 9:15 or 11am; otherwise, the only way to get in, and to see the marble slab beneath which Boleyn and Grey's decapitated bodies were entombed, is with a Yeoman Warder Tour—salacious tales of gory fates are spun virtually on top the graves of the people who suffered them, which by any measure is tacky. It's a shame the cheap histrionics of the interpretation strip this ancient Tower of so much depth and dignity.

Tower Hill, EC3. www.hrp.org.uk. ② **084/4482-7777.** Admission £25 adults, £19 students and seniors, £12 children 5–15 (higher posted prices include a "voluntary donation"), cheaper if purchased online. Mar–Oct Tues–Sat 9am–5:30pm and Sun–Mon 10am–5:30pm; Nov–Feb Tues–Sat 9am–4:30pm and Sun–Mon 10am–4:30pm; last admission 30 min before closing. Tube: Tower Hill or Tower Gateway DLR.

Other Attractions in The City

Bank of England Museum ★ MUSEUM   The intermittently compelling tale of the B of E is recounted in appealingly patronizing but generous detail, accompanied by plenty of antiques from the vaults. That's fine if you understand finance, but most people lose the plot pretty quickly. Along the way are some fun oddities, including a million-pound note, printed in the early 19th century for internal accounting, and reimbursement claims from families of *Titanic* victims. There's lots of expensive swag, such as a primitive safe from 1700, heaps of silver treasures, and a gold bar so pure (1 part in 10,000 impure) that it was given to Queen Elizabeth as a coronation gift. Guess she didn't need it. It's also fun to watch Her Majesty age on the money over the years. The most popular exhibit is probably a 28-lb. standard gold bar encased in a clear plastic box, that you're challenged to lift. The rest of the

GREAT art GALLERIES

Hayward Gallery ★ The principal exhibition space of the Southbank Centre, hidden on its back rampart, hosts terrific blockbuster shows along the lines of Ansel Adams, 1920s Surrealism, and a 60-artist panorama of modern African art. It takes itself quite seriously, which can be good for a laugh. A major show in 2018 is on German photographer Andreas Gursky. South Bank Centre, Belvedere Rd., SE1. www.southbankcentre.org.uk. ⓒ 087/1663-2501. Charge for exhibitions. Mon noon–6pm; Tues–Wed and Sat–Sun 11am–7pm; Thurs–Fri 11am–8pm. Tube: Waterloo.

House of Illustration ★ This gallery-cum-museum is dedicated to the art of illustration—sometimes the children's book kind (world-famous Roald Dahl illustrator Quentin Blake is on the board), sometimes the magazine kind, but always well-selected. You'll find two changing exhibitions at a time plus a fantastic little gift shop. 2 Granary Sq., N1. www.houseofillustration.org.uk. ⓒ 020/3696-2020. Free admission to 1 gallery; charge for exhibitions. Tues–Sun 10am–6pm, last admission 5:30pm. Tube: King's Cross St Pancras.

Saatchi Gallery ★ This landmark, the only resident in the three-story, 6,500-sq.-m (70,000-sq.-ft.) former Royal Military Asylum building (1801) in Chelsea, used to be unmissable for avant garde contemporary art; now exhibitions are too often shills for luxury brands (Hermés, Rolls-Royce). Only commit if the current fare is a true artists' showcase. Duke of York Square, SW3. www.saatchigallery.com. ⓒ 020/7811-3070. Free admission. Daily 10am–6pm. Tube: Sloane Square.

Stephen Wiltshire Gallery ★★ Stephen Wiltshire, an autistic artistic savant, can draw huge, twisting, intricately detailed ink-and-paper landscapes after seeing the real view for just a few seconds. This collection is located in the **Royal Opera Arcade** off Pall Mall, which dates to 1818—it's the world's oldest shopping arcade, essentially the first indoor shopping mall. 5 Royal Opera Arcade, Pall Mall, SW1. www.stephenwiltshire.co.uk. ⓒ 020/7321-2622. Free admission. Mon–Fri 10am–5:30pm, Sat appointment only. Tube: Charing Cross or Piccadilly Circus.

Whitechapel Gallery ★★ Since 1901, the Whitechapel has reliably led the development of new artistic movements. In 1939, it brought to Britain Picasso's newly painted *Guernica* as part of an exhibition protesting the then-current Spanish Civil War. Later it introduced Jackson Pollock's abstracts There's always a challenging exhibition, talk, or screening going on. 77–82 Whitechapel Rd., E1. www.whitechapelgallery.org. ⓒ 020/7522-7888. Free admission. Tues–Sun 11am–6pm (Thurs until 9pm). Tube: Aldgate East.

Bank isn't open, but you can peek inside with the free Bank of England Virtual Tour app.

Threadneedle St., EC2. www.bankofengland.co.uk/museum. ⓒ 020/7601-5545. Free admission. Mon–Fri 10am–5pm, last admission 4:30pm. Tube: Bank.

The Charterhouse ★★ HISTORIC SITE Opened in 2017 after being off limits since 1348, this once-powerful vestige of Medieval London is hard to explain. It has been a monastery, school, mansion, a home for the poor, and a burial ground—in fact, you'll meet the skeleton of one longtime resident, a victim of the Black Plague in the 1300s, discovered in the digging for the new

Elizabeth Line. A journey so winding makes for a hodgepodge of ancient things to amaze you: gardens and cobbled courtyards, a chamber where young Queen Elizabeth I held court, a paneled Jacobean chapel, palpable evidence of the Dissolution of the Monasteries by Henry VIII. It's a miracle that such a pocket of timelessness should still exist in the middle of the city. The museum is free to see, but you want to book ahead for a tour sponsored by the retired Brothers who still take shelter here—they take you into areas you can't otherwise see.

Charterhouse Square, EC1. www.thecharterhouse.org. © **020/3818-8873.** Free admission. Tues–Sat 11am–4:45pm. Standard tours £10 (11:30am, 1:45pm, and 2:45pm Tues–Sat), Brothers' Tours £15 (2.15pm Tues, Thurs, Sat). Tube: Barbican or Farringdon.

Dr. Johnson's House ★ HISTORIC HOME A rare surviving middle-class home from the 18th century (built in 1700), this slouching and brick-faced abode happens to be that of famous lexicographer Samuel Johnson, who lived here from 1748 to 1759. If you're hoping to learn a lot about him, you'll have to spring for a book in the gift shop. Little substance is provided in the house itself, which fortunately merits some mild interest on its own terms (the corkscrew latch on the front door, which prevented lock-picking from above, is an example). The rooftop garret in which Johnson and six helpers toiled to publish the first comprehensive English dictionary was burned out in the Blitz, ironically, by a barrel of burning ink which flew out of a bombed warehouse; you can still see some scorch marks on the ceiling timbers. Ink defined the house and nearly destroyed it, but it also saved it, because the printers who used it in the intervening years boarded up the walls, preserving them. While you're here, pop round the corner to the wonderful Ye Olde Cheshire Cheese pub (p. 107). Dr. Johnson sure liked to.

17 Gough Sq., EC4. www.drjohnsonshouse.org. © **020/7353-3745.** Admission £6 adults, £5 seniors and students, £2.50 children 5–17. May–Sept Mon–Sat 11am–5:30pm; Oct–Apr Mon–Sat 11am–5pm. Tube: Blackfriars.

The Monument ★ LANDMARK Back in 1677, it was the tallest thing (61m/200 ft.) in town and it made people gasp. Today, it's hemmed in by personality-free glass buildings. The Monument was erected to commemorate the destruction of the city by the Great Fire in 1666. Its height also represents the distance east from its base to the site of Thomas Farynor's bakery in Pudding Lane, where the conflagration began. There's only one thing to do in this fluted column of Portland stone: Climb it. The spiral staircase of 15cm (6-in.) steps, which has no landings, gradually narrows as it ascends to the outdoor observation platform—a popular suicide spot until 1842, when a cage was installed. They'll tell you it's 311 steps to the top, but they're lying—it's 313, if you count the two steps before the box office. Check out the metal band snaking down the north side; it's a lightning rod, and it crosses along a Latin inscription blaming Catholics for starting the fire (the insult was chiseled off in 1831). Tickets are discounted in combo deals with the Tower Bridge Exhibition (p. 164). Go on a pleasant day (unless you'd like a good wind whipping), be prepared to leave large bags downstairs, and ask for your free certificate of accomplishment before you go.

Monument St. at Fish St. Hill, WC4. www.themonument.info. © 020/3627-2552. Admission £5 adults, £3.30 seniors and students, £2.50 children 15 and under (cash only). April–Sept daily 9:30am–6pm; Oct–Mar daily 9:30am–5:30pm; last admission 30 min before closing. Tube: Monument or Bank.

EAST LONDON & DOCKLANDS

The part of London east of the City encompasses many square miles and dozens of separate neighborhoods, but most visitors will only hear it referred to broadly as "East London." It starts around Shoreditch and Whitechapel and, as you go east, begins to incorporate rehabbed former industrial wastelands. **Docklands,** the area bordering the river, is rich in upscale condos and corporate offices. **Greenwich** is a gorgeous villagelike neighborhood on the southern bank of the Thames. And in Stratford, the biggest population center of East London, everything seems newly made, including the Queen Elizabeth Olympic Park.

Dennis Severs' House ★★★ MUSEUM   This 1724 town house was dragged down by a declining neighborhood until the 1970s, when eccentric Californian Dennis Severs purchased it for a pittance, dressed it with antiques, and delighted the intelligentsia with this amusingly pretentious imagination odyssey—he called it "Still Life Drama." Other museums are unrealistically neat and cordoned off, but his house looks lived-in, so the past feels as real as it truly was. As Severs, who died in 1999, put it, "In this house it is not what you *see,* but what you have only just *missed* and are being asked to imagine." You could go during the day, but it's best on Monday, Wednesday, and Friday after dark for "Silent Night." As you approach, the shutters are drawn and a gas lamp burns. You're admitted by a manservant who speaks little. He motions you to explore the premises, silently and at your own pace. Suddenly, you're in the parlor of a prosperous merchant in the 1700s; the owners seem to be home but in the next room. Candles burn, a fire pops in the hearth, the smell of food wafts in the air, and a black cat dozes in the corner. Out on the street, you hear footsteps and hooves. Room by dusky room, you silently explore corners overflowing with the implements of everyday life. It's as if the residents were just there, leaving toys on the stairs, beds rumpled, mulled wine freshly spilled, tea growing cold. By the time you explore the attic, you'll have accompanied the house and its occupants through its decay into a collapsing slum. "Silent Night" is one of London's most invigorating diversions.

18 Folgate St., E1. www.dennissevershouse.co.uk. © 020/7247-4013. Admission £10 Mon daytime or Sun visits, £15 Silent Night visits (£18 for Christmas period). Day visits: Sun noon–4pm; selected Mon noon–2pm; last admission 45 min before closing. Silent Night: Mon, Wed, Fri 5–9pm (reservations required). Tube: Liverpool St.

Geffrye Museum ★★ MUSEUM   This complex, a U-shaped line of dignified brick houses built in 1714 for ironworkers, feels removed from the rush of the East End. Inside is a walk through the history of the home:

Docklands & Greenwich Attractions

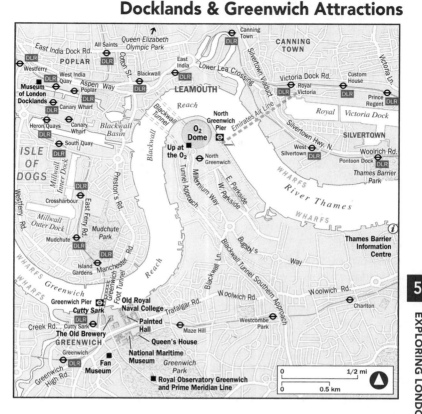

re-creations of typical middle-class London abodes from the 1600s to the late 20th century, artfully arranged to appear lived-in. Complete explanations of each item on display include illuminating information about which pieces were necessary and which were merely trendy. To some, they're just rooms full of furniture; to others, the Geffrye is a chance to understand how people of the past lived. You know which person you are. One building here is a restored almshouse for the poor; book timed tours to see how charity cases lived back in the day (check the website for the schedule; £3 adults, free for children 15 and under). On weekends, curators plan discussions, lectures, and kid-oriented crafts workshops, which gives the place much more energy than you'd expect from a design-based attraction. Especially on fine days from April to October, the grounds are an exceptional place to relax. The walled herb garden encourages touch, to release scents, and its period plots are historically accurate, cultivated with plants used in several eras, including Elizabethan and Victorian times.

136 Kingsland Rd., Shoreditch, E2. www.geffrye-museum.org.uk. (C) **020/7739-9893.** Free admission, including audio tour. Tues–Sun 10am–5pm. Tube: Hoxton.

Museum of Childhood ★★ MUSEUM   The awesome V&A Museum (p. 148) chronicles kid-dom through the ages in this location, pulling from a considerable archive of toys, clothing, dollhouses, books, teddy bears, and games. Objects are placed at kids' eye-level with simplified descriptions. Some young ones don't grasp the concept—toddlers burst into tears when they see a crib behind glass that they can't climb into—but if they're too young for exhibits, bring them to one of the daily kids' activities, such as stories or drawing. Child-rearing history is also addressed; look for the "Princess Bottle" of 1871, which had a reservoir shape that allowed for quick milk dispensing but also incubated bacteria, a fact that wasn't realized until countless babies died. The MoC's double-galleried glass-and-steel hall, which has a cafe, is itself an artifact; it began its life in South Kensington as the home of the nascent V&A collection but was re-erected here in the 1860s—the fish-scale mosaic floor was assembled by female prisoners, many of whom (in an ugly irony) weren't allowed to see their own kids.

Cambridge Heath Rd., E2. www.museumofchildhood.org.uk. ℰ **020/8983-5200.** Free admission. Daily 10am–5:45pm. Tube: Bethnal Green.

Museum of London Docklands ★★★ MUSEUM   Most of the city's museums would have you believe that London was always a genteel bastion of refined gentlemen. The real story lies in working men who shortened their own lives to put teacups into more privileged, manicured hands, and in the labor that circulated profits from slavery into banks and onto City gallery walls. Housed in a brick rum-and-coffee warehouse from 1804, the three-floor museum, strong on plain-speaking explanations, traces the history of working on the Thames, starting with Anglo-Saxon times and ending now. You can inspect an intricate model of the medieval London Bridge, which like the Florentine Ponte Vecchio was stacked with homes and businesses but clogged the river's flow so drastically that it was a threat to life. You'll also roam Sailortown, a creepy warren of quayside alleys, all shanties and low doorways, meant to evoke the area's early-19th-century underworld. Finally, the spotlight shifts to the harrowing Blitz, when the East End, taking the brunt of the Reich, was obliterated by fire from the sky and forced to reinvent itself as a corporate citadel. The whole circuit takes 2 to 3 hours. There's also an interactive, river-themed play area for kids, Mudlarks.

No. 1 Warehouse, West India Quay, E14. www.museumoflondon.org.uk/docklands. ℰ **020/7001-9844.** Free admission. Daily 10am–6pm, galleries close 5:40pm. Tube: West India Quay DLR or Canary Wharf.

Ragged School Museum ★ MUSEUM   The Victorians weren't very nice people. Although in 1883, as many as 60,000 families lived in a single room, church-run schools still charged a penny a week and had a dress code, and the many kids who couldn't manage ended up on the street. Thomas Bernardo was headed for missionary work abroad when he realized East London kids needed him more than foreigners did; he took in the "ragged" children who couldn't even muster shoes, gave them an education, and made them his "home kids," feeding and nurturing them. From 1877 (when one in four

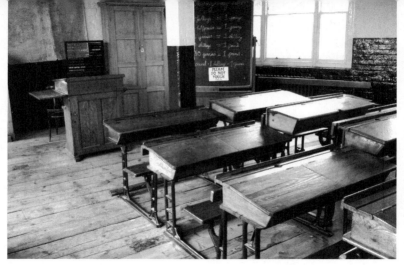

The Ragged School Museum is a time capsule of a Victorian charity school.

children who lived around here died) to 1908, he used this canalside warehouse as a school—playground in the basement, classrooms (now re-created) up top—and he worked to help the most desperate kids emigrate for better lives. One in 11 Canadians can trace their ancestry to "home" children who went to ragged schools like this one. This little museum is like Bernardo's school: homegrown, rough around the edges, run as a labor of love, and welcoming.

46–50 Copperfield Rd., E3. www.raggedschoolmuseum.org.uk. *© **020/8980-6405.*** Free admission (suggested donation). Weds–Thurs 10am–5pm, first Sun of the month, 2pm–5pm. Tube: Mile End or Limehouse DLR

The Royal London Hospital Museum ★ MUSEUM The Royal London Hospital has been central to London life since 1740, when it was established—supported by donations—to help the desperate condition of the poor. That history has put a lot of cool material in its hodgepodge archive, including letters by unfairly forgotten hero nurse Edith Cavell, forensic files from the Jack the Ripper case, a portion of George Washington's false teeth, and personal belongings of Joseph "The Elephant Man" Merrick, the sweet but luckless soul who lived in rooms on the premises until his death at age 27. You'll see it all, plus lot of skin-crawling archaic medical instruments that will fascinate anyone who works in modern healthcare. This place can keep funky hours; it's always smart to call ahead.

St Augustine with St Philip's Church, Newark St., E1. bartshealth.nhs.uk. *© **020/7377-7608.*** Free admission (suggested donation). Tues–Fri 10am–4:30pm Tube: Whitechapel or Aldgate East.

Up at the O₂ ★★ TOUR Built on a toxic peninsula wasteland on the Thames in the '90s, the Millennium Dome was conceived as a showplace for what turned out to be a poorly attended turn-of-the-century exposition. It's

supported by a dozen 100m-tall yellow towers, one for each hour on the clock, in honor of the nearby Greenwich Prime Meridian—a preening and meaningless symbolism that cost £789 million, and then stood empty for half a decade. In 2007, however, it was finally reborn as the city's finest performance arena, with 20,000 seats (p. 242). Now, Londoners can stomp on it like they always wanted. Climbers, about 10 at a time, hook into a safety rigging system and follow a guide over a tensile fabric catwalk laid a few feet over the Dome's roof, to an observation platform at the zenith of the structure. There they pause for 15 minutes of photos of East London (the City is mostly hidden behind Canary Wharf's towers). Beneath them, humming like a ship at sea, is a Dome conquered. The excursion isn't for the height-averse—at your highest, you're 52m (171 ft.) above the ground—and it's not for big eaters or children, either (the weight cutoff is 130kg/286 lb., and you have to be at least 10 years old). But it's also not scary, since you're tethered and the shoes they lend you grip well. If the weather's bad, you get matching jumpsuits like Ooompa-Loompas. The climb, which is more like a stroll up a steep hill, takes 45 minutes; the rest of the 90-minute experience consists of getting harnessed and psyched up.

Peninsula Sq., SE10. www.theO2.co.uk. © **020/8463-2680.** Weekday climbs £28; weekend/holiday/sunset/twilight climbs £35. 10am to 6–10pm, depending on season. Tube: North Greenwich or North Greenwich ferry.

Greenwich Attractions

Situated on a picturesque slope of the south bank of the Thames, Greenwich once was home to Greenwich Palace, where both Henry VIII and Elizabeth I were born. The last part of the palace to be constructed, the **Queen's House** (1616, Inigo Jones, p. 177), still stands, but most of the grounds were rebuilt in the late Georgian period as the equally palatial Royal Hospital, a convalescence haven for disabled and veteran sailors now known as the **Old Royal Naval College** (p. 176). High on the hill, in Greenwich Park, is the **Royal Observatory** (p. 177), and between them stands the **National Maritime Museum** (p. 175). Many of these treasures are owned by the state, so most entrance fees are waived; you can play the whole day without paying more than a few pounds. Most tourists come to get a photo straddling the **Prime Meridian,** the line that slices through the Observatory and marks zero degrees longitude. Stop by the **Discover Greenwich visitor center,** alongside the *Cutty Sark,* for background information and to pick up a walking tour from the Greenwich Tour Guides Association (www.greenwichtours.co.uk; © **0757/577-2298**). Greenwich offers a Meridian Line tour at noon, or town highlights at 2:15pm. Tours costs £8 adult, £7 seniors/students/kids, and last about 90 minutes.

Cutty Sark ★★ HISTORIC SHIP   The only clipper ship left in the world was launched in 1869; by the end of its 52-year career, it had traveled the equivalent of to the moon and back, carrying cargos including tea, wool, and furniture. By the sunset of its sailing life, it was a decrepit old thing, renamed *Ferreira,* having survived hurricanes in America and the loss of its mast in Cape Town. It was eventually drydocked in Greenwich to show off for

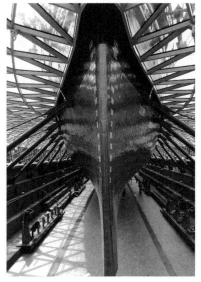
The brass keel of the *Cutty Sark*.

tourists, but worse indignities were yet to come: A 2007 fire twisted its iron frame and devastated its hull planking (fortunately, sails, masts, prow, figurehead, and deckhouses had been safely stored for a restoration). As you tour its hold, climbing stairs and weaving across decks (and accidentally banging your head on low thresholds), note that the white-painted framework you see is original, while the grey is new. Restoration provided an opportunity for the present lavish presentation: Today, it's as gorgeous as when Britain dominated the seas, and instead of floating in the Thames, it floats 3.6m (11 ft.) over a dry dock skirted by a glass canopy. At the end of a full ship tour, visitors can peep beneath the streamlined brassed keel. It's a slight cheat, because the hull originally was coated with Muntz metal, bitumen, and felt, but hey, it looks incredible. It'll never be speedy again, but it's never looked hotter. If you're also entering the Royal Observatory (p. 177), buy a combo ticket and save a few pounds.

King William Walk, SE10. www.rmg.co.uk/cuttysark. (C) **020/8312-6608.** Admission £14 adults, £12 seniors and students, £7 children 5–15 (higher posted prices include a "voluntary donation"). Daily 10am–5pm; last admission 4:15pm. Tube: Cutty Sark DLR, Greenwich river ferry, or Greenwich National Rail.

The Fan Museum ★ MUSEUM   This is as niche as museums get, but it's classy and it truly has the best of what it claims to honor—some 4,000 artful specimens, many of them precious, going back a millennium. Fans were necessities in the centuries before air-conditioning, when flames generated constant heat and corsets severely restricted breathing; these tools were the only things that helped ladies remain conscious. There are regular exhibition of the little lifesavers, such as collections of Christmas-themed imagery, Biblical themes, and so on. The museum also offers a reasonably priced afternoon tea at 2:15pm and 3:45pm (reservations required)—don't faint, but it's just £8.

12 Crooms Hill, SE10. www.thefanmuseum.org.uk. (C) **020/8305-1441.** Admission £4 adults, £3 seniors and students. Tues–Sat 11am–5pm, Sun noon–5pm. Tube: Cutty Sark DLR, Greenwich river ferry, or Greenwich National Rail.

The National Maritime Museum ★★ MUSEUM   Don't be put off by the topic. The world's largest maritime museum is extraordinarily kid-friendly, brimming with buzzy set-piece toys such as steering simulators and a giant play area that looks like a world map. So it's not as, ahem, dry as most would

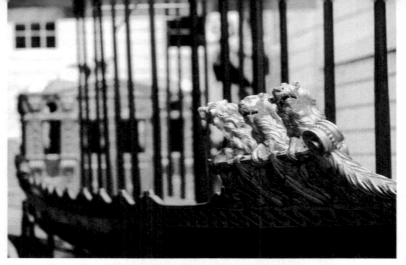
Gold details on a boat on display at the National Maritime Museum.

expect. Because so much of Britain's history from the 17th to 20th centuries was transacted via the high seas, this place isn't just about boats and knots. The facility has an endless supply of Smithsonian-worthy artifacts that would do any museum proud. Highlights include a musical stuffed pig clutched in a lifeboat by a *Titanic* passenger; and, most ghoulishly, the bloodstained breeches and bullet-punctured topcoat that Admiral Lord Nelson wore on the day he took his fatal shot (in a new gallery devoted to the man). Get the creeps from relics from Sir John Franklin's ill-fated 1848 Arctic expedition, including lead-lined food tins that likely caused the explorers to go mad and probably eat each other. Also excellent is the Atlantic Worlds display, which plumbs the British role in the slave trade, something few London museums touch upon. The museum also presents the oft-ignored viewpoint that through the East India Company, England looted India—in fact, the English word *looted* has Hindi origins. It's not all so gloomy, though; there are big set pieces such as figureheads, models, antique instruments, and entire wooden vessels. Weekends are full of free kids' events (storytelling, treasure hunts) that bring suburban London families pouring into the gates, and the fun Greenwich Market is running nearby then, too. Maps cost £1.

Romney Rd., Greenwich, SE10. www.nmm.ac.uk. ℂ 020/8858-4422. Free admission. Daily 10am–5pm. Tube: Cutty Sark DLR, Greenwich river ferry, or Greenwich National Rail.

Old Royal Naval College ★ HISTORIC SITE/LANDMARK   This 1696 neoclassical complex, primarily the work of Christopher Wren, is mostly used by a university but offers two main sights: the Painted Hall and the Chapel. The **Painted Hall,** fresh off a major conservation, is adorned with 40,000 square feet of incredible paintings by Sir James Thornhill that took nearly 2 decades to complete. It was the setting for the funeral of Admiral Nelson, but it may never have looked more glorious than today, because recent restoration removed years of candle grime and even crusty food splatters from rowdy pensioners' banquets. Through September 2018, something special is afoot: You can climb the restoration's scaffolding (adults £10, £5 kids 6–17; book ahead online) and inspect the work close up on 60-minute guided tours. The **Chapel,** in the Greek Revival style, is the work of James Stuart. 90-minute tours by accredited guides run daily at 11:30am and 2pm. If the ORNC's stately symmetry rings a bell, that's because it was used as a stand-in for Paris in the movie musical *Les Misérables.* It's also where you'll find the **Old Brewery** (p. 106), with plenty of garden space where you can kick back with very stiff pints.

Greenwich, SE10. www.ornc.org. ✆ **020/8269-4747.** Free admission. Grounds daily 8am–6pm; buildings daily 10am–5pm; Royal Chapel Sun at 11am for worship. 90-min tours (reservation line ✆ **020/8269-4799**) £5 adults, free for children 15 and under. Tube: Cutty Sark DLR, Greenwich river ferry, or Greenwich National Rail.

The Queen's House ★ HISTORIC HOME   Viewed from the river and framed by the newer Old Royal Naval College, the Queen's House enjoys as elegant a setting as a building could wish for. Inigo Jones took 22 years to come up with a then-revolutionary Palladian-style summer retreat for Charles I's wife, Henrietta Maria. It was completed only in 1638—just before the Civil Wars cut both Charles and his building schemes off at the head, and Henrietta scurried off to France. The house has a few pleasant galleries and displays, including Orazio Gentileschi's *Joseph and Potiphar's Wife,* which, after the house's 2016 restoration, was returned to these walls for the first time since around 1650. The nautilus-shaped Tulip staircase, plus other rooms, are considered to be haunted by an unknown specter, so have a camera ready.

Romney Rd., SE10. www.rmg.co.uk. ✆ **020/8312-6565.** Free admission. Daily 10am–5pm. Tube: Cutty Sark DLR, Greenwich river ferry, or Greenwich National Rail.

The Royal Observatory ★ HISTORIC SITE/MUSEUM   Commanding a terrific view from the hill in Greenwich Park, with the towers of Canary Wharf spread out in its lap, the Observatory is yet another creation of Christopher Wren (from 1675), and the place from which time zones emanate. Historically the Empire's most important site for celestial observation, it houses significant relics of star-peeping, but the paid areas aren't worth the money. Most of the good stuff—marked on the map in red—is free, including a small Astronomy Centre and an exhibition on time. The only things admission buys you are an unremarkable ceiling-projection planetarium and the sparsely furnished, borderline-interesting Flamsteed House by Wren, which has a collection of 18th-century clocks once used to crack the mystery of measuring longitude (an advance that ushered the English Empire to worldwide dominance). Most people plunk down admission not because they care about those but to gain access to the Meridian Courtyard. The Prime Meridian, located at precisely 0° longitude (the equator is 0° latitude), crosses through the grounds, and hordes of coach tourists pay to wait an hour for an Instagram moment of straddling the line with a foot in two hemispheres at once—but the secret is they don't have to. The line continues down the wall on the walkway north of the courtyard, where the Meridian is free and there's never a wait. In the old days, the red Time Ball fell precisely at 1pm daily so that the city could synchronize its clocks; it still rises at 12:55pm and drops 5 minutes later. You could set your watch by it, but technically, you already do. If you're also visiting the *Cutty Sark* (p. 174), a combo ticket will save you a few pounds.

Greenwich Park, Greenwich, SE10. www.rmg.co.uk. © **020/8312-6565.** Free admission for most of grounds. Flamsteed House and Meridian Courtyard: £9.50 adults, £7.50 seniors and students, £5 children 15 and under. Planetarium: £7.50 adults, £6.50 seniors and students, £5.50 children 5–15. Combination ticket: £13 adults, £9.50 seniors and students, £6.50 children 15 and under. Daily 10am–5pm; last admission 4:30pm. Tube: Cutty Sark DLR, Greenwich river ferry, or Greenwich National Rail.

OUTER LONDON

Dulwich Picture Gallery ★★ MUSEUM   A 15-minute train ride from Victoria and an 8-minute walk lands you in a pretty villagelike enclave of South London, where a leafy stroll acclimates one to contemplation and appreciation. Here you'll find one of the world's most vital collections of Old Master paintings of the 1600s and 1700s, kept in just a few rooms. Magnanimous donors made it England's first public gallery (opened 1817), designed with a surplus of light by Sir John Soane (who also left us his own cramped museum; p. 126). A visit is almost indescribably serene, the better to stare into the Cheshire Cat face of one of its star masterpieces, Rembrandt's *A Girl at a Window*—how did he capture her bemusedly frank expression? A handheld video tour unspools fascinating backstories of 10 works you might otherwise pass by, such as the portrait of young Venetia Stanley, which exists because she was discovered dead in bed and her distraught husband summoned Van Dyck to capture her beautiful corpse. Twist ending: Her beloved might have poisoned her. At the airy cafe, grab tea with Devon clotted cream for £6.

Gallery Rd., Dulwich Village, SE21. www.dulwichpicturegallery.org.uk. © **020/8693-5254.** Admission £7 adults, £6 seniors and students, free for children 17 and under; special exhibitions cost more. Tues–Sun 10am–5pm, last entry 4:30pm. National Rail: West Dulwich Station.

Eltham Palace and Gardens ★ HISTORIC HOME   Eltham (*ell*-tum) was once a palace on the level of importance with Hampton Court or Greenwich—Henry VIII was a boy here. Time was not kind to the grounds, though, and by the 1920s, Stephen and Virginia Courtauld, a wealthy childless couple, bought the Tudor ruin to rebuild into an ocean liner-inspired mansion for entertaining their movie-industry friends. The guided tour provides a delightful peek into the eccentricity and insularity of the wealthy—while it worships their entertaining skills, the evidence uncomfortably suggests they were awful people. Stephen was prone to sulking, and their obnoxious pet lemur, Mah-Jongg, liked to bite guests—it bit one Arctic explorer so badly an artery was severed, which postponed his exploration by three months. (Note Jongy's likeness carved into various architectural details.) Most country houses drive home stiff Georgian elegance, but Eltham is about the excesses of Art Deco living and a capsule of Britain between the wars. After tearing down sections that might have had Tudor origin, the Courtaulds lived here only 11 years. The surrounding moat and 19 acres of greenery and gardens, however, still feel like they must have 400 years ago.

Court Yard, Eltham, Greenwich, SE9. www.english-heritage.org.uk. ℂ **020/8294-2548.** Admission £14 adults, £13 seniors and students, £8.60 children 5–15. Apr–Sept Sun–Fri 10am–6pm, other periods daily noon–5pm (hours shift seasonally). National Rail: Eltham from Charing Cross.

The Freud Museum ★ HISTORIC HOME   In a hilly Hampstead neighborhood of spacious brick-faced homes, Sigmund Freud, having just fled the Nazis, spent the last year of his life here. His daughter Anna, herself a noted figure in psychoanalysis, lived on in the same house until her own death in 1982. Sigmund's study and library, which came from the doctor's famed offices at Berggasse 19, Vienna, were left precisely as they were on the day he died—which he did on a couch, of course.

20 Maresfield Gardens, NW3. www.freud.org.uk. ℂ **020/7435-2002.** Admission £8 adults, £6 seniors, £4 students, free for children 11 and under. Wed–Sun noon–5pm. Tube: Hampstead.

Hampton Court Palace ★★ PALACE   A 35-minute commuter train ride from the center of town, Hampton Court *looks* like the ideal palace because it *defined* the ideal. The rambling redbrick mansion was a center for royal life from 1525 to 1737, its forest of chimneys standing regally in 24 hectares (59 acres) of achingly pretty riverside gardens, now painstakingly restored to their 1702 appearance. Visitors come seeking vibrations left by Henry VIII during the 811 days he spent here (yes, that's all; he had more than 60 houses, partly because his court devoured so much food it kept exhausting local resources). The Crown still stocks precious art in many of the 70 public rooms, which start out Tudor and end up Georgian. It can take a whole day to see properly.

The entrance at Hampton Court Palace was definitely built to impress.

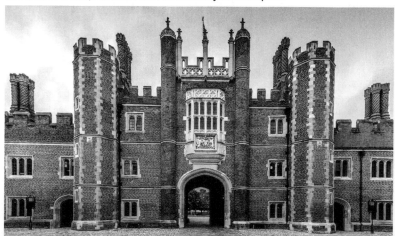

The inflexibly programmed audio guide, which follows a handful of themed trails (Young Henry VIII's Story, Henry VIII's Apartments, etc.), is free, but it harps endlessly on the same old stories about King Henry's wives; if you're looking for deeper explanations, research beforehand. What you're told panders to Tudor scandals because curators apparently think it makes history more interesting. On a surface level it does, but ultimately, it reduces this famous location to little more than a stereotypical set of a tawdry bygone play. The staff can't even adequately describe the paintings on the walls because the Royal Collection, which loans them, keeps switching their locations at a whim. Days are full of live events, which may include re-enactments of gossipy events by costumed actors; traditional cooking using bygone methods in the **Tudor Kitchens** (a popular stop); bizarre spoken-word performances in the hammer-beamed **Great Hall;** or ghost tours. Whatever you do, don't neglect the 26.7-hectare (66-acre) **gardens**—regally planted with historical accuracy (topiaries, sculpted yews, 300-year-old trees); they're half the reason to visit. Make time to lose yourself in the Northern Gardens' 500-year-old shrubbery **Maze,** installed by William III; kids giggle their way through to the middle of this leafy labyrinth. The well-mannered **South Garden** has the Great Vine, the oldest and largest vine in the world, planted in 1768; its black grapes are sold in the gift shop in early September. Wear strong shoes because the grounds are cobbled. Seeing this consumes half a day; if I had to choose between it and Windsor (p. 286), I'd choose Windsor.

East Molesey, Surrey. www.hrp.org.uk. © **084/4482-7777.** Admission £21 adults, £17 seniors and students, £10 children 5–15 (higher posted prices include a "voluntary donation"), £2 cheaper if bought online. Mar–late Oct daily 10am–6pm; late Oct–Mar daily 10am–4:30pm; last admission 1 hr before closing. National Rail: Hampton Court from Waterloo Station.

Royal Botanic Gardens, Kew ★★ PARK/GARDEN   The 121-hectare (300-acre) gardens, with many expansive lawns, earned a spot on the UNESCO list of World Heritage Sites in 2003. As you'd expect, the glasshouses are world-class—there are 2,000 varieties of plants, many descended from specimens collected in the earliest days of international sea trade. Of the seven conservatories, the domed **Palm House,** built from 1844 to 1848 and jungle-warm, is probably

TAKE THE thames TO HAMPTON OR KEW

From April to September daily, you can take **London River Services** (www.wpsa.co.uk; © **020/7930-2062;** £17 adults, £8.50 children 5–15, cash only) all the way from Westminster in central London to Hampton Court, the way Henry VIII did on his barges. It can be a commitment of 3 hours, however, and tides sometimes play such havoc with

schedules that you may arrive too late to see much. You will have to take the train the other way. Trains go twice an hour from Waterloo, take 35 minutes, and let you off across the river from the Palace: much easier. Kew is simpler: The ferry's round-trip fare is £25 adults and £13 children. It goes four times a day and takes 90 minutes.

the world's most recognizable greenhouse, while the **Temperate House** is the world's largest glasshouse containing the world's largest indoor plant (the 17.7m/58-ft.-tall Chilean wine-palm, planted in 1843—and that's not a typo). It's undergoing a £34 million restoration until 2018, but they've relocated most of the plants (except the *Encephalartos woodii* cycad, extinct in the wild and too fragile to move). Other attractions include a bamboo garden, a water lily pond, **Treehouse Towers** (a tree-themed play area for children 3–11), and, it must be said, a heartwarmingly charming village outside the gates. The gardeners are champs; in 1986, they coaxed a bloom from a portea that hadn't flowered in 160 years. Kew's contributions to botanical science are ongoing since 1759, but not mired in the past; it also provides a free app that lets you scan labels to learn more and find blooms. Unless you're a fevered horticulturalist, however, it will ultimately feel like a park you have to pay for—and pay a lot, at that. Also be aware that many of the goodies clamp down in winter (including Kew Palace, included in the price, p. 183), so this is best in the summer.

Kew, Richmond, Surrey. www.kew.org. ✆ **020/8332-5655.** Admission £17 adults, £16 seniors and students, £3.50 children 16 and under; discounts sometimes available online. Daily 9:30am–6:30 (closes at 6pm in fall and 5:15pm in winter). Tube: Kew Gardens.

Warner Bros. Studio Tour London—The Making of Harry Potter ★★★ MUSEUM London's most popular new family outing is like a DVD extra feature that comes to life; it's a full day out, and as gripping as the fine museums can be. On the very lot where the eight movies of history's most successful film franchise were shot, it seems that every set, prop, prosthetic, wig, and wand—and I mean every last thing—was lovingly saved for this polished, informative, and exhaustive walk-though feast. You could spend hours grazing the bounty, from the students' Great Hall to Dumbledore's roost to Dolores Umbridge's den to the actual Diagon Alley. There's not much filler, so book your entry time for early in the day so you'll have time to wander. Even if you care nothing about the movies, you will be blown away by the craftsmanship of items that got barely 2 seconds of screen time. The finale, an astounding 1:24 scale model of Hogwarts Castle embedded with 2,500 fiber optic lights, is 50 feet across and takes up an arena-size room, lit to simulate day and night. Midway through the tour, in an outdoor area containing 4 Privet Dr. and the actual Knight Bus, you'll find one of only four places on Earth where you can taste Butterbeer and Butterbeer ice cream. And you won't *believe* the gift shop. Easy 15-minute trains (don't get on one that takes 40 min.) go three times an hour from Euston Station—but not, fans sigh, from Platform 9¾ at King's Cross. (Although there, an enterprising Potter souvenir stall affixed a sign and sells people pictures.) You will wait just outside the Watford Junction station for the shuttle bus.

Warner Bros. Studios Leavesden, Aerodrome Way, Leavesden, Hertfordshire. www. wbstudiotour.co.uk. ✆ **08450/840-900.** Admission £37 adults, £29 children 5–15, free for children 4 and under, £118 family of 4. Return train ticket £10–20. Reservations required. Open daily. First tours 9–10am, last tours 4–7pm depending on day, closes 2½ hr after last tour time. National Rail: Watford Junction, then a £2.50 return shuttle bus that meets trains.

Other Outer London Attractions

Fuller's Brewery Tours ★ FACTORY TOUR Beer has been made on this Thameside property in West London since the 1600s, and Fuller's has been in charge of the brewing since 1845. Now this steampunk-feeling brick complex supplies some 380 pubs with its products, particularly its popular London Pride. They refuse to move to cheaper digs because a new water supply would change the flavor. Its tour is professional and engaging, more educational than bacchanalian—these people are passionate about their heritage. Free samples once you're done!

Chiswick Lane South. www.fullers.co.uk/brewery/book-a-tour. ℐ **020/8996-2000.** Tours £20. Mon–Sat hourly 11am–3pm. No children under 16, no tasting under age 18. Reservations required. Tube: Tube: Turnham Green, then a 20-minute walk.

Home of Charles Darwin—Down House ★★ HISTORIC HOME Charles Darwin made one of history's most important voyages, but once back in England, he barely left his home here in the idyllic parish village of Downe. Upstairs you'll find out about the man and his life (did you know the scientist who theorized about mutation married his own first cousin?) and downstairs, guided by an audio tour narrated by Sir David Attenborough, you'll explore his study, his greenhouse, and his enchanting garden of lawns and breezy fields. No wonder he never left again. There are two charming country pubs to enjoy while you wait for the bus back; your Oyster card will get you here.

Luxted Rd., Downe, Kent. www.english-heritage.org.uk. ℐ**0370/333-1181.** Admission £12 adults, £11 seniors and students, £7.10 children 5–15. Apr–Sept daily 10am–6pm; Oct–Nov daily 10am–5pm; Nov–mid-Feb Sat–Sun 10am–4pm; mid-Feb–Mar Weds–Sun 10am–4pm. National Rail: Bromley South, then bus no. 122 and 7-min. walk.

Horniman Museum ★ MUSEUM A rich Victorian dilettante collected crazy stuff from all over the world, and rather than let it gather dust, he built a museum in South London. This repository of some 350,000 items has since blossomed into a wild educational ride, with something for everyone, particularly children. To wit: a cherished collection of 7,000 musical instruments (Boosey & Hawkes, once the U.K.'s largest instrument maker, donated its archive) and a huge range of items regarding anthropology (masks, puppets, folk art) and natural history (stuffed creatures galore). There's even a modest aquarium, a cafe, and some gorgeous gardened grounds on a hill with a panorama of London 6 miles north.

100 London Rd., Forest Hill. www.horniman.ac.uk. ℐ**020/8699-1872.** Free admission. Daily 10:30am–5:30pm. Tube: Forest Hill Overground.

Kenwood ★★ HISTORIC HOME Bask in a country-house high without leaving the city. Kenwood is a sublime 18th-century job by Robert Adam with a sigh-inducing southern view across Hampstead Heath, from within the green embrace of 112 acres. Inside, the walls are hung with paintings that would be the envy of the National Gallery, including Vermeer's *The Guitar Player,* a John Singer Sargent, and a Rembrandt self-portrait. The title

Outer London

EXPLORING LONDON

character of the 2014 film *Belle* was raised by Lord Mansfield in this house, and the film was shot here. There's no better place to enjoy an English summer than on its acres of lawns or alongside its ornamental pond.

Hampstead Lane, NW3. www.english-heritage.org.uk. © **020/8348-1286.** Free admission. House: daily 10am–5pm (summer until 6pm); grounds: 8am–dusk. Tube: Archway or Golders Green, then bus no. 210.

Kew Palace and Queen Charlotte's Cottage ★ PALACE   Remember George III? He's the dilettante ruler who, during his reign from 1760 to 1820, lost the American colonies and went crazy from suspected porphyria: see the movie *The Madness of King George* for the tragic tale. Kew Palace is where he spent his childhood and later went insane, and you can tour a piece of his vanished palace, recently restored with scientific exactitude. It's only the size of a standard manor house and lacks interpretation except for some ill-advised histrionic audio enactments that no one pauses to endure. Across Kew Gardens, the little Queen Charlotte's Cottage is an imitation of a humble village home. Its Picnic Room is painted with vines across its vaulted ceiling—work attributed to King George's daughter, Princess Elizabeth. In late April, the Cottage, which is at Kew's southwest end, is surrounded by bluebells in bloom.

Royal Botanic Gardens, Kew, Richmond. www.hrp.org.uk. © **020/8332-5655.** Included in Kew Gardens admission: £15 adults, £14 seniors and students, £3.50 children 16 and under; discounts sometimes available online. Kew Palace: Apr–Oct 10am–5:30pm; closed Nov–Mar. Cottage: Sat–Sun and bank holidays 10am–4pm. Tube: Kew Gardens.

Mandir ★ TEMPLE   The breathtakingly pretty, many-pinnacled Mandir in northwest London is the largest Hindu temple outside of India. This fabulous concoction was completed in 1995, after some 5,500 tons of Italian Carrara marble and Bulgarian limestone were carved in India and assembled by volunteers. Its dome was built without using steel or lead. The interior is as white and lavishly detailed as a doily—it's apt to amaze even people generally unimpressed by such virtuosity. Tourists are welcome—try to be there to witness the musical wick-lighting Arti ceremony at 11:45am. If you're entering, shorts or skirts must fall at least to the knee (although ankle-length is preferable and sarongs are available to borrow); visitors must also remove their shoes.

105–119 Brentfield Rd., NW10. londonmandir.baps.org. © **020/8965-2651.** Free admission. Daily 9am–6pm. Tube: Wembley Park, then bus no. 206, or Stonebridge Park, then bus no. 112.

Thames Barrier Visitor Centre ★ LANDMARK/MUSEUM   People forget that London floods. Parliament has been under water, and in 1953, surges killed 307 people in the U.K. At least, London *used* to flood. The Thames Barrier is the city's primary defense against it, comprised of ten 20m (66-ft.) steel-and-concrete gates that can be raised to block the 520m (1706-ft.) span of the river in just 10 minutes. Most of the time you can't see the gates, which rest on the riverbed, but the piers that raise and lower them are always visible, strung across the river like a row of mini-Sydney Opera

Houses. At the visitor center you plumb the Barrier's construction and, if you're lucky, see a test raise.

1 Unity Way, Woolwich, SE18. www.gov.uk/guidance/the-thames-barrier. ☎ **020/8305-4188.** Admission £4 adults, £3.50 seniors and students, £2.50 children 5–15, free for children 4 and under. Thurs–Sun and bank holiday Mon 10:30am–5pm. Rail: Woolwich Dockyard or Charlton.

Wimbledon Lawn Tennis Museum ★★ MUSEUM   Most of us can't get into the tournament (see "Netting Wimbledon Tickets," p. 185), and there's an 11-year waiting list to become a member to the All England Lawn Tennis & Croquet Club, the official name of Wimbledon. But for us, there's still something worth seeing the rest of the year. The museum is like a Hall of Fame, with an emphasis of course on Wimbledon, with artifacts going back to 1555. The climax, most times of year, is the hallowed room shimmering with the silver men's "Challenge-Cup" and women's "Challenge-Plate," which are the actual Championships trophies inscribed with every winner's name. (The British have never been prouder than they are now that Scotsman Andy Murray brought home the trophy after 77 years.) There is no other museum in the world where a ghostly video apparition of John McEnroe appears in a locker room to vent about opponents. (He comes in peace. No need to duck.) Tennis fans should absolutely spring for the tour of the grounds, too, which is truly all-access, including entry into the Competitors' Complex reserved for players, a photo op in the press conference room where they meet the media, and the all-important Centre Court, where Finals are always played, and always on grass. The guides are fantastic and challenge you to stump them.

Church Rd., SW19. www.wimbledon.com/museum. ☎ **020/8946-6131.** Museum admission £13 adults, £11 seniors and students, £8 children 5–16. Museum with tour: £25 adults, £21 seniors and students, £15 children 5–16 (one free child for each paying adult). Apr–Sept, daily 10am–5:30pm, Oct–Mar daily 10am–5pm. Tube: Southfields, then 15-minute walk or bus no. 493; or National Rail from Waterloo to Wimbledon Station, then bus no. 493.

OVERRATED ATTRACTIONS

In every city, you invariably find attractions that are heavily publicized but, once seen, are revealed to be time poorly spent. London provides a variety of overpriced pursuits catering to people who seem content to ignore its true treasures—there's even an elaborate attraction by the London Eye devoted to the movie *Shrek,* which needless to say you can safely skip. Take our advice: Don't be suckered by the hype.

ArcelorMittal Orbit OBSERVATION TOWER   This 114.5m-tall (376-ft.) vertical scribble, a publicity exercise by a steel concern that is now failing, has observation decks at 76m (249 ft.) and 80m (262 ft.), but it barely matters when there's not much to look at. It originally overlooked the Olympics, but with the torch and the games gone, it now peers into a stadium many miles from town. So tragic have attendance numbers been than in 2016 it desperately

Netting Wimbledon Tickets

It's easy watching the Wimbledon Championships on TV for 2 weeks in late June and early July, but seeing it in person is a trickier matter. High hotel prices are just the beginning. Because tickets for the final matches go to VIPs, you're more likely to catch famous players during the early rounds, when the club's 19 grass courts are all in use. For the price of a "ground pass" (£15–£25, cash only) you can get roaming access to all but three courts (surcharges of £29–£175 are levied for Centre, No. 1, and No. 2 courts, and those tickets are distributed by lottery the previous summer). Around 6,000 ground passes are distributed each morning starting at 7:30am, so arrive many hours before that to camp in Wimbledon Park, Church Road side (no large luggage allowed). If you snag one, you'll probably be inside by noon, before matches begin. You can wander around to your heart's content, drinking Pimm's Cup and eating strawberries and cream, and watching matches on giant screens, but you'll still need to get into the three most important courts. You can try by ballot, but that closes in December. Meanwhile, Ticketmaster (and no one else; ticketmaster.co.uk) may release several hundred tickets for Centre Court and Court 3 the day before play. Another clever way to get in is to bum tickets off people as they get tired and leave for the day; just don't offer money—the organizers hate that because they sell unused tickets, too, for charity. Those are resold after 3pm to those already on the grounds (£5–£10). On weekdays and rainy days, your chances of getting unfilled seats for the best courts are better, since people are working or huddling indoors. And after 5pm, ground-pass rates dip to, at most, £18, which isn't such a bad deal since matches continue until 9pm. It's all ridiculously complicated—the English love complicated admission schemes—so check ahead on Wimbledon.com to ensure rules remain the same.

added a 40-second tube slide, the world's longest and tallest—narrow enough to bonk your head and fast enough to smash your phone—that drops from one of the observation levels, wrapping around the structure 12 times. They put a helmet and elbow pads on you, tuck your feet into a cubby at the end of a mat, and send you screaming. It also offers an abseil thrill from 80m/262 feet high (www.wireandsky.co.uk; ✆ 020/3198-0407; £85; minimum age 14, maximum weight 120kg/264 lbs.). Wear a jacket because it gets windy in the exposed areas. And no, it doesn't orbit.

Queen Elizabeth Olympic Park, E20. arcelormittalorbit.com. ✆ 0333/800-8099. Admission £18 adults, £11 children 3–6 (tower without slide: £13/£7.50). Slide restricted to people taller than 4'2"/1.3m. Mon–Fri 11am–5pm, Sat–Sun 10am–6pm; last admission 30 min before closing. Tube: Stratford.

Emirates Air Line OBSERVATION GONDOLA   Opened for the Olympics as a Thames crossing between the ExCeL convention center and the O₂ dome, it's simply an enclosed, 10-person gondola with recorded commentary that shuttles between two places most tourists never go. It's too far from the City to be a good panoramic substitute for the Eye or the Shard. Don't let them sucker you into spending over £10 for the "Experience" package that includes a touristy flight simulator/Emirates PR puffery on the ground. The ride takes 5 to 10 minutes.

Emirates Cable Car Terminal, Edmund Halley Way, E10, or Royal Docks side 27 Western Gateway, E16. www.emiratesairline.co.uk. ℘ **0843/222-1234.** Admission £4.50 adult, £2.30 children (without Oyster card); or £3.40 adults, £1.70 children 5–15 (with Oyster card). Mon–Fri 7am–9pm; Sat 8am–9pm; Sun 9am–9pm, closed at 8pm in winter. Tube: North Greenwich or Royal Victoria DLR.

The Household Cavalry Museum MUSEUM   Along Whitehall, where guards try mightily to ignore buffoonish tourists who try to get them to crack a smile, this tiny museum pays soporific tribute to the martial ceremonies of the Queen's Life Guard. You might see troopers groom horses through a glass partition or regard cases of uniforms and regalia with glazed eyes, but—nothing against these dedicated men—you won't get much back on your investment. On the hour, mounted dutymen change, and at 11am, the Life Guard changes, but you can see those outside for free.

Horse Guards, Whitehall, SW1. www.householdcavalrymuseum.co.uk. ℘ **020/7930-3070.** Admission £7 adults, £5 seniors and children 5–16. Apr–Oct 10am–6pm; Nov–March 10am–5pm. Tube: Embankment.

The London Dungeon ATTRACTION   Avoid it like the plague. This sophomoric gross-out, with locations in nine cities, sops up overflow from the London Eye. Costumed actors bray at you as you're led through darkness from set to set, each representing a period of English history as a 13-year-old boy might define them. The climax is a pair of indoor carnival rides. If you dread being picked on by bad stand-up comics, you're going to hate this place. Booking ahead may not save you having to queue. If you can't resist, at least bundle it with a ticket on the London Eye for a discount.

County Hall, Westminster Bridge Rd., SE1. www.thedungeons.com. ℘ **0871/243-2240.** Admission £30 adults, £24 children 5–15, £7–£8 cheaper booked online. Times change but roughly daily 10am–5pm. Tube: Westminster or Waterloo.

London Sea Life Aquarium AQUARIUM   Sure, it's fun to see sharks under your feet and penguins on a faux floe. But sorry Charlie, the truth is there is nothing here you can't see at other fish zoos. There are more than three dozen other locations worldwide by Sea Life, the McDonald's of fish tanks, and this one feels as cramped as a 16th-century galleon.

County Hall, Westminster Bridge Rd., SE1. www.sealifelondon.co.uk. ℘ **0871/663-1678.** Admission £26 adults, £21 children 3–15, free for children 2 and under, 10% discount online. Mon–Thurs 10am–5pm; Fri–Sun 9:30am–6pm; last admission 1 hr before closing. Tube: Waterloo or Westminster,

The London Zoo ZOO   Yes, it has an esteemed history going back to 1828 as a menagerie for members of the Zoological Society of London. It's just that it's ultimately only a zoo, and a smallish one at that, with few large animals. Sumatran tigers and baby penguins are not enough to justify the high ticket price, especially for first-time London visitors who could be exploring the city instead.

Outer Circle Rd., Regent's Park, NW1. www.zsl.org. ⓒ **020/7722-333.** Admission £24 adults, £22 seniors and students, £18 children 3–15. Daily 10am–6pm. Tube: Camden Town, then bus no. 274.

Madame Tussauds ATTRACTION   Have you ever heard of Katrina Kaif? Zoe and Alfie? Jessica Ennis-Hill? If your answer is no, you won't get much joy out of this ferociously priced, miserably crowded wax trap. The execution of its doppelgangers, which you can usually touch (Harry is behind ropes, girls), is generally superb. But the focus of this world-famous wax-works is on British celebrities. A 5-minute, Disney-esque ride, "The Spirit of London," invokes every conceivable London stereotype, from the Artful

ritual ABUSE

I'm only telling you this because I love you: **Changing the Guard,** sometimes called Guard Mounting, is an underwhelming use of your time, even if admission is free. Arrive at Buckingham Palace at least 45 minutes before the 11:30am ceremony if you don't want to face the backs of other tourists. A marching band advances from Birdcage Walk (often, playing themes from Star Wars, West Side Story, or ABBA—so much for traditional English customs), then members of the Queen's Life Guard—two if the queen's away, three or four if she's in—do a change around their sentry boxes behind a heavy fence. And that's it, give or take additional prancing. Buckingham Palace (www.royal.gov.uk) sells a $1 smartphone app that will help decode the ritual. It takes place daily May–July, every other day the rest of year, and it gets cancelled in heavy rain (St James's Park, Victoria, or Green Park tube).

Guards patrol all day, without crowds, at both Buckingham Palace and at Horse Guards Arch on Whitehall (which does its own, uncrowded change daily at 11am, or 10am Sun). Or park yourself at **Wellington Barracks,** just east of the Palace

along Birdcage Walk, by 11am, and catch the Inspection of the Guard that happens before the same guards march over to the Palace for the main event. Then use the day's golden hours for something less touristy.

Ceremony of the Keys at the Tower of London (www.hrp.org.uk; ⓒ **020/3166-6278;** Tower Hill tube or Tower Gateway DLR), is held every night at 9:53pm as the Yeomen lock up the Tower of London. It's been a routine for more than 700 years—not even German bombs cancelled it. But it's an awful lot of work for not much payoff: You must enter the Tower at 9:30pm (several hours after closing time, so you can't combine it with a day's visit) and leave around 10:05pm, even though the whole show takes less than 7 minutes—plus, photos aren't allowed. As for the event, the Chief Yeoman Warder approaches the heavy wooden gate with keys and a lantern, is asked "Halt, who comes there?," passes muster, and locks up the gates to a bugle call. The end. If you want to see that, apply for tickets online (admission is free), with a nightly maximum of six places April to October. It sells out 11 months in advance.

Dodger to plague victims. As you glide through, you'll suddenly wonder if you're the real dummy here.

Marylebone Rd., W1. www.madame-tussauds.com/london. ℂ **0871/894-3000.** Admission based on time of year and time of day, peaks at £29 adults, £24 children 4–15. Daily 9:30am–5:30pm, slightly longer Sat–Sun and holidays. Tours continue at least 45 min. past posted closing time. Tube: Baker St.

Ripley's Believe It or Not! ATTRACTION   Like foot fungus, the worthless rip has spread wherever tourists stagger. Now it's in London. Its halls of oddities (sample: a portrait of Diana made from lint) are useless and not worthwhile even for the kitsch value. This is the definition of a tourist trap. And it costs more than Westminster Abbey! Fortunately, "or Not" is an option.

1 Piccadilly Circus, W1. www.ripleyslondon.com. ℂ **020/3238-0022.** Admission £28 adults, £28 seniors and students, £21 children 5–15; £4 discount online 1–13 days ahead, half price booked 14+ days ahead. Daily 10am–midnight. Tube: Piccadilly Circus.

The Sherlock Holmes Museum ATTRACTION   Set up a house as if it were really the home of a fictional character, prop up some shabby mannequins, and then charge tourists to see it. That's the scheme and it has worked for years, so well there's often a line and it recently hiked prices 50%.

221b Baker St., NW1. www.sherlock-holmes.co.uk. ℂ **020/7224-3688.** Admission £15 adults, £10 children 15 and under. Daily 9:30am–6pm. Tube: Baker St.

OUTDOOR LONDON

Buildings come and go, but London's open spaces have remained unchanged for centuries—they're the city's oldest places. There are often walks and tours scheduled, so check websites to see what's coming.

Epping Forest ★★★ PARK/GARDEN   Mostly because its soil is unsuitable for farming, for a millennium this remained a semi-virgin woodland—it's the best place to get a feel for what Britain was like before humans denuded its land. It's the largest open space in London, 6,000 acres, 12 miles long by 2½ miles wide, and it contains a universe of diversity—650 plant species, 80 ponds where waterfowl splash, and even some 1,500 species of fungi. Getting lost in the woods is feasible, but not likely, since it stretches in a single direction. Henry VII built a timber-framed hunting lodge in 1542 that was inherited by his daughter Elizabeth and, astoundingly, still stands: **Queen Elizabeth's Hunting Lodge** (reach that via the Chingford rail station).

Rangers Rd., Chingford, E4. www.cityoflondon.gov.uk. ℂ **020/8529-6681.** Free admission. Daily 6am–dusk. Lodge: daily 10am–5pm. Tube: Snaresbrook or Wood St. National rail: Chingford.

The Green Park ★★ PARK/GARDEN   The area south of Mayfair between Hyde Park and St James's Park was once a burial ground for lepers, but now is a simple expanse of meadows and light copses of trees. It doesn't have much to offer except pastoral views, and most visitors find themselves crossing it instead of dawdling in it, although its springtime flower beds

FAMOUS graves

London's top tombs don't just belong to royalty. Visit these historic area cemeteries for a tranquil day out and to say hello to some major figures.

Bunhill Fields (Old St. tube): *The Pilgrim's Progress*'s John Bunyan, poet William Blake, author Daniel Defoe

Golders Green Crematorium (Golders Green tube): Ashes of writers Bram Stoker, Doris Lessing, and Seán O'Casey; musician Keith Moon; dancer Anna Pavlova, actor Peter Sellers; Sigmund Freud

Highgate Cemetery (www.highgate cemetery.org; Archway tube): **Karl Marx,** authors **Douglas Adams** and **George Eliot** (East Cemetery, £4 entry), actor **Ralph Richardson,** artist **Lucian Freud** (West Cemetery), and in a private area, **George Michael.**

Kensal Green Cemetery (www.kensal greencemetery.com; Kensal Green tube and National Rail): Writers **Terence Rattigan, Anthony Trollope, Harold Pinter, Wilkie Collins, J. G. Ballard, William Makepeace Thackeray;** engineers **Marc Isambard Brunel** and **Isambard Kingdom Brunel**

Royal Hospital Chelsea (Sloane Square tube): **Margaret Thatcher**

St Mary's Church, Battersea (Clapham Junction National Rail): Lapsed rebel **Benedict Arnold** (his crypt is now used as a kindergarten)

St Mary Magdalen Roman Catholic Church Mortlake (Mortlake National Rail): adventurer **Sir Richard Burton** (under a tent made of Carrera marble)

St Nicholas Church, Chiswick (Stamford Brook tube): Artists **William Hogarth** and **James McNeill Whistler**

St. Nicholas Church, Deptford Green (Deptford National Rail): Writer **Christopher Marlowe**

(which bloom brightest Mar–Apr) are marvelous. Don't sit in one of those picturesque striped deck chairs unless you've got a few quid to pay as rent. Piccadilly, SW1. © **030/0061-2350.** Free admission. Daily 24 hr. Tube: Green Park.

Greenwich Park ★★ PARK/GARDEN   Decently sized (74 hectares/183 acres), it was once a deer preserve maintained for royal amusement; a herd of them still have 5 hectares (13 acres) at their disposal. It's been a Royal Park since the 15th century, although the boundary wasn't formally defined until the early 1600s when James I erected a brick wall around it, much of which still survives. On top of its clean-swept main hill are marvelous views of the Canary Wharf district, and the world-famous **Royal Observatory** (p. 177), commissioned in 1675 by Charles II, serves as the intersection point for the Prime Meridian, making it the center of Greenwich Mean Time. Most people combine a visit here with the many other museums of Greenwich (p. 174).

Greenwich Park, SE10. www.royalparks.gov.uk. © **030/0061-2380.** Free admission. Daily 6am–9pm. National Rail: Greenwich or Maze Hill, or Cutty Sark. DLR or Greenwich ferry.

Hampstead Heath ★★★ PARK/GARDEN   Some 7 million visitors a year come to the 320-hectare (791-acre) Heath, in northwest London, to walk on the grass, get enveloped by thick woods, and take in the view from the magnificent Pergola, a beguiling overgrown Edwardian garden and a true

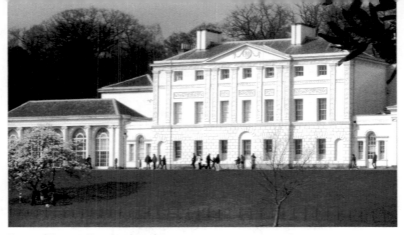

Kenwood House at Hampstead Heath.

London secret. The Heath is a perennial locale for aimless strolls and (it must be confessed, George Michael) furtive trysts. The Heath has several sublime places to rest, including the just-restored **Kenwood House** (p. 182), a sumptuous neoclassical home from 1640; and the inviting and woody **Spaniards Inn** (Spaniards Rd. at Spaniards End, NW3; www.thespaniardshampstead.co.uk; ℂ **020/8731-8406**). The Heath's hilltop is another favored lookout point. The Heath isn't considered a park by locals, but a green space. The difference is irrelevant. It's transporting.

www.cityoflondon.gov.uk/hampstead. ℂ **020/7332-3505.** 7:30am–dusk. Tube: Hampstead or Hampstead Heath Overground.

Hyde Park & Kensington Gardens ★★★ PARK/GARDEN Bordered by Mayfair, Bayswater, and Kensington, these two conjoined areas are the largest park in the middle of the city. Hyde Park is home to a meandering lake called the Serpentine, the famous **Speakers' Corner** (p. 141), and the **Diana Fountain** (p. 144). The most famous promenade is Rotten Row, probably a corruption of "Route de Roi," or King's Way, which was laid out by William III as his private road to town; it runs along the southern edge of the park from Hyde Park Corner. Kensington Gardens, which flows seamlessly from Hyde Park, only opened to plebes like us in 1851, and it hasn't yet shed its country-manor quality. You'll also find the **Serpentine Gallery** (west of W. Carriage Dr. and north of Alexandra Gate; www.serpentinegallery.org; ℂ **020/7402-6075;** free admission; Tues–Sun 10am–6pm; South Kensington tube), a popular venue for its modern art exhibitions and an art bookshop. Each summer, a leading architect creates a fanciful pavilion there. Volunteers sometimes run guided tours of the park's quirks; check the bulletin boards at each park entrance to see if one is upcoming. Borrow a Boris Bike and cruise around this giant green playground, and don't forget to look for Sir George Frampton's marvelous bronze statue of Peter Pan (1912) near the west shore of the Long Water.

Hyde Park, W2. www.royalparks.org.uk. ℂ **0300/061-2000.** Free admission. Daily 5am–midnight. Tube: Hyde Park Corner, Marble Arch, or Lancaster Gate.

THE hidden park

Sure, everybody knows about London's famous green spaces, but there's one recreation area, stretching from London's northwest to its east through gentrified lanes and industrial wasteland alike, that few tourists are told about. It's the **Regent's Canal,** which threads from Paddington through Camden, Islington, and East London before joining with the Thames (26m/86 ft. lower) just before Canary Wharf. It was completed in 1820 to link with canals all the way to Birmingham and feed the city's massive seagoing trade. In those days, barges were animal-drawn and the districts along the waterway were rat-infested and perilous, but today, it's one of the frontiers for development; many of the horse tracks are leafy promenades, shadowy warehouses have become affluent loft condos, and the use of houseboats has soared 60% over the last half-decade. A new development north of King's Cross station is revealing even more glories. Along the shore, you'll pass docks where houseboat barges tie up; their owners

can be found topside, making conversation with passersby. The most popular segment is probably the crescent just north of Regent's Park. Set in a former icehouse, the **London Canal Museum** (12–13 New Wharf Rd., N1; www.canal museum.org.uk; ℭ **020/7713-0836;** admission £4; Tues–Sun 10am–4:30pm; Kings Cross St Pancras tube) is devoted to the waterway and operates tours of its towpath and boat tours of the Islington Tunnel, which stretches for 1.2km (¾ mile) under the streets. **London Waterbus** (www.londonwaterbus.com; ℭ **020/7482-2550**) and **Jason's Trip** (www.jasons.co.uk; no phone) ferry riders in longboats through the 270-foot Maida Hill Tunnel and the glorious villas that line the canal between Little Venice (Warwick Ave. tube) and Camden's markets (Camden Town tube). Ferries run in either direction, year-round; a ride costs £8.50 for adults, £7 seniors and children 3–16. There are no tourist boats that currently ferry riders east of the locks at Camden.

Queen Elizabeth Olympic Park ★ PARK/GARDEN   A dearth of trees and a usual bracing wind make this park feel a lot like a theme park in which all of the attractions got up and left. Most of the amenities are things that only attract locals, who remember when it was an industrial wasteland. The Pringle-shaped Aquatics Centre and Velopark make for striking architecture, but this park is mostly of interest if you want to see the place you saw on TV—yet the torch is gone, the stadium has been downgraded for a soccer team, and the ArcelorMittal Orbit tower (p. 184) is ultimately pointless. If you do go, Stratford station dumps into a mall (one of the nicest in the city); to find the park, go up one level and exit near the John Lewis.

Stratford, E20. www.queenelizabetholympicpark.co.uk. ℭ **020/3288-1800.** Free admission. Daily 24 hr. Tube: Stratford.

The Regent's Park ★★★ PARK/GARDEN   It's the people's park (195 hectares/487 acres), best for sunning, strolling long expanses—it can take a half-hour to cross it—and darting into the bohemian neighborhoods that fringe it. Once a hunting ground, it was very nearly turned into a development for the buddies of Prince Regent (later King George IV), but only a few of the private terrace homes were built. You will notice Winfield House, on 5

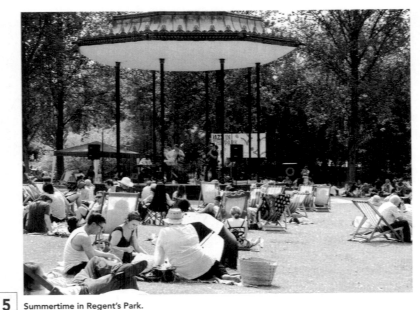

Summertime in Regent's Park.

hectares (12 acres) near the western border of the park, which has the largest garden in London after the queen's; the American ambassador lives there—surprised? The most breathtaking entrance is from the south through John Nash's elegant Park Crescent development, by the Regent's Park and Great Portland Street Tube stations. North of the park, just over the Regent's Canal and Prince Albert Road, **Primrose Hill Park** (Chalk Farm or Camden Town tubes) affords a panorama of the city from 62m (203-ft.) high.

Regent's Park, NW1. www.royalparks.gov.uk.ⓒ **030/0061-2300.** Free admission. Daily 5am–9pm. Tube: Baker St., Great Portland St., or Regent's Park.

St James's Park ★★ PARK/GARDEN   The easternmost segment of the contiguous quartet of parks that runs east from Kensington Gardens is bounded by Whitehall to the east and Piccadilly to the north. James I laid it out in 1603 and Buckingham Palace redeveloped it a century later. Its little pond, St James's Park Lake, hosts ducks and other waterfowl. The Russian ambassador made a gift of pelicans to the park in 1667; six (three of them a 2013 gift from the city of Prague) still call it home, and are fed their 13kg (28 lb.) of whiting daily at 2:30pm at the Duck Island Cottage. The park has a fine view of Buckingham Palace's front facade, where royal couples smooch on balconies (but live in a section of the building you can't see). The real draw is people-watching, since a cross-section of all London passes through here. It's not a place for picnics or ball throwing, and there's little in the way of amenities or activities—unless you count voyeurism, and why wouldn't you?

The Mall, SW1. www.royalparks.org.uk.ⓒ **0300/061-2350.** Free admission. 5am–midnight. Tube: St James's Park.

Victoria Park ★★ PARK/GARDEN   This was the largest and finest open space in East London when it opened in 1845, the capital's first public park. Bordered by canals and divided in two by Grove Road, it covers an area of just under 87 hectares (220 acres) and contains two lakes, formal gardens, sports facilities, and a bandstand. Other notable features include a Grade II-listed 1862 drinking fountain and two arches from the pre-1831 London Bridge—now turned into benches. In summer, big music events such as Lovebox come here. The park also forms the central section of the **Jubilee Greenway Walk,** a route marked out in 2009 with glass paving slabs in honor of the queen's Diamond Jubilee, and stretching for exactly 60km (37 miles)—1 kilometer for each year of her reign—from Buckingham Palace to the Olympic Park. She doesn't use it.

Grove Rd., E3. www.towerhamlets.gov.uk/victoriapark. © **020/7364-7971.** Free admission. Daily 7am–dusk. Tube: Mile End/Overground, Hackney Wick, or Homerton.

ORGANIZED TOURS

Walking Tours

There are so many guides to choose from—the best ones are led by government-accredited "Blue Badge" professionals, so always look for the Blue Badge—that you could fill a week with walking tours alone. Plenty of qualified operators cater to custom business (many only cater to groups), but these will let you join individually. Also check that online compendium of day tours, Viator (www.viator.com).

City of London Guided Walks ★★   The government gives written and performance-based exams to the experts who lead its excellent weekly tours. The experience is less theatrical and denser with facts than what London Walks (see below) generally provides, and group sizes tend to be smaller, too. There are 17 from which to choose, including ones on Dickens, the City's top 10 sights, and Roman London. Tours are 1½ to 2 hours. Pre-booking is advised, but not essential.

City Information Centre, St Paul's Churchyard, EC4. www.cityoflondonguides.com. Tours £7 adults, £6 seniors and students, free for children 11 and under. Tube: St Paul's.

City of Westminster Guides ★★   Westminster, the area of London west of the City that includes the theater district, also contracts officially tested guides to lead tours there. Advance booking isn't required, but tours sometimes only go in summer. Tours are 1½ to 2 hours; locations vary.

www.westminsterguides.org.uk. Tours £12 adults, £9 seniors and students, free for children 11 and under.

The Classic Tour ★   If you don't have all day, this 75-minute whirlwind of the major sites gives you as much style as possible in a limited window of time: You ride on a modified double-decker 1960s Routemaster bus—for decades the standard for commuting Londoners—as a somewhat hammy *take it for 1st day?*

guide gives you the quick lowdown on everything you pass, from Buckingham Palace to the famous Tower Bridge (which you'll cross).

www.theclassictour.com. © **0844/318-7655.** Tours £15 adults, £15 seniors and students, £12 children 5–15.

Context Travel ★   Leave the greasepaint in the hotel room—these tours are for those with intellectual leanings. Context bills them not as hammy storytelling sessions but as "walking seminars," some several hours long and for premium rates, hosted by professors, historians, and other scholars. For example, one of its 2014 additions was about London's role in the colonial slave trade, a topic most museums ignore. Some tours are only available to groups, but inquire about availability. Locations vary.

www.contexttravel.com. © **800/691-6036** (U.S.).

Dotmaker Tours ★★   Dotmaker's clever weekend walks delve into offbeat topics such as chimneys, tunnels, the story of sounds like St Paul's bells, where the city dumps its rubbish, and where London's past geniuses have found their inspiration. Tours are 2 hours; locations vary.

www.dotmakertours.co.uk. Tours £18 adults, £15 seniors and students.

Eating London Tours ★★   I recommend this 3½-hour, stuff-yourself-silly walking romp though some of the greatest victuals in the East End. You'll get to try eight tastings of flavors that are truly East End and not faked for tourists, from fish and chips to Brick Lane curry to Beigel Bake salt beef to a pint in an old-fashioned pub—all while getting a solid lay of the land from an entertaining guide. It also does a more expensive evening tour of Soho (£94; no kids on that one), of the pubs in Docklands, and of the Indian grub on Brick Lane. Locations vary.

www.eatinglondontours.co.uk. © **020/3289-6327** or 215/688-5571 (U.S.). Tours £69 adults, £54 children 13–18, £42 children 12 and under.

Footprints of London ★★★   Truly passionate, accredited guides with a depth of knowledge both own and operate this company, and they come up with topics that are much more diverse and surprising than rivals': hidden maritime artifacts, neighborhood explorations by the famous "poverty maps" of the 1890s, great paintings of London, Charlie Chaplin's Kennington, and even a sing-along combining suffragettes with Winston Churchill and wartime music. Great stuff! Have a look to see what they've concocted for when you visit.

www.footprintsoflondon.com. Tours £12 adults, £9 seniors and students. Reservations recommended but not required.

Greenwich Guided Walks ★   Like London, Greenwich operates its own official tours with carefully vetted guides. There are usually two basic 90-minute tours daily from the Greenwich Tourist Information Centre

(Discover Greenwich) taking in the main sights plus the Royal Observatory and the Meridian Line.

www.greenwichtours.co.uk. ✆ **07575/772-298.** Tours £8 adults, £7 seniors and students, free for children 13 and under. Tube: DLR: Cutty Sark.

London Walks ★★★ Undoubtedly one of the city's best tourist services, London Walks' tour list is inspiring. On weekdays, there are often more than a dozen choices, and on weekends, nearly 25, which means that if you ever find yourself with a few hours to kill, you can always find instant occupation. Every tour (most are £10) departs from a Tube stop, and none require reservations, which makes arrangements easy. The marquee tour is probably "Jack the Ripper Haunts," which heads out to the streets of Whitechapel around sunset and, in the pursuit of ghoulish entertainment, employs considerably more grotesquerie than uncontested facts. Many of the group's other walks are more informative, including "The Blitz," "Old Mayfair," Harry Potter filming sites, and even guided tours of the British Museum. Other topics can supply authoritative tours on lesser-visited areas such as Hampstead village or the "Little Venice" near Regent's Canal, places few other touring companies touch. The group also provides guidance (and discounts) for Westminster Abbey, as well as "Great Escapes!" of Bath, Stonehenge, Cambridge, Canterbury, and other day-trip favorites (entry fees and train transit are included in the price, £22–£53); they may go weekly or seasonally. If there's any fault with London Walks, it's that some groups swell to untenable sizes, and many of the guides, although proven knowledgeable when pressed, rely too commonly on canned performance shtick (in fact, many are actors, but then again, histrionics are preferable to a narcotic delivery). The best way to remedy both problems is to pick a tour with narrower appeal; you'll have a better chance to ask questions. Tours are 2 hours; prices and locations vary.

www.walks.com. ✆ **020/7624-3978.** Tours £10 adults, £8 seniors and students.

Muggle Tours ★★ Although it's based on a mass-appeal trend, it's worthy. This well-assembled tour dispenses reams of Harry Potter trivia, from the books to the movies and locations from the movies. Groups of 20 start at London Bridge, near Borough Market (p. 95), and wind up in Leicester Square. Because so much London history is folded in, there's enough for non-Potterheads. Book online. Tours are 2½ hours.

www.muggletours.co.uk. ✆ **07917/411-374.** Tours £13 adults, £11 children 11 and under. Tube: London Bridge.

Unseen Tours ★★★ London is more than kings, art, and canned tall tales. See it from a raw angle, and plumb its modern issues, on a walk guided by homeless and former homeless residents. Walks go on six different routes—around Shoreditch, Brick Lane, Covent Garden, London Bridge, Brixton, and Camden/Primrose Hill. Tours last 2 hours; locations vary.

www.sockmobevents.org.uk. ✆ **0751/426-6775.** Tours £12 adults, £8 seniors and students.

Escorted Tours

take on 1st night

There are many reasons to lean against those hop-on, hop-off bus tours. First, they're expensive. Also, after 10 minutes of rolling down the streets in these tourist-processing machines, everything you've seen will blend into a miasma of antiquity. Third, these tours are like playing Russian roulette, because your experience depends on the skill and brains of your guide and/or the quality of the amplification system, over which you have no control.

Narrated bus tours often make you wait 15 to 30 minutes to catch your next leg, which can add up to hours wasted, and although your ticket will be good for 24 hours, don't expect to catch anything from 6pm or so until after 9am the next morning. Day tickets may come with a free walking tour (Changing the Guard, Jack the Ripper) and a hop-on, hop-off pass for the river shuttle boat (although some report that paying customers may crowd out passholders like you). Unfortunately, both of those perks must often be used during the same 24 hours as the bus ticket's validity, demolishing their usefulness.

In sum, London is a walker's city, and you're better off getting an overview on foot or, if you really want a ride, from a window seat on a real double-decker bus, which is £4 for the whole day if you use Oyster pay-as-you-go (see p. 314 for the best routes for sightseeing), or £21 for the whole week. But if you insist on perceived convenience, you can buy tickets at any marked bus stop.

HOP-ON, HOP-OFF

It's also possible to buy all-day tickets for hop-on, hop-off access to regular ferry boats on the Thames. Head to p. 317 in the last chapter for those.

Big Bus Tours Like its competition, it offers three circuitous routes, although two of them (Red and Blue) cover much of the same ground and narration is frequently prerecorded (it's live on Red, recorded on Blue) with out-of-date information. It doesn't matter at which of the 50-odd stops you get on, but since drivers often change at Green Park on Piccadilly, you can avoid that wait by starting there. Most people get on at Marble Arch, Regent Street south of Piccadilly Circus, Charing Cross Road north of Trafalgar Square, or under the South Bank Lion at Westminster Bridge. Prices can be a few pounds higher if you don't book ahead.

48 Buckingham Palace Rd., SW1. www.bigbustours.com. © **020/7808-6753.** 24-hr tours £26 adults, £13 children 5–15 (including City Cruise tour and 3 walking tours); 48-hr tickets additional £7 adults/£5 children. Daily 8:30am–8pm.

Golden Tours Open Top Bus Tours The discount option. Golden Tours is one of the big machines in town, offering every permutation of bus tour and day-trip excursion you can imagine. None are particularly special, but they get the job done at low-ish prices, which means crowds. Its main product is a system of routes granting 24-hour access to a network of nearly four dozen stops (which can be a waste of money since stops are generally only open from 8am–4:30 or 5pm), plus one free walking tour and one free river boat ride. Its Classic Tour covers most of the core city including South Kensington, and the Essential Tour forgoes South Ken but is the only line with a live narrator. Tickets are good for any line. Commensurate with the lower prices, buses can be shabby.

11a Charing Cross Rd., WC2, 156 Cromwell Rd., SW7, and 4 Fountain Sq., 123–151 Buckingham Palace Rd., SW1. www.hoponhopoffplus.com. ✆ **020/7630-2040** (U.K.) and 800/509-2507 (North America). One-day tickets £26 adults, £12 children 5–15, £66 for family of 2 adults and 2 children; 24-hr tickets £2–£4 more and include 1 river cruise and 1 walking tour. Add £6 adults, £3 children for 2nd 24-hr. period. Daily 9am–4:30pm.

The Original Tour London Sightseeing   Tours, conducted on open-top coaches, are covered for 24 hours with a ticket, so you can go around five times if your feet hurt. You can catch the bus (three interconnecting circuits that supply solid coverage of the main sights) at any of the 80-odd stops on the routes, but most people begin at Piccadilly Circus, Trafalgar Square, Embankment Station, near Victoria Station, or outside Madame Tussauds. Live narrators appear, without much vigor or inspiration, on the Yellow Line, which covers the broadest swath of town, while other lines are likely to have digital spiels, sometimes too quiet to hear. Two of its routes come with audio/booklet packs for kids, but you have to pick them up at its office.

17–19 Cockspur St., SW1. www.theoriginaltour.com. ✆ **020/8877-1722.** Tours £30 adults, £15 children 5–15; £4 adults, £2.50 children discount online (including river cruise). Mar–Oct daily 8:30am–5:20pm; Nov–Feb Fri–Sun 8:30am–5:20pm and Mon–Thurs 8:30am–4:50pm.

OTHER TOURS

Brit Movie Tours   Increasingly, people feel more connection with movies and TV than with the history that actually wrought them. For them, Brit Movie Tours hosts an array of excursions ranging from walking tours to full-day coach, including an 8-hour *Downton Abbey* visit (£80 adults, £70 children 15 and under) that sells out months ahead, and tours for James Bond, *Doctor Who,* and Harry Potter locations (£12–£27 adults/£10–£20 children 15 and under).

www.britmovietours.com. ✆ **020/7118-1007.**

City Cruises   When you take a standard trip on these generously glass-sided and -topped boats, live narrators point out details of interest. The "Red Rover" ticket allows you to hop on and off all day. Boats, which have café-bars, depart every 30 minutes, generally between 9am and 9pm, from five piers: Westminster, London Eye, Bankside, the Tower, and Greenwich, which covers a lot of the area tourists like seeing. Using it to get to Greenwich can save money off buying several one-way tickets on standard ferries, but simple return tickets are cheaper on *Thames Clippers.* The 40-minute **London Eye River Cruise** (londoneye.com; ✆ **0870/500-0600;** £13 adults, £6.50 children 5–16; daily 11:45am–4:45pm), from London Eye pier is less of a value because you can't get off to explore.

www.citycruises.com. ✆ **020/774-0400.** Tours £13 single, £17 return. 24-hr. passes: £19 adults, £13 seniors and students, £9.25 children 5–16, £37 for 2 adults and 3 children; 72-hr. passes about £3 more;10% online discount.

London Helicopter Tours   Six-seated choppers take off from Battersea and supply an epic bird's-eye view of the city, following the Thames to Greenwich, back to Hammersmith, and returning to Battersea in 12 to 18 minutes (the "Buzz" route covers less ground). Your pilot is pressed uncomfortably into double duty as a guide, dispensing dubious information such as dating the *Cutty Sark* 300 years before its actual construction. Never mind; the view is the thing, and it's an unbeatable view. You'll see the Shard from above, the ligature of countless rail lines binding the city together, and flights at 11:30am will spy Changing the Guard in the distance at Buckingham Palace. One downside: There are two seats in the front at the dashboard and four in a row along the back, so on shared flights, those two middle passengers are getting a poorer view for the same money.

London Battersea Heliport, Bridges Court, Battersea, SW11. www.thelondonhelicopter. com. ℂ **020/3811-4655.** Tours £150–£220. Daylight hours only. Tube: Clapham Junction.

Thames RIB Experience   Touristy to the core and annoying to everyone except passengers, this outfit loads groups of about a dozen in semi-inflatable RIB speedboats with twin 245-horsepower engines and flits downriver to Canary Wharf, around the O_2, or Greenwich from three far-flung piers. Try in vain to make a lasting memory of St Paul's flying past, your eyes blurry from estuary spray. Tours are 50 to 75 minutes. Its competition, offering similar thrills: **London RIB Voyages** (www.londonribvoyages.com; ℂ **020/928-8933;** £39–£53), which goes from close to the London Eye and from St Katharine's Pier near the Tower of London all the way to the Thames Barrier; and **Thames Jet** (www.thamesjet.com; ℂ **020/7740-0400;** £34–£39).

Victoria Embankment, WC2. www.thamesribexperience.com. ℂ **020/3613-2323.** Tours £27–£55 adults, £24–£39 children 15 and under; prices depend on tour length. Tube: Embankment or Charing Cross, Tower Hill, or North Greenwich.

LONDON SHOPPING

B lame Elizabeth I. Sure, the old girl loved her baubles and gold-embroidered bodices, but her biggest contribution to English consumerism was defeating the Spanish Armada. That established England as the dominant player on the high seas, which opened channels of international trade, and soon the Thames was more jammed with bounty than the parking lot at the mall on Christmas Eve. Ever since then, London has had a hankering for the finer things. Grease up your credit card!

Stores across the city generally open at 9 or 10am daily and close at 7 or 8pm, although boutiques may close at 6pm and the department stores and Oxford Street shops are often open as late as 9pm. On Sunday, relatively new terrain for British shopping, 11am or noon to 6pm is common (although arcane laws mean some stores won't make a sale until noon); very few places stay open past then. Expect crowds on weekends, when people pour into town from the countryside.

THE GREAT SHOPPING STREETS

Appropriately for a city obsessed with class, London's prime shopping streets aren't usually defined so much by what they sell as by how much you'll spend to bring home their booty.

The Arcades of Piccadilly & Old Bond Street

Tube: Green Park: There are several iron-framed, skylighted "arcades" (closed Sun), built by 19th-century blue bloods for shopping along these streets in any weather. The best include the longest one, **Burlington Arcade,** a block-long parallel to Old Bond Street at Piccadilly (silverware, cashmere, handbags, Ladurée *macarons*); the **Royal Arcade,** south of Burlington Gardens (antiques, shoes, watches, and Budd Shirtmakers, in residence since the arcade's 1910 opening); and **Piccadilly Arcade,** across from Burlington Arcade (men's tailoring; it leads to Jermyn St. [p. 201], a heart of haberdashery).

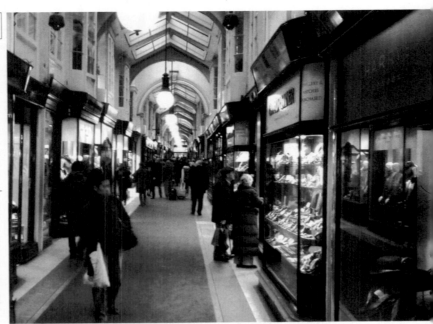

The Burlington Arcade is the longest arcade, running parallel to Old Bond Street.

Carnaby Street

Tube: Oxford Circus or Piccadilly Circus: This used to be for the mod crowd, but today its legendary hyper-alternative looks are mostly found on Memory Lane. Instead, expect mainstream sporty choices such as North Face and Vans. Better for browsing is **Kingly Court,** a former timber warehouse converted into a mini-mall for 30-odd upcoming designers. carnaby.co.uk.

Cecil Court

Tube: Leicester Square: Distinguished by original glazed-tile Victorian storefronts, matching green-and-white shop signs, and a refreshing lack of cars, Cecil Court (it and St Martin's Court just north are said to have inspired Harry Potter's Diagon Alley) was once the cradle of British cinema, but today it's a holdout of the antiquarian book trade that used to dominate Charing Cross Road. Favorites are Marchpane, at 16, a trove of vintage children's literature; Pleasures of Past Times' David Drummond, at 11, an "ephemerist" collecting theatrical memorabilia; and Travis & Emery, at 17, specializing in music and books about music. www.cecilcourt.co.uk.

Seven Dials

Tube: Covent Garden: Every lane around Covent Garden is an obvious shopping drag, full of the usual brands but increasingly some one-off names.

Check out **Neal Street** for shoes, **Long Acre** for big clothing stores, and **Floral Street** for designers. www.coventgardenlondonuk.com.

Jermyn Street

Tube: Piccadilly Circus or Green Park: The quintessential street for the natty man is home to several multi-named haberdashers that have been in business for more than a century. Try Harvie & Hudson, Hilditch & Key (since 1899), Hawes & Curtis, and mahogany-lined Turnbull & Asser (1895)—dresser of Chaplin, Churchill, Prince Charles, Ronald Reagan, William, Harry, and James Bond. There's also a growing number of shoemakers, such as Tricker's, which tend to be better as you move toward St. James's Street. It connects to Piccadilly via Princes Arcade, which is also strong on shoes.

Kensington High Street

Tube: High Street Kensington: London's coolest department store street in the '60s is less mod now. The big tickets have since decamped for the malls, and it's now a hodgepodge of upmarket brand names, young trendy stuff on the east end, plus some boutiques on **Kensington Church Street.**

King's Road

Tube: Sloane Square or South Kensington: The Chelsea avenue where affluent "Sloaneys" spend is where you go to dream—increasingly, about what King's Road used to be. Most of the truly unique stores have recently been elbowed aside by the same old names, but amid the familiar (Ted Baker, Rag & Bone, Anthropologie), you'll find a few independent boutiques, high-end mommy wear, and some designer furnishings. That doesn't mean the French cafes on Sloane Square aren't prime real estate for watching those happy rich kids pass by.

New Bond Street

Tube: Bond Street or Green Park: The ultimate high-end purchasing pantheon runs from Oxford Street to Piccadilly, partly as Old Bond Street. Every account-draining trinket maker has a presence, including Sotheby's, Van Cleef & Arpels, Graff, Harry Winston, Tiffany & Co., Chopard, and Boucheron. Asprey, at 165–169, sells adornments few can afford, but its Victorian facade is a visual treat for all incomes. A short walk west, **South Molton Street** continues the luxury, but at a half-step down in expense. Check out Browns (p. 210), which gave Alexander McQueen and John Galliano early validation.

Oxford Street

Tube: Marble Arch, Bond Street, or Oxford Circus: The king of London shopping streets supports the biggest names, including Topshop, H&M, the ever-mobbed Primark, and a few lollapalooza department stores like Selfridges, John Lewis, and Marks & Spencer. Boy, are weekends crowded! www.oxfordstreet.co.uk.

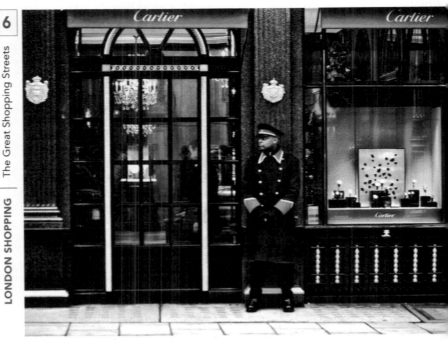

New Bond Street offers high-end shopping with stores such as Cartier's.

Redchurch Street

Tube: Shoreditch High Street: This 3-block Shoreditch stretch, once rammed with cabinetmakers, today is at the forefront for stylists. The 150-year-old menswear brand Sunspel opened its first retail shop here; Labour and Wait (p. 218) vends desirable kitchen toys; Maison Trois Garçons does slick interiors; and Terence Conran's super-chic hotel/restaurant/café complex Boundary, including the café Albion, seals the deal for scenesters. Around the corner, **Boxpark,** a hipster mall comprised of five dozen rehabbed shipping containers, hosts both emerging names and not-really slumming corporate brands, while **Cheshire Street** is ideal for vintage discoveries.

Sloane Street

Tube: Knightsbridge: Offshore millionaires come here to feast at the top of the consumerist food chain: Bulgari, Valentino, Miu Miu, Prada, Armani, and everything else haute and showy. And no farther than you can throw a chocolate truffle, Harvey Nichols and Harrods. www.sloane-street.co.uk.

Tottenham Court Road

Tube: Tottenham Court Road or Goodge Street: Locals sniff, but Tottenham Court Road's lower half, from Oxford Street north to Store Street, is their drag for cut-rate electronics (including voltage converters). North to

Torrington Place, pickings shift to brilliantly designed housewares and furnishings at Habitat (p. 218) and London's grande dame of smart styling, Heal's (p. 218).

Upper Street

Tube: Angel: Islington's chief avenue is emerging as a low-key location for boutiques, vintage outfits, and kitchen-sink junk shops, all pleasantly spelled by unpretentious pubs and cafes. While you're south of the Green, explore the sidewalks of **Camden Passage** (p. 207), known for antiques and bric-a-brac.

THE SHOPPING PALACES

Fortnum & Mason ★★★   So venerable is this vendor, which began life in 1707 as the candle maker to Queen Anne, that in 1922 archaeologist Howard Carter used empty F&M boxes to tote home the treasures of King Tut's tomb. The quintessentially British, modestly sized department store, which has a focus on gourmet foods, is renowned for its glamorous food hampers, which were first distributed in the days before World War I, when soldiers' families were responsible for feeding their men on the field. Picnic sets now come with bone china and can cost £300, but you can also pack your own. For the full experience, which will leave your family with no inheritance, head to

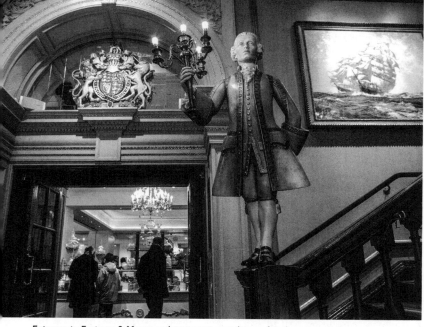

Entrance to Fortnum & Mason, a department store known for elegant picnic hampers.

the first floor to peruse its famous wicker hampers, which you can then fill with goodies from the ground-floor Food Hall and have shipped. Select from a cornucopia of such tongue-teasing triumphs as jarred black truffles and fresh Blue Stilton cheese in ceramic pots. In addition to a huge selection of tea packaged in distinctive canisters (*so* much tea), F&M makes its own "parlour ice" (ice creams), "royal game pie" (loafs of seasonal game meats layered with cheese), and something called Rubies in the Rubble (chutney made from fruits obtained in London's markets). Content yourself, as most do, with a wander through the carpeted upper-floor departments, which are lit by chandelier, serenaded by classical music, and illuminated by a lotuslike atrium skylight. The fragrance department smells like a rose garden. High tea can be taken in the top-floor St James's tearooms, among the city's most sumptuous (reservations ✆ **0845/602-5694**), while lunching ladies can be found in the banquettes of the Fountain Restaurant. When the clock strikes the hour over the store's Piccadilly entrance, two modern mechanical representations of Mr. Fortnum and Mr. Mason emerge, bow to each other approvingly, and return to business inside.

181 Piccadilly, W1. www.fortnumandmason.london. ✆ **020/7734-8040.** Tube: Green Park or Piccadilly Circus.

Harrods ★   Now owned by the Qatari royal family's financiers, a miraculous holdover from the golden age of shopping has been retooled into a bombastic mall appealing largely to free-spending out-of-towners. Few London-born people bother with it, yet it thrives, proof of just how awash with foreign fortunes the city truly is. Its thronged Food Hall rooms are a glut of exorbitantly priced meats and cheeses, its ornate seven-floor facade emblazoned like a Christmas tree after dark, its jewelry hall attended by robotic staff plying the husbands of spoiled wives with champagne until they give in. But much floor space, where too-loud rock music blares nonstop, is devoted either to brands you'd find for a third of the price at your local mall or to One-Percenter nonsense such as £150,000 sculptures. The artificial environment, from the overpriced razzmatazz to the clerks wearing straw hats, would be more authentic at Disneyland than in London of old. In the souvenir "emporium" on the second floor (£17 for sandwich-size gusset bags; £15 mugs; teddy bears aplenty), I sense the air has been pumped with the same scent you smell at Disney wherever the company wants to coax customers into purchasing (a trick called "olfactory coding"). Of the many escalator banks, the most interesting is the uproarious Egyptian-themed one at the store's center. At its base is a tacky brass fountain memorial to Dodi Al-Fayed and Princess Diana, who died together in Paris in 1997—his father owned Harrods at the time and campaigned to prove Prince Philip ordered the murder of Diana lest she marry a Muslim. A lipstick-smudged wine glass from the couple's final tryst is preserved along with a ring with which al-Fayed claims his son intended to propose to Diana. Tacky! If you crave a real British department store, visit Fortnum & Mason or Selfridges; if you want to be flabbergasted by the pompous excesses of the jet set, Harrods is the overly shellacked circus for you, but don't be fooled into thinking it's something traditional.

87–135 Brompton Rd., SW1. www.harrods.com. ℗ **020/7730-1234.** Tube: Knightsbridge.

Harvey Nichols ★ *Absolutely Fabulous*'s shallow anti-heroines Patsy and Edina spoke of it with the same breathless reverence most people reserve for deities. You'll need the income of a god to afford a single thread of Harvey Nick's women's and men's fashions, and although the British-owned store isn't as popular as it used to be—it's been here since the 1880s—a stroll through this eight-floor spendthrift's heaven is entertaining. Note the lunching ladies on display in the fifth-floor restaurant—think of it as a zoo for old money.

109–125 Knightsbridge, SW1. www.harveynichols.com. ℗ **020/7235-5000.** Tube: Knightsbridge.

John Lewis ★★ Every Englishman knows that if you want a sound deal, you go here, where there's a price guarantee; it employs an army of people to scout for the lowest prices in the area, which it matches. That may sound like the gimmick of a low-rent wannabe, but John Lewis, established in 1864, is in fact a respected cooperative owned by its employees, and their interest in its success shows in their attentive service and seemingly limitless product line. It also has some exceptional buyers; you'll find things here no other store carries (the bedding department is renowned). Art fans shouldn't miss the building's eastern face, upon which is mounted an abstract cast-aluminum sculpture, *The Winged Figure* (1960), by one of the most important artists of the 20th century, Dame Barbara Hepworth, whose work is in the Tate Britain (p. 132).

Oxford St. at Holles St. www.johnlewis.com/oxfordstreet. ℗ **0844/693-1765.** Tube: Oxford Circus.

Liberty ★★ Founded in 1875, Liberty made its name (and earned some mockery) as an importer of Asian art and as a major proponent of Art Nouveau style. Now its focus is distinctly British. The timber-and-plaster wing looks Tudor, but is actually a 1924 revival constructed from the salvaged timbers of two ships, HMS *Impregnable* and HMS *Hindustan;* the length of the latter ship equals the building's length along Great Marlborough Street. The store's stationery and scarf selections are celebrated, as are its fabrics (many of which are designed in house or only available briefly), and the beauty hall is one of the best. The soft wooden spaces are creaky and seductive, while the staff service is so obsequious it evokes a bygone era.

210–220 Regent St., W1. www.liberty.co.uk. ℗ **020/7734-1234.** Tube: Oxford Circus.

Marks & Spencer ★★★ The beloved M&S is the country's favorite midlevel department store for good-looking clothing staples. Its own-brand looks, once shoddy and ill-fitting, have been re-envisioned as affordable riffs on well-tailored fashions, and it sells the go-to suit for many a young man starting out in life. M&S is particularly beloved for its underwear, and its bathrobes are preternaturally soft. But its crowning achievement is its giant **food**

halls ★★★ (usually tucked underneath the store but sometimes a stand-alone shop called **Simply Food**), which sell an astonishing array of prepared meals, soups and sandwiches, and well-selected yet inexpensive wines. M&S is a national treasure, with nothing like it in other countries, and it's about time the English remembered that.

Flagship: 458 Oxford St., W1. www.marksandspencer.co.uk. ℃ **020/7935-7954.** Tube: Marble Arch.

Selfridges ★★★   Selfridges fills the real-life role in London life that many tourists think Harrods does; aside from Harrods' olive drab sacks, no shopping bag speaks louder about your shopping preferences than a canary yellow screamer from Selfridges. It's unquestionably the better of the two stores, since it's not merely a sprawling sensory treat, but also sells items you'd actually buy. Since its 1909 opening by Harry Gordon Selfridge, an immoderate American marketing genius from Marshall Field's in Chicago (the building was designed by Daniel Burnham, of Manhattan's Flatiron Building fame), Selfridges has pioneered many department store practices. Placing the perfumes near the front door, filling its 27 ground-floor windows with consumerist fantasias, coining the phrase "the customer is always right"—all Selfridges inventions. Some one million products are for sale, and the beauty department is Europe's largest. The thicket of food counters on the ground floor gets busy at lunchtime, and the rest of the store is just as popular at other times; some 17 million visits are recorded each year. Selfridges has traded in history, too; the first public demonstration of television was held on the first floor in 1925, and 3 years later, the store sold the world's first TV set. During much of the Blitz, Churchill's transatlantic conversations with FDR were encoded via a scrambler stashed in the cellar. The store's popularity is enjoying a goose thanks to the series *Mr. Selfridge,* with Jeremy Piven barking his way through the title role, which gives the store the soapy treatment.

400 Oxford St., W1. www.selfridges.com. ℃ **0800/123-400** (U.K.) or 113/369-8040 (overseas). Tube: Bond St. or Marble Arch.

RECOMMENDED STORES

For a city world-famous for shopping, where people from around the world arrive with one fat wallet and leave with 10 stuffed suitcases, there's no way to give proper celebratory due to everything that is wonderful and for sale. Some stores, though, are so original and site-specific that they can sweeten the experience of being in London, even if you don't buy a thing.

Art & Antiques

After Noah ★   More like an upscale junk shop with restoration chops, it makes its name on vintage toys, crockery, bathroom fittings, cheerful celluloid jewelry, and wooden desks and bedsteads (sadly, those are too large to get home). 121 Upper St., N1. www.afternoah.com. ℃ **020/7359-4281.** Tube: Angel.

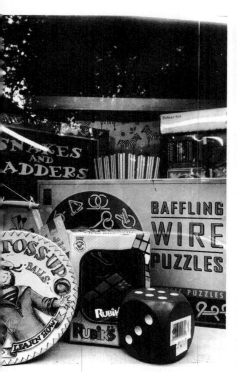

Window display at After Noah, which resembles an upscale junk shop.

Blue Mantle ★ For dream renovations back home, the largest antique fireplace showroom in the world salvages the good stuff with warm English touches when developers knock down classic buildings—which is happening more than we like. 306–312 Old Kent Rd., SE1. www.bluemantle.co.uk. ℗ **020/7703-7437.** Tube: Borough.

Camden Passage ★★ Plenty of tourists swing through the booths, so bargains aren't always easy to come by. Still, shimmering examples of china, silverware, cocktail shakers, military medals, coins, and countless other hand-me-downs overflow the cases. Despite the name, it's in Islington. Off Upper St., N1. www.camdenpassageislington.co.uk. Market on Wed, Sat, smaller one Sun. Tube: Angel.

Grays ★★ Not the place to go if you're looking for the lowest deal (it's in Mayfair), but it's definitely a source for variety. There are some 200 vendors, many experts registered in the official antiques societies, split among two buildings, selling everything from Victorian jewelry to toys to strange bric-a-brac and collectible silverware. Weekdays are best. Head into the basement of the Mews building to see the River Tyburn, which was buried by 18th-century redevelopment but now feeds into Grays' goldfish trough. 58 Davies St., W1. www.graysantiques.com. ℗ **020/7629-7034.** Closed Sun. Tube: Bond St.

LASSCo ★★ From stained glass to paneling and faucets to wood flooring, you'll get an incredible selection of fittings and furniture rescued from museums, churches, pubs, and homes at LASSCo (the London Architectural Salvage and Supply Company). 41 Maltby St., SE1. www.lassco.co.uk.℗ **020/7394-8061.** Tube: Bermondsey. Also at Brunswick House: 30 Wandsworth Rd., SW8; ℗ **020/7394-2100.** Tube: Vauxhall.

Books

The territorial nature of publishing means that many books that are for sale in London won't be in print back home. Take time to trawl the used-book stores along **Charing Cross Road** and, off that, the collectibles of **Cecil Court** (p. 200), which runs to St Martin's Lane. The major art museums are strong on titles in their respective disciplines, especially **Tate Modern** (p. 155),

Museum of London (p. 159), and the biographies of the National Portrait Gallery (p. 124). Now that the Samuel French bookstore has closed, performing artists turn to the bookshop at the National Theatre, Southbank, SE1; shop.nationaltheatre.org.uk; ℗ 020/7452-3456; Waterloo tube).

Daunt Books ★★ Lined with oak galleries and lit by a long, central skylight, Daunt prides itself on its travel collection, which is located down a groaning wooden staircase. Everything is arranged by the country it's about—Third Reich histories under Germany, Tolstoy under Russia. It's no slouch in the general interest categories, either. Clerks seem to know what will interest the vaguest browser, and the cashier's desk is always piled with choice curiosities. 83 Marylebone High St., W1. www.daunt books.co.uk. ℗ **020/7224-2295.** Tube: Baker St.

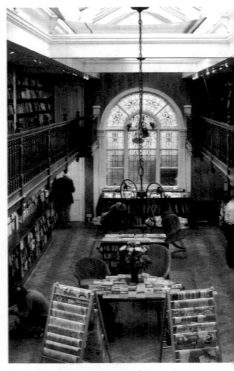

Daunt Books on Marylebone High Street has an extensive travel collection.

Foyles ★★ In business since 1903, this institution has thus far navigated the onslaught of high rents and low readership. After the 1999 death of its off-putting and tyrannical owner, the store was once again passed to the next generation of the Foyle family, and it finally caught up with modernity just in time to avoid closure. Its huge inventory of 200,000 titles straddles both popular and specialty topics. There are small outlets at Waterloo Station and the Royal Festival Hall on Southbank, but this beloved HQ is more like a theme park for readers, full of talks, special events, and signings. If you sign into its free Wi-Fi, you can get walking directions to the shelf containing the title you want. 107 Charing Cross Rd., WC2. www.foyles.co.uk. ℗ **020/7437-5660.** Tube: Tottenham Court Rd.

Hatchards ★★ Although the Duke of Wellington and the queen herself are counted among its customers, Hatchards, the oldest bookseller in the city (1797), is noted for its signed first editions, as well as for its famous shoplifters: An 18-year-old Noël Coward was apprehended as he stuffed a suitcase full of books. (Characteristically, he talked his way out of trouble.) It has been trading since 1801 at its current location, which means it was selling books before Hardy, Dickens, or the Brontës were writing them. Virginia Woolf wrote about it, too, in *Mrs Dalloway*. You'll find it not far west of Waterstones (p. 209). 187 Piccadilly, W1. www.hatchards.co.uk. ℗ **020/7439-9921.** Tube: Piccadilly Circus.

Housmans Booksellers ★ London supports a vibrant protest community—don't forget this is where Karl Marx fashioned his views that changed the world—and since 1945, the city's preeminent store for radical books has been Housmans. It also boasts the United Kingdom's largest collection of magazines and newspaors, with some 200 titles on offer at any time, plus stationery and a cafe (free trade all the way). You're not going to find most of the stuff here published back home. Wednesdays at 7pm, an author speaks. 5 Caledonian Rd., N1. www.housmans.com. ✆ **020/7837-4473.** Tube: King's Cross St Pancras.

Persephone Books ★ Persephone rediscovers and reprints works by forgotten mid-20th-century writers, most of them female—it was responsible for reintroducing *Miss Pettigrew Lives for a Day,* which then became a movie. The shop, on a street brimming with other boutiques, is charming. 59 Lamb's Conduit St., WC1. www.persephonebooks.co.uk. ✆ **020/7242-9292.** Tube: Russell Square.

Stanfords ★★★ Marvelous since 1901, Stanfords trades in globe-trotting goodness, from guides to narratives to fiction with a worldview. Should you accidentally leave your map in your hotel room, beeline to the basement; the floor there is covered with an oversized reproduction of the London A-Z map as well as reams of maps for purchase, especially for walking trails across Britain. 12–14 Long Acre. www.stanfords.co.uk. ✆ **020/7836-1321.** Tube: Covent Garden.

Waterstones ★★★ In a location opened in 1936 as Simpson's clothiers—the Art Deco model for Grace Brothers in the saucy Britcom *Are You Being Served?* (the show's creator was a clerk)—this branch of the giant chain is now Europe's largest bookshop. Even if Waterstones is a Big Gorilla of bookselling, it handles the stewardship of that dubious title with dignity; there

The Royal Warrant

When you're snooping around the stuffy shops of St James's or Mayfair, keep an eye out for a royal crest near the store's sign. That insignia is a seal of approval—its presence means that the business counts a member of the royal family as a customer and has done so for at least 5 years. To earn Prince Charles's plumed crest, stores have to do even more and prove they abide by a sustainable environmental policy. The queen is represented by a lion and a unicorn, but William doesn't have any warrants registered yet. Once a business wins a warrant—about 800 have done it, from chandeliers to elevator repair—it's extraordinarily rare to see it withdrawn (to its humiliation, Harrods lost its seal in 2000). Which hotel does the queen prefer? The Goring (p. 47), which earned its warrant in 2013. More great retailers: Anderson & Sheppard (Prince Charles's clothing), Corney & Barrow (wine), Jeroboams (cheese), and Dewar's (the queen's quaff). But don't ask what specific items businesses are delivering to the Palace; shopkeepers aren't permitted to tattle. To learn which companies supply the Windsors—say, where the queen buys her corgis' dog food—search the current warrant holders at www.royalwarrant.org.

are six sweeping floors, an enormous London section, plenty of easy chairs for freeloaders, scads of discount offers, and a dedicated events space for visiting authors. The top floor's panoramic cafe, 5th View, hops after work and into the evening. 203 Piccadilly. www.waterstones.com. ⓒ **0843/290-8549.** Tube: Piccadilly Circus.

Clothing & Accessories

The clothes you find in the U.K. will not be the same as in major stores elsewhere. Site **Dressipi.com** tracks the current pulse of English High Street women's fashions.

Albam ★★   Unusually, this men's boutique seeks out well-constructed, honest clothing (most made in the U.K.) but doesn't mark it up by insane factors. Although its prices are similar to those of high-casual chain stores, the store has a following among guys because its clothing lasts so long. 23 Beak St., W1. www.albamclothing.com. ⓒ **020/3157-7000.** Tube: Piccadilly Circus or Oxford Circus.

Beyond Retro ★★   A one-stop for classic items (jeans, jackets, boots, and other casuals), it's a haunt of the poor and stylish, who can put together an off-margin look without overdrawing. There's a branch in Soho (58–59 Great Marlborough St., W1; ⓒ **020/7434-1406;** Oxford Circus tube), but this is the location with the cat Tiny, who lives in the store and has become a local mascot. 110–112 Cheshire St., E2. www.beyondretro.com. ⓒ **020/7613-3636.** Tube: Shoreditch High St. or Whitechapel.

Blitz London ★★   Blitz has crowned itself Europe's largest vintage shop, a boast I cannot authenticate, but it's true you'll be spoilt for choice. 55–59 Hanbury St., E1. www.blitzlondon.co.uk. ⓒ **020/7377-8828.** Tube: Shoreditch High St.

Browns ★★   Some 100 designers, all of them for higher-end purchasers, fill these five connected shops at the top of Mayfair. For four decades, it's been a marketplace for upscale women, but increasingly, it's pitching to a younger and more casual set. 24–27 S. Molton St., W1. www.brownsfashion.com. ⓒ **020/7514-0016.** Tube: Bond St.

Burberry Factory Outlet ★   Although its East London location is charmless and somewhat laborious to reach, it's worth it for overstock prices that dip 30% to 70% lower than what's on sale in the brand's high-end stores—still expensive, but a lot less than the usual damage. 29–31 Chatham Place, E9. ⓒ **020/8328-4287.** Tube/National Rail: Hackney Central.

Cordings ★★   Britain's top manufacturer of Wellington boots, which were invented for the first Duke of Wellington, can be found at this well-heeled and very English emporium of field clothing, suits, waistcoats, tweeds, and knitwear that cost a pretty pound. It has traded here since 1877. 19 Piccadilly, W1. www.cordings.co.uk. ⓒ **020/7734-0830.** Closed Sun. Tube: Piccadilly Circus.

Diverse ★   One of the first boutiques to move into Islington's Upper Street, Dicerse has moved to a more affordable 'hood but keeps stock changing even as it spotlights white-hot labels, many of which go on to greatness.

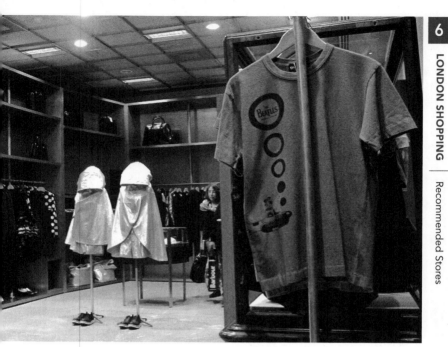

Dover Street Market offers couture and a bakery on the top floor.

Clothes tend toward arty, which is to say interesting but not irresistible. 148 Fortress Rd., NW5. www.diverseclothing.com. ℂ **020/7813-7425.** Tube: Tufnell Park.

Dover Street Market ★ A high-minded multidesigner concept, heavy on pretentious industrial architecture, is supported by couture (all of Comme des Garçons' lines) fused with multimedia art installations, all in a six-story department store–like space with a bakery on the top floor. 17–18 Dover St., W1. www.doverstreetmarket.com. ℂ **020/7518-0680.** Tube: Green Park.

The Goodhood Store ★★ Consummately East End, the clothing and "life store" products sold in this popular, half-serious two-story emporium are all about what it means to feel cool. Don a faux-vintage T-shirt printed with inscrutable gibberish, carry home a "The Masses are Asses" mug for your latte, and stock up on the latest on-trend grooming products. Independent, self-knowing—but it only *looks* secondhand. 151 Curtain Rd., EC2. www.goodhood store.com. ℂ **020/7729-3600.** Tube: Old St.

Herbert Johnson ★★ This hatter, in business since 1889, made Indiana Jones' famous fedora, called The Poet Hat, for Steven Spielberg in 1980. That's so awesome, not much more needs to be said, except that it can make a cool hat for you, too. In the Swaine Adeney Brigg store, 7 Piccadilly Arcade, SW1. www.herbert-johnson.co.uk. ℂ **020/7409-7277.** Closed Sun. Tube: Green Park or Piccadilly Circus.

Jack Wills ★★ "Fabulously British," it brags, but this line still comes off a bit like American Eagle Goes to Eton. It goes for a sporty prep school look with rugby shirts, tweeds, cute striped trunks, and brightly hued jumpers. It has expanded internationally, but here's the three-story flagship. 136 Long Acre, WC2. www.jackwills.com. ℗ **020/7240-8946.** Tube: Leicester Square.

James Smith & Sons ★★★ This shop out of time, hung from the outside with old-style high Victorian lettering, is rattling the rafters inside with handmade umbrellas and walking sticks. That's all it makes, as it has done since 1830, so you can imagine the wonders: handles of hazelnut wood, ebony, buffalo horn, and antler, from £25 to more than £300. Clerks can also fashion a box so you can check your purchase onto the plane. Hazlewood House, 53 New Oxford St., WC1. www.james-smith.co.uk. ℗ **020/7836-4731.** Tube: Holborn or Tottenham Court Rd.

Jimmy Choo ★ The legendary Malaysian cobbler started his luxe line in 1996 with a fashion editor from the British edition of *Vogue*. Today, he designs a couture line that is sold by appointment only at 18 Connaught St. (℗ **020/7262-6888**), a location so exclusive it's not posted on the corporate website. If you're not a celebrity or MP's wife, you'll have to content yourself with the 3-level flagship store. 27 New Bond St., W1. www.jimmychoo.com. ℗ **020/ 7493-5858.** Tube: Bond St.

Joules ★★ Tongue-in-cheek, summery British clothing in whites and brights for a jaunty day out (especially for women). Unit 15, Waterloo Station, N1. www.joules.com. ℗ **020/7928-1323.** Tube: Waterloo.

Levisons ★★ In an old storefront with the vintage smell of bygone closets, find early-era men's jackets and suits you could only locate in England— Harris tweeds, school uniforms, tailored peacoats. The stock changes weekly. In fact, all of Cheshire Street is lined with boutiques for unusual vintage finds. 1 Cheshire St., E2. www.levisons.co.uk. ℗ **020/3609-2224.** Tube: Shoreditch High St.

Lock & Co. ★ Exquisitely crafted classic British hats (Panamas and bowlers, for men, women, and kids, too) are made by this hatter dating to 1765. Their hats have been favored by Wilde, Churchill, Prince Charles, Oddjob from *Goldfinger,* and even the queen—it tailors the inside of her crowns. 6 St James's St., SW1. www.lockhatters.co.uk. ℗ **020/7930-8874.** Tube: Green Park.

Mango ★ Take the cream of high fashion and make it accessible for the typical English young woman—that's the formula at this slightly upmarket label, which does well when you want your look to be colorful, casual, and maybe even beachy. 225–235 Oxford St., W1. mango.com. ℗ **020/7534-3505.** Tube: Oxford Circus.

Monsoon ★ One of the favored High Street brands for women, Monsoon's outfits are for independent dressers who favor bright hues and aren't afraid of a few embellishments. It also does good eveningwear. 498–500 Oxford St., W1. monsoon.co.uk. ℗ **020/7491-3004.** Tube: Marble Arch.

New Look ★★   Another reliable and very successful High Street chain, New Look does a huge amount of cute casual wear fashionably and cheaply. Its specialty is women's clothes, but it does a few men's, and it captures trends without going overboard. 500–502 Oxford St., W1. www.newlook.co.uk. ℭ **020/7290-7860.** Tube: Marble Arch.

Nick Tentis ★   This London-born men's designer (favored by Eddie Red-mayne and Martin Freeman) revitalizes the Savile Row neighborhood's fusty looks with ready-to-wear suits in youthful, Mod-culture cuts and modern, sometimes daring, fabrics. 37 Savile Row, W1. www.nicktentis.com. ℭ **020/7287-1966.** Tube: Piccadilly Circus or Oxford Circus.

Office ★★★   The H&M of footwear rips off designer styles cheaply but effectively. You'll find it everywhere in town, but one of the most convenient locations is here, in the Seven Dials area of Covent Garden. Office's major competition **Schuh,** found around town, mostly stocks other brands (although it has its own sub-line). 57 Neal St., WC2. www.office.co.uk. ℭ **020/7379-1896.** Tube: Covent Garden.

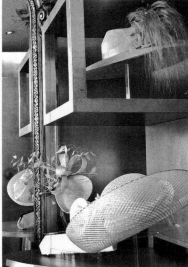

Hats at Philip Treacy.

Philip Treacy ★★   If you're invited to Ascot, it would be churlish not to be seen in one of Philip Treacy's world-famous designs in *haute couture* hats, bonnets, or fasci-nators. If you're not, you're welcome to go home with a £1,200 white ele-phant. 69 Elizabeth St., SW1. www.philip treacy.co.uk. ℭ **020/7730-3992.** Closed Sun. Tube: Victoria or Sloane Square.

Primark ★★★   The most intense, most crowded, most oppressive store on Oxford Street roils with young families stuffing baskets with cheap-as-chips fashionable outfits, shoes, luggage, and outrageously lowballed accessories. Unfortunately, we're also talking about a clientele that discards garments wherever they want, staff that deals with the rubble using big push brooms, no washrooms, and products that won't last a year. But the bar-gains! Oh, the bargains—most stuff is less than £10, and £1 deals are common. You just can't help leaving with sacksful. "The devil wears Primark," mutter the snobs. 213 Oxford St., W1. www.primark.co.uk. ℭ **020/7495-0420.** Tube: Marble Arch. Also at 14–18 Oxford St., W1. ℭ **020/7580-5510.** Tube: Tottenham Court Rd.

River Island ★★   Another of the popular, affordable women's High Street fashion brands, River Island is headquartered in West London and designs most of its wares in-house. Dresses are affordable, shoes are cool, leather jackets well-cut, and there's a kid's line. In 2013, Rihanna tried her hand at formulating a collection for the brand. Police had to restrain the crowd. The course of fashion did not change. 301 Oxford St. (✆ **0844/826-9835**), 207–213 Oxford St. (✆ **0844/847-2666**), and 309 Oxford St. (✆ **0844/395-1011**), W1. www.river island.com. Tube: Oxford Circus.

Rokit ★★   Because it's been cool for longer than many of its competitors have been in business, Rokit has a strong following. Probably the largest collection in the city, it sells retro and vintage threads, shoes, and accessories that are funky and hipster-prone, from 1950s industrial uniforms to tracksuits. 42 Shelton St., WC2. www.rokit.co.uk. ✆ **020/7836-6547.** Tube: Covent Garden. Also in Whitechapel (101 and 107 Brick Lane, E1, ✆ **020/7375-3864,** Shoreditch High St. tube) and Camden (225 Camden High St., NW1, ✆ **020/7267-3046,** Camden Town tube).

Topshop ★★★   At this 8,361-sq.-m (90,000-sq.-ft.) store, some 1,000 employees are on hand, many charged expressly with helping shoppers put together a smashing new outfit. The range of accessories is dizzying—you can even get tattooed or pierced if you're so inclined. It's not just women, either,

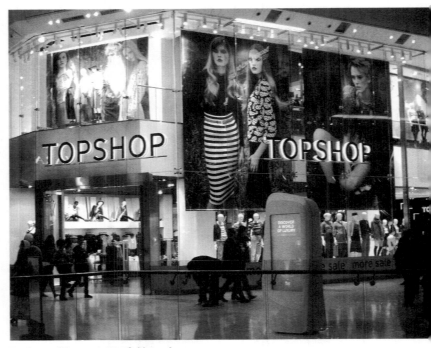

Topshop and Topman in Westfields London.

WHAT CAN I bring home?

Although you should always claim edibles when you pass through Customs, very few things will be confiscated. Most stuff, including baked goods, honeys, vinegars, condiments, roasted coffee, teas, candy bars, crisps, pickles, and homemade dishes are good to go. And Cadbury chocolate! Stores can't import it to the U.S. now, so grab all you can! Always check your country's requirements, but these things are certain to make the inspector dog's nose twitch:

o Meat and anything containing meat, be it dried, canned, or bouillon.
o Fresh fruit and vegetables.
o Runny cheeses, but not firm ones (rule of thumb: If you have to keep it chilled, leave it behind).
o Rice. As if you would import rice.
o Plants, soil, wood, and seeds (non-edible). Ask the nursery whether you need paperwork, because many varieties are permitted. And be warned that officers in Australia respond to wood like it's kryptonite.

because the incorporated **Topman** is crammed with deal seekers, too, and its colorful socks are legion and fun. Designs are at the vanguard of youth fashion, yet the prices are defiantly low, which makes this forward-thinking store a primary stop. 214 Oxford St., W1. www.topshop.com. ✆ **020/7636-7700.** Tube: Oxford St.

Uniqlo ★★★ Savvy and of unexpectedly low prices, the Japan-based, rapidly multiplying megastore is another staple on any sensible Oxford Street shopping spree. The first renter to pay £1,000 per foot in rent for its £40,000-square-foot store on Oxford Street, it does jeans and tops extremely well, but it's also known for cool socks and sweaters, though its hallmark is poppy colors and sporty casuals. 311 Oxford St., W1. www.uniqlo.co.uk. ✆ **020/7290-7701.** Tube: Oxford St.

World's End ★ For a few years in the 1970s, Vivienne Westwood's shop was the coolest place on the planet. The clock at this guerilla boutique still runs backwards, but London's punk heyday is long over, and Westwood went from rebel to royalty. Never mind the bargains—her Anglomania label is a living museum, but it's not cheap. Still, the fanciful couture inventions, flowing with fabric, are outlandish enough to enchant. 430 Kings Rd., SW10. www.worldsendshop.co.uk. ✆ **020/7352-6551.** Closed Sun. Tube: Fulham Broadway.

Food

Don't neglect the outdoor markets (p. 219), **Borough Market** (p. 95 in chapter 4), or the food halls of the shopping palaces (earlier in this chapter). One warning: Don't buy tea from a touristy shop. Stick to the reputable sellers like **Twinings** (p. 217) or **Fortnum & Mason** (p. 203).

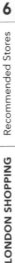

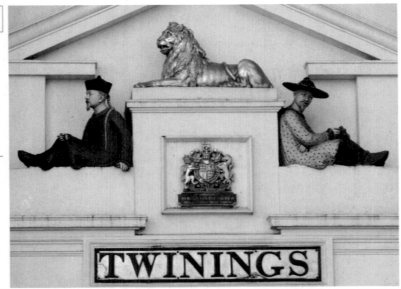

Twining's, the queen's tea and coffee merchants.

A. Gold ★★   English food has been a punch line for so long that even the British were starting to believe the reputation. A. Gold looks longstanding because of its vintage fittings, but it's actually a newcomer. It peddles country comfort food that you can't even find at the English supermarkets anymore, such as Cornish salted sardine filets, Romney's Kendal mint cakes, Geo. Watkins Anchovy Sauce, and Yorkshire brack—okay, those names aren't helping, are they? 42 Brushfield St., E1. www.agoldshop.com. *C* **020/7247-2487.** Closes 4pm. Tube: Liverpool St.

Dark Sugars Cocoa House ★★   Sublime handmade chocolates and truffles (gin and lime, stem ginger and honey, and more) sourced from a family farm in Ghana are the addictive wares at this Brick Lane success story. The golden "pearl" orbs containing smooth hazelnut nougat are delicate and divine, and the shop makes incredible hot chocolates—try it with chili—and even vegan versions. They don't deliver to North America, so indulge here. There's a small shop at 141 Brick Lane, but this flagship is larger. 124–126 Brick Ln, E1. www.darksugars.co.uk. *C* **074/294-7260.** Tube: Liverpool St. or Shoreditch High St.

The SAvanna ★   For a taste of South Africa, try *biltong* or *droëwors,* two flavorful jerkies made of local beef. SAvanna will also sell you antipodean candy (Lunch Bar) and sodas—the Stoney ginger beer curls your toes. There are locations in Victoria, Paddington, and Liverpool Street stations, testament to the number of expats from former Empire nations who live here. Multiple locations. www.thesavanna.co.uk. *C* **020/8971-9177.** Tube: London Bridge.

Twinings ★★   Does this tea boutique rely on tourist traffic? Definitely. But it's still steeped in tradition, having taken over from a coffee shop in this narrow, portrait-lined location in 1706. Here you can sample, taste, mix-and-match, and savor the leaf in all its varieties—or just peruse its little tea museum. 216 Strand, WC2. www.twinings.co.uk. ℂ **020/7353-3511.** Tube: Temple.

Health & Beauty

Boots ★   Do I dare suggest you patronize the ubiquitous High Street brand that has devoured all other drugstores? Yes, I certainly do. Something like 80% of fragrance sales in the U.K. are conducted over Boots' counters, and the chain's endless 3-for-2 promotions almost always include something worth taking home, be it Berocca vitamins or other hard-to-get items. Makeup costs a few pounds less than at most other stores. It's authentically British, too—its founder, John Campbell Boot, the second Baron Trent, has his picture in the National Portrait Gallery. Multiple locations. www.boots.co.uk.

Neal's Yard Remedies ★★★   At the forefront of Britain's powerful green movement, this shop supplies beauty aids, holistic treatments, massage oils, and even make-your-own-cosmetics ingredients, all cruelty-free, clear of toxins, and naturally formulated. Its products—London's answer to the New York beauty boutique Kiehl's—are respected for their quality. The namesake store was squeezed out of gentrified Neal's Yard, so the location you're most likely to visit is at Borough Market. 4 Stoney St., SE1. www.nealsyardremedies. com. ℂ **020/7407-4877.** Tube: Covent Garden.

Penhaligon's ★★★   I don't enjoy the mental image of Prince Charles lighting a Lily of the Valley candle and anointing his body with English Fern eau de toilette, but the fact is that Penhaligon's, established in 1870, is listed as an official supplier of "toilet requisites" to the Prince of Wales, so it may be happening right now. The company hand-squeezes and custom designs its own fragrances for both men and women—generally floral-based and gentle—and sidelines in luxury shaving and grooming products. Another

Humidorable

Cigars are big business in London, and not just because the city was once the capital of the world tobacco trade. Many wealthy visitors from Arab countries are not permitted to drink alcohol by dint of their religion but they may enjoy a fine stogie, so most finer hotels offer humidors as well as cocktail bars. Dating to 1787, **James J. Fox** claims to be the oldest cigar merchant in the world, and its pedigree is peerless:

Oscar Wilde indulged himself here, and Winston Churchill slouched in its weary brown leather armchair while he perused the Coronas. Come to inhale the rich, musky aroma, to select one of its fine bowl pipes, or even to smoke— the city's public smoking ban does not apply here. (19 St James's St., SW1. www.jjfox.co.uk. ℂ **020/7930-3787.** Tube: Green Park.)

picturesque location is at 16–17 Burlington Arcade (Green Park tube). 41 Wellington St., WC2. www.penhaligons.co.uk. © **020/7836-2150.** Tube: Covent Garden.

Housewares

Conran Shop ★★　Gorgeous, contemporary, smartly selected pieces made Conran's name in housewares; its flagship store is a master class in elegant urban furnishings and desirable home accessories. Its building is just as worthy: the 1911 Art Nouveau headquarters of the Michelin Tire Company, coated with decorative tiles of era racing cars and the Michelin Man (aka Bibendum). The newer location in Marylebone, however, is more convenient (55 Marylebone High St., W1; © **020/7723-2223;** Baker St. tube). 81 Fulham Rd., SW3. www.conranshop.co.uk. © **020/7589-7401.** Tube: South Kensington.

Habitat ★★★　Consider it not for furniture but for its cheerful linens, kitchen tools, and bath fabrics. In pursuit of this department store's mandate (set by founder Sir Terence Conran) to bring high design to the masses at affordable prices, A-list artists (Tracey Emin, Manolo Blahnik) have been recruited to contribute temporary items, and products are always peppy and practical. Although this store is Habitat's showpiece, a nice-size outpost is at 208 King's Road in Chelsea (Sloane Square or South Kensington tubes). 196–199 Tottenham Court Rd., W1. www.habitat.co.uk. © **084/4499-1122.** Tube: Goodge St.

Heal's ★★　A stalwart since 1810, but not stuffy like one, Heal's (like Liberty, p. 205), was instrumental in forwarding the Arts and Crafts movement in England. Its furniture and housewares, which are usually defined by chic shapes, have proven so influential that in 1978 it donated its archive to the Victoria & Albert museum. The kitchen department is popular. 196 Tottenham Court Rd., W1. www.heals.co.uk. © **020/7636-1666.** Tube: Goodge St.

Labour and Wait ★★　The most expensive dustpan you'll ever own will be the envy of dirt everywhere. This store's gorgeously designed kitchenware, bathroom items, gardening tools, and stationery—from vintage enamel to new sculptural metalwork—will put some chic into your chores. Even its location, an emerald-tiled former pub, is functionally fabulous, and its neighbors along Redchurch Street, selling clothes and interior items, are just as stylish. 85 Redchurch St., E2. www.labourandwait.co.uk. © **020/7729-6253.** Closed Mon. Tube: Shoreditch High St.

Pitfield London ★★　Funky and smart homewares and kitchenwares that are, as the kids say, "carefully edited." This means they're often one-offs or artist-made (bamboo cups and plates, for example) or hard-to-find (vintage Bakelite radios). Find it here and no one will have anything like it back home. 31–35 Pitfield St., N1. www.pitfieldlondon.com. © **020/7490-6852.** Tube: Old St.

Stationery

Paperchase ★★★   Paperchase does for stationery what Habitat does for chairs and tables: imbues them with infectious style, bold colors, and wit. Its journal selection is incomparable. Starting in summer, stock up on holiday cards, not only since they're much cheaper in the U.K. than abroad, but also because some proceeds go to charity (but be aware that the non-standard envelope sizes may require extra postage back home). There are many so-so branches, but this three-floor flagship is a big paper cut above. There's even a cafe. 213–215 Tottenham Court Rd., W1. www.paperchase.co.uk. ℂ **020/7467-6200.** Tube: Goodge St.

Ryman Stationery ★   If you're into office supplies (admit it—it's time to come out of the supply closet), the ubiquitous chain, which makes an appearance on almost every busy U.K. shopping street, is a good place to stock up on hard-to-find English-size A4 paper, clamp binders (not common in the U.S.), and convenient "box files" (also absent from other countries' stationers), available in a spectrum of sprightly colors. Multiple locations. www. ryman.co.uk.

Smythson of Bond Street ★★★   In addition to a line of leather journals, organizers, and handbags, this firm does stationery impeccably. The queen, a one-woman thank-you note industry, buys her paper here. The cotton-fiber content is probably higher than in your bedsheets. 40 New Bond St., W1. www.smythson.com. ℂ **020/7629-8558.** Closed Sun. Tube: Bond St.

Toys

Hamleys ★★★   Remote-control helicopters in your hair, magicians at your elbow, rugrats at your knees. This high-octane toy store is run by a gaggle of cheerful young floor staff, themselves kids at heart, who giddily demonstrate the latest toys. The experience will send you into sensory overload. Seven floors are stuffed with amusements—the fifth floor is nothing but sweets. Depending on when you go, there may be free pirate face painting, a caricaturist, or even a beach party. It's one of the world's few department stores devoted just to children, and the only must-see toy store in London— even if you don't have kids. 188–196 Regent St., W1. www.hamleys.com. ℂ **0871/ 704-1977.** Tube: Oxford Circus.

LONDON'S GREATEST MARKETS

Unfortunately, with the inexorable spread of megastores, outdoor markets that have been feeding Central Londoners since the Dark Ages are finding themselves extinguished. The following markets soldier on. Not every market sells something you can take home, unless you count memories: For example, the **Columbia Road Flower Market** (Sun at 8am; Old St. tube), is an Eden for

English blooms, which get cheaper around 2pm, near closing time. **Borough Market,** which is fully described on p. 95, is all about prepared foods or things you can't get past Customs. Even if you aren't keen to buy anything, however, stroll down one of these market lanes. Whether for gourmets, tourists, or locals, it's like a front-row seat to the ongoing opera of everyday life, and a taste of London as it once was.

> **Market Hours**
>
> Unless otherwise noted, markets are mostly outdoors and generally kick off at around 8 or 9am in the morning and start packing up at around 3pm.

Berwick Street Market ★

Berwick St. around Broadwick St. www.berwickstreetlondon.co.uk. Daily 9am–6pm except Sun. Tube: Piccadilly Circus.

Good for: The last daily street market in the West End, dating to the crowded days of the 1840s, is now being produced by developers. Gone are the Cockney calls, in are the overpriced baked goods and hipster coffee—convenient, but false.

Also check out: The gourmand-pleasing specialty shops lining the route.

Brick Lane Markets ★★★

Brick Lane at Buxton St. www.bricklanemarket.com. ℂ **020/7770-6028.** Tube: Shoreditch High St.

Good for: The Vintage Market (Fri–Sun, clothes), Backyard Market (Sat–Sun, crafts), Boiler House (Sat–Sun, food), and Tea Rooms (Sat–Sun, antiques). As you can see, Sundays are a banner day: UpMarket does trendy fashions then, too, food stalls are everywhere, and Spitalfields Market (p. 223) is also in full swing.

Also check out: The Beigel Bake (p. 100) for London's version of a bagel.

Brixton Market ★

Electric Ave. at Pope's Rd. brixtonmarket.net. Mon–Sat. Tube: Brixton.

Good for: Exotic produce, spices, halal meats, music from soul to reggae and hip-hop.

Also check out: Brixton Village, stalls selling African and Caribbean clothes, foods, and housewares; Ritzy's Art Fayre, a designer market, every Saturday.

Camden MARKETS ★★

Camden High St. at Buck St. www.camdenlock.net. Daily (weekends best). Tube: Camden Town.

Good for: A rambling warren of 700 stalls for vintage wear, sunglasses, leather, goth gear, and fast foods, partly in a canal-side setting, and favored by tourists. Between the Lock Market, the Market Hall, the Horse Stables, and Camden Lock Village across the street, options seem never-ending, but the crowds are utterly exhausting.

Also check out: Stables Market, on the other side of the railway off Chalk Farm Road, sells vintage clothes, antiques, and pop culture knick-knacks; Electric Market (on Camden High St.) is an indoor fair of vinyl, programs, and film posters (Sat) and retro and punk clothes (Sun).

Chapel Market ★★

Islington. Tues–Sun. Tube: Angel.

Good for: Cheese, dumplings, meat pies, toiletries—a real catch-all working-class market that actually feeds workaday Londoners.

Also check out: The antithesis of a market, the gleaming N1 Islington mall, dominates the eastern end of the street; it's New London versus Old London.

Greenwich Markets ★★

11A Greenwich Market. www.greenwichmarketlondon.com. Tues–Sun (weekends best). Tube: Cutty Sark DLR or Greenwich National Rail.

Good for: 40 stalls of antiques (Tues, Thurs, Fri), plus crafts, honeys, breads, and cakes under a historic market roof.

Also check out: The cafes lining the covered Craft Market.

Leather Lane Market ★

Leather Lane between Clerkenwell Rd. and Greville St. Mon–Fri 10:30am–2:30pm. Tube: Farringdon.

Good for: Local flavor. Hot and ready-to-eat food, be it Jewish (latkes, salt beef), Mexican (burritos), or universal (salads); sweat suits and skirts, jeans.

Also check out: Ye Olde Mitre pub (p. 108), a street away.

Maltby Street Market ★★★

Maltby St., SE1. www.maltby.st. ℭ **020/7394-8061.** Sat 9am–4pm, Sun 11am–4pm. Tube: London Bridge or Bermondsey.

Good for: Food stalls run by vendors who decamped from overrun Borough Market, purveying gorgeous flavors such as gooey "bad brownies," mugs of horseradished Bloody Marys, and "African volcano" hot sauce. Located on the railway vaults of Ropewalk, south of the Tower Bridge.

Also check out: Historic pie and mash vendor M. Manze (p. 96) is nearby.

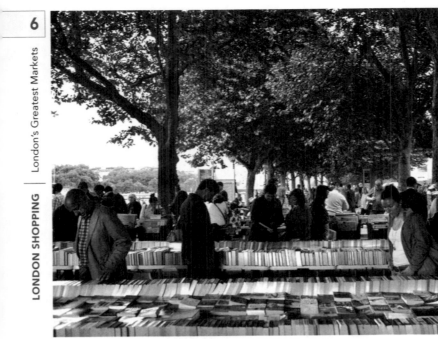

Southbank Centre's outdoor used-book market.

Portobello Road Market ★

www.portobelloroad.co.uk. ⓒ **020/7727-7684.** Fri–Sat. Tube: Notting Hill Gate or Westbourne Park.

Good for: Antiques, hot foods, jewelry, vintage clothes, tourist tat by the ton. Overcrowded and overrated, but thanks to the movies, it's not going anywhere.

Also check out: The packed pubs along the route; the galleries and antiques shops in the storefronts, where prices can be better than at the stalls.

Queen's Market ★

Green St. at Queen's Rd. www.newham.gov.uk. ⓒ **020/8475-8971.** Tues and Thurs– Sat. Tube: Upton Park.

Good for: 80 stalls and 60 local stores for ingredients from Asia, Africa, Russia, the Caribbean, and elsewhere; international clothes and rugs. Although it's not very posh, it is very Everyday London. Sunday is a quieter day.

Also check out: Its defenders' website, www.friendsofqueensmarket.org.uk, which has argued their market is half as expensive as Walmart.

HACK THE tax attack

First, the good news: When you see a price in England, that's the full price. Tax is always included. Now, the bad news: That tax is usually charged at a rate of 20%. It's called VAT (Value-Added Tax), and it goes to enviable programs such as national health care, so that any British citizen who needs health care doesn't have to go into debt to get it.

And more good news: Tourists can often get a little of that back. As long as the store you're patronizing participates in the VAT Retail Export Scheme (many don't) and you get the paperwork from them while you're there (stores have varying minimum-purchase requirements), you can apply for a refund, minus a dismaying chunk for administrative fees. The only purchases it doesn't work for are vehicles, unmounted gemstones, and anything requiring an export license (except antiques). The system mostly benefits those who spend hundreds or thousands of pounds, not tourists with casual purchases.

To get money back:

○ Be a non–European Community visitor to the U.K.

○ Obtain stamped tax refund documents from each retailer. At big stores, you may have to wait in line with I.D. and receipts for as long as a half-hour and the store may take a cut of several pounds as a processing fee.

○ On the day you leave Britain, present that document to the VAT refund desk at the airport. The line may be extreme. You must also have the goods on hand, which means a) you must put them in your carry-on, or b) you pack the goods in your baggage but first check in at your airline to pick up your travel documents, then bring your yet-to-be checked baggage for inspection, and then submit your baggage at the airline counter once that is finished. This process can take up to 2 hours, and even then you may only get £7 back for every £100 spent, so decide if it's really worth the hassle.

Britain maintains information via www.hmrc.gov.uk. or ℂ **029/2050-1261.**

Riverside Walk Market ★★

Southbank under the Waterloo Bridge. Daily noon–7pm in good weather. Tube: Waterloo.

Good for: Tables of used books, maps, lithographs, and wood engravings.

Also check out: Lower Marsh Market on Lower Marsh between Westminster Bridge and Baylis roads (south of Waterloo station), a classic produce market.

Spitalfields Market ★★

Commercial St. between Brushfield St. and Lamb St. www.visitspitalfields.com. Daily. Tube: Liverpool St.

Good for: Up-and-coming designers and artists, prepared world food, handmade housewares, jewelry, vintage posters. It's the most gentrified market in town, and especially on Saturdays, there are one-of-a-kind clothing items, not all of them affordable. Sit-down restaurants surround the covered market. The market's success was a linchpin in East London's revitalization.

Also check out: Visit the Style Market for fashions on Saturday afternoons.

Walthamstow Market ★

Walthamstow Market St. Tues–Sat. Tube: Walthamstow.

Good for: 450 non-touristy stalls selling everything from knockoff clothes to junky food to Chinese-made batteries—it's the longest market street in Europe.

Also check out: You may not have the energy to see much else in this multi-cultural neighborhood—the market itself is a kilometer long.

LONDON NIGHTLIFE

et no one tell you that London tucks itself into bed early. Perhaps that was true in your grandfather's day—now, the U.K. rocks 'til dawn. The Tube may shut down after midnight on weeknights, but the main lines now go all night on weekends, so for the intrepid, the entertainment can rollick until morning. With hundreds of theaters, nightclubs, cinemas, and music halls, London has more to offer on a single night than many cities can muster in an entire year, and its output influences the whole world.

That said, London's nights aren't perfect. The city's prevailing liquor laws force places to sometimes unceremoniously dump their clientele on the streets in mid-toast. Whereas in Spain, Greece, and New York, the night rarely begins before 1am, that's usually when the DJ packs up even at many of London's top clubs. If you require just one more cocktail to close the deal, a very few clubs will serve until 3am, and they come and go; ask your new friends at the bar which place is the cool one right now. The Night Bus system (p. 316) assuages some financial pain, but it's a buzzkill to end a festive night of drinking with your legs crossed on a slow-moving bus.

GETTING THE SCOOP Complete listings information for entertainment is published Saturdays in the London papers, but you don't have to wait until you arrive. Excellent online sources for things to do include **Londonist.com, LondonCalling.com, Time-Out.com, Townfish.com,** and the Twitter accounts Everything London (**@LDN**), **@LeCool_London** (nightlife). **@SkintLondon** and the app **Frugl** help with finding cheap or free activities. These sources are good, too:

- **Visit London** (www.visitlondon.com): "What's On" in the "Things to Do" section is assiduously updated and, even better, it's free
- *Metro* (www.metro.co.uk): Free in racks at Tube stations, most copies of this newspaper are gone by mid-morning, but commuters leave copies behind on the trains; it's considered green to recycle a pre-read newspaper.
- The *Evening Standard* (www.standard.co.uk): This free paper appears at Tube stop entrances in midafternoon—some days, there's an accompanying lifestyle magazine in a nearby stack. *ES* is also available online for free.

THEATER

If you leave London without seeing at least one stage show, then you'll have missed one of this city's most glittering attractions: This is where Shakespeare defined great writing and Gilbert and Sullivan shaped modern musical theater. London's influence isn't just in antiquity, either; the great work continues to this day, and if you doubt it, look at the lists of Oscar, Emmy, and Tony winners from the past decade.

Whenever you hear the phrase "West End" in relation to shows, think of the term as describing the 60-odd top-tier theaters in the middle of town. These are the shows that most tourists flock to see, but that doesn't mean they're always the best—the West End is increasingly clogged with mediocre dramas propped up by Hollywood names and by so-called "jukebox" musicals that are the intellectual equivalent of bubble gum.

A great many West End shows begin their lives at companies found elsewhere in town, which most tourists don't hear about. For challenging work mounted by producers intent on taking artistic risks, look to them. Many of them have designed and built facilities expressly for pumping out fresh projects, and each of them has a devoted following of fans and donors. What's more, you're just as likely to catch stars—all at prices that are half what you'd shell out for a West End megamusical that was created by committee.

Standard curtain times range from 7:30 to 8pm for evening shows; matinees start anywhere between 2 and 4pm. Every theater is different, so check your ticket. Nearly all shows are closed, or "dark," on Sundays.

It's easy to make a night of it. Every theater has its own bar, and many sell ice cream and snacks at intermission ("interval"). Companies with their own buildings might even run their own mid- to high-end restaurants.

Theater Tickets for Less

If you are desperate to see a specific show, book tickets before you leave home to ensure you won't be left out. Check with the **Society of London Theatre** (www.officiallondontheatre.co.uk), the trade association for theater owners and producers (established in 1908), for a rundown of what's playing and soon to play, as well as discount offers. Keep in mind that many links, including Visit London's, will deliver you to ticket sellers who'll hit you for a premium of as much as 20% for your booking. Only use that method if you'd be heartbroken to miss a particular show.

Given a lead time of a few weeks, the established **LastMinute.com** sells tickets for half price, as does **LoveTheatre.com** (click "Special Offers"). BroadwayBox.com's **www.theatre.co.uk** posts the known discount codes for the West End shows.

Once you get to London, grab a copy of *The Official London Theatre Guide,* dispensed for free in nearly every West End theater's lobby and at countless brochure racks; it tells you what's playing, where, for how much and how long, and the location of each theater. **TKTS** (south side of Leicester

saving ON THE STAGE

Apart from using TKTS, how can you save on a show?

- **Matinees are often cheaper than evening shows.** Unfortunately, they also cut into your daylight touring time.

- **Ask about standing room tickets and "day seats."** Many theaters sell standing room for a tenner (£10–£20). "Day seats" are a daily allotment of cheap seats, but you'll have to queue at the theater in the morning. *The Book of Mormon* begins a fun lottery for £20 seats 2½ hours before curtain.

- **Buy at the box office** to avoid paying booking fees.

- **In one of the older theaters, you can often settle for a restricted-view seat.** You may have to crane your neck to see around the edge of a balcony or a pillar, but you'll be in the room. They cost about a third of top-price seats. **Theatremonkey.com** posts theater-specific ratings.

- **If you're a student, some box offices (but not TKTS) may offer you discounts of 20% to 40%.** Carry a recognized ID card.

Square; www.tkts.co.uk; Mon–Sat 10am–7pm, Sun 11am–4:30pm; Leicester Square tube), operated by the Society of London Theatre, sells same-day seats for as much as half off—the best stuff is sold in the first hour of opening. While the white-hot shows won't be represented here, about 80% of West End shows are—TKTS posts a list of its available shows on its website so you can know ahead of time. When musicals are half off, they're around £30 to £40, and plays cost £20 to £30, although the prices fluctuate per production with up to a £3 per ticket service charge. Come armed with a magazine or a newspaper that lists what the shows are about, because TKTS offers no descriptions. Also put the free app **TodayTix** on your phone—it also discounts shows in the days and hours before curtain and it's a terrific source for deals.

The West End is dotted with closet-size stalls hawking tickets to major shows and concerts. Don't deal with them. They are for audiences who simply *must* get tickets to their chosen show regardless of the fees—as high as 25% over cost. Before you give your money to any of these outfits, check with the self-policing **Society of Ticket Agents and Retailers** (www.star.org.uk; ✆ **01904/234-737**) to find out who is reputable. Scalpers, called **touts** here, often issue counterfeit tickets or abscond with your cash before forking over anything at all. Some sightseeing discount cards also brag about discounts, but their deals are mostly for the longest-running, touristy shows and they don't save you nearly as much as TKTS would—only around £20 off the top price.

London's Landmark Performance Places

The Barbican Centre ★★ In the 1950s, earnest but misguided city fathers turned their attentions toward redeveloping a bombed-out crater. The end result was a forbidding mixed-use concrete complex that took more than

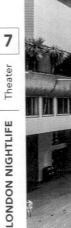

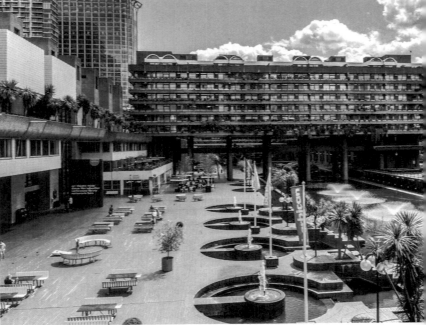

The Barbican Centre was built in a bombed-out crater.

20 years to finish. They optimistically planned for lively crowds by adding Europe's largest arts and conference center, too, with a concert hall, two theaters, three cinemas, and two galleries, and now they're the best thing about the place—and one of the best things about London arts in general. You can't always find something going on in all of its venues, and even when things are rocking full-tilt, the bunkered Barbican is so windswept it makes *Blade Runner* look like Candy Land, but what does play here is rarely dull. It's nearly impossible to classify the Barbican's fare, since it hosts a wide range of the world's great orchestras (including the London Symphony Orchestra), singers, and composers, plus a handful of banner festivals each year, particularly in the realm of contemporary music and experimental theater. Its cinemas often screen films fresh from major festival triumphs. Silk St., EC2. www. barbican.org.uk. © **020/7638-8891.** Tube: Barbican.

The Bridge Theatre ★   In late 2017, a major new venue was opened by City Hall, south of Tower Bridge, with an emphasis on well-produced new work. The Bridge was instantly A-list, attracting heavy-hitting talent such as Ben Whishaw, Rory Kinnear, and Simon Russell Beale in productions including *Julius Caesar* directed by former National Theatre director Nicholas Hytner. One Tower Bridge, SE1. www.bridgetheatre.co.uk. © **0843/208-1846.** Tube: London Bridge.

The Bush Theatre ★★★   The Bush, which for more than 40 years has showcased a formidable output from new writers, started as a pub theater; in 2011, thanks to a lifesaving campaign that rallied support from the likes of Judi Dench and Daniel Radcliffe, it got its own facility in a disused Victorian library. Besides attracting exciting writers, it brings in stars (like Kate Beckinsale and the late Alan Rickman) who want to connect with audiences. 7 Uxbridge Rd., W12. www.bushtheatre.co.uk. ℂ **020/8743-5050.** Tube: Shepherds Bush.

Donmar Warehouse ★★★   You can't often snag a last-minute ticket to this 250-seat house without standing in line for returns. Its productions, mostly limited runs of vividly reconceived revivals, are edgy and buzzy. Past coups for this comfortably converted brewery warehouse include the *Cabaret* revival that introduced Alan Cumming to the world, as well as appearances by world-class performers such as Ian McKellen and Nicole Kidman. The front row of full-price tickets are dished out each Monday at 10am sharp for performances 2 weeks later, with a maximum of two tickets per person. 41 Earlham St., WC2. www.donmarwarehouse.com. ℂ **0844/871-7624.** Tube: Covent Garden.

Menier Chocolate Factory ★★   In an intimate setting among exposed beams and cast-iron columns, a converted you-know-what from the 1870s is

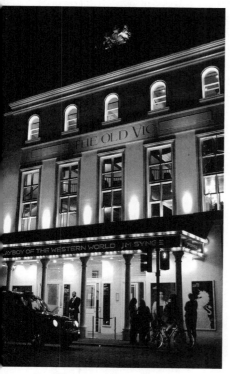

where some of the city's hottest musical revivals have been mounted. Its *Sunday in the Park with George* and *A Little Night Music* transferred to the West End and later to Broadway. This company, which also does non-musical plays, is one of the few to do Sunday shows; it's dark on Mondays. 51–53 Southwark St., SE1. www.menierchocolatefactory.com. ℂ **020/7378-1713.** Tube: London Bridge.

Old Vic ★   Hitmaking director Matthew Warchus (*Matilda*) is now in charge, drawing celebrities like Vanessa Redgrave, Kim Cattrall, and, last season, *Star Wars*'s John Boyega; acting legend Glenda Jackson was even coaxed back on stage here after a quarter century in Parliament. The place is known for mounting intellectual, meat-and-potatoes drama—stuff actors love to sink their teeth into—as well as lively fare such as the musical *Groundhog Day,* which it exported to Broadway. The 200-year-old building

The Old Vic is home to intellectual dramas.

is pulling bigger crowds than ever before, and The Pit Bar, downstairs, is a stylish pre- and post-show hangout. The Cut at Waterloo Rd., SE1. www.oldvic theatre.com. ℃ **0844/871-7628.** Tube: Waterloo or Southwark.

Royal Court Theatre ★★ The preeminent writer's theater, the Royal Court has fought censorship and unveiled international brilliance for so long that it's now a preeminent actor's theater as well. On the east side of jaunty Sloane Square, it devotes a hefty portion of its schedule to important pre-mieres by the likes of Bruce Norris and Caryl Churchill and performances from fierce actors such as Ben Whishaw and Fiona Shaw. Among the plays it gave the world include *Look Back in Anger, The Rocky Horror Picture Show* (in its upstairs studio theater), George Bernard Shaw's *Major Barbara* and *Heartbreak House,* and Mike Bartlett's *Cock.* Sloane Square, SW1. www.royal courttheatre.com. ℃ **020/7565-5000.** Tube: Sloane Square.

Royal National Theatre ★★★ The government-subsidized power-house people simply call The National is the country's, and possibly the world's, most noted showpiece for top-flight drama and classical acting. Lau-rence Olivier was its first director, and the tradition of world-class perfor-mances has been unerring: Judi Dench, Ralph Fiennes, Anthony Hopkins, Maggie Smith, and Benedict Cumberbatch have been regulars. The National always mounts a diverse repertoire of British works in its three permanent (and one temporary) theaters, spanning Shakespeare to classic musicals (the *Oklahoma!* that made Hugh Jackman a star) to emotional spectacles (*War Horse* began here) to world premieres of well-made plays by the world's best playwrights. The 2018 season includes Bryan Cranston in an adaptation of *Network, Pinocchio* with the support of Disney songs, and a re-mounting of the classic play *Amadeus.* A recent renovation made the brutalist riverside

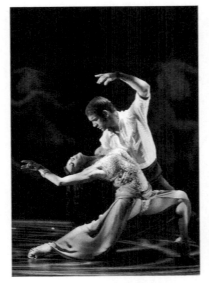

complex a pleasure to spend time in, having added several places to eat, caffeinate, or tipple. The fascinating (and free) Sherling High-Level Walk-way allows anyone off the street to watch the activity backstage; there's even a periscope so kids can peer over railings into the scenery shops. To find that, head down the eastern side road toward the Dorfman, go inside, and take the lift to the second level. As the people's theater, the National's pricing is populist. Some 100,000 tickets a year are discounted to £15 for the Travelex season (℃ **020/7452-3000**). Catch one of the 75-minute tours (£10–£13) showing off the inner workings or costume

Sadler's Wells is home to ballet and dance.

department, or shop in the lobby bookstore, a performing arts nirvana. South Bank, SE1. www.nationaltheatre.org.uk. ℂ **020/7452-3000.** Tube: Waterloo.

Sadler's Wells ★ Sadler's Wells has been a part of the fabric of London life for so long (since 1683) that its current two-house home, dating to 1998, is actually the sixth. You can turn to this Islington establishment to catch some of the world's greatest companies in movement- or rhythm-based performances that transcend language. Its specialties are ballet (Matthew Bourne is a frequent guest artist), contemporary dance, and daring opera (Rufus Wainwright's *Prima Donna* premiered here). It also programs the Peacock Theatre on Portugal Street near the Holborn Tube. Rosebery Ave., EC1. www.sadlerswells. com. ℂ **020/7863-8198.** Tube: Angel.

Shakespeare's Globe ★★ One would think that a reconstruction of an Elizabethan theater on the Thames (see p. 155 for architectural details) would support mostly kitschy productions for tour groups. That it is, in fact, a serious concern that attracts the finest classically trained performers is thanks partly to its founding artistic director (1995–2005), Oscar-winning actor Mark Rylance. The tone for quality that he set is maintained today—in 2017, the artistic director was fired, in part, for the anachronistic sin of using artificial lighting. "Groundling" tickets to stand for the show have been £5 for 20 years

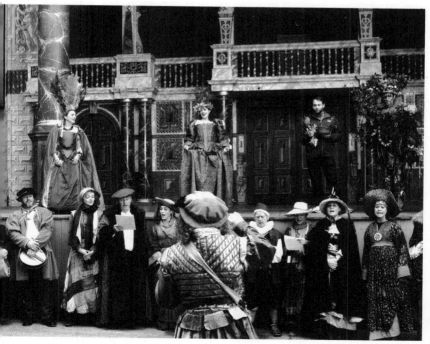

Performers at Shakespeare's Globe.

THE QUIRKS OF LONDON theatergoing

London theater can be a strange experience for outsiders:

○ Programs are not free; they cost from £3 (for plays) to £5 (for musicals). Big productions may only sell a glossy souvenir brochure, for £7 to £10.

○ Some seats are equipped with plastic opera glasses, which can be rented for the show with a 50p or £1 coin.

○ What North American theaters call "orchestra" seats, London houses call the "stalls." And instead of a "mezzanine," they have a "Dress Circle," and above that, "Upper Circle" or "Royal Circle." If there happens to be a third, topmost level, that is the "balcony," or sometimes, the "gallery." And because many theaters were constructed in a class-obsessed era, there may be a separate street entrance for each area.

○ The break between acts is called an "interval," not "intermission."

○ The big snack? Ice cream, sold by ushers (or "attendants").

○ Older theaters are required to deploy the "fire curtain," which seals the stage from the auditorium in the event of flames, once during every performance. It's usually done discreetly during the interval.

○ Leave big bags at the hotel, because these old seats can be knee-knockers. And ladies, cover your knees, because in the Circles, they will likely be at head-level of the person sitting in front of you.

now. The season at the open-air Globe is spring through fall, but in a 340-seat Jacobean indoor theater, the Sam Wanamaker (named in honor of the American actor who fought to reconstruct the Globe), there's something happening year-round. In the candle-lit Wanamaker, actors are so near that you could reach out and touch them. 21 New Globe Walk, Bankside, SE1. www.shakespeares globe.com. ⓒ **020/7401-9919.** Tube: Southwark or Mansion House.

Southbank Centre ★★★ Like the Barbican, this is a bleak canvas-colored slab architects don't know quite how to fix. It was conceived as a postwar pick-me-up, but age was not kind; despite a peerless Thames location, it's a forbidding architectural scowl, looking more like a pile of sidewalk curbs than an artistic capitol. It's perkier on the inside, however. Some 1,000 programs a year go down at its three concert venues, as well as in its huge central hall, which has a cafe and is open to everybody. Dance, film, classical and contemporary music, and the London Jazz Festival fill the bill, which is prolific if self-important. Don't miss the Undercroft, the hideous concrete negative space under the building along the Thames. When the Centre went up, this area was thought to be useless, so skateboarders and street artists claimed the architectural mistake. Recently, landlords tried to evict them for shops, but too late—the skaters proved too beloved. Belvedere Rd., SE1. www. southbankcentre.co.uk. ⓒ **020/7960-4200.** Tube: Waterloo.

London's Great Smaller Theaters

Almeida Theatre ★★   The inviting Almeida, which has its own contemporary pub, sticks to its guns, mounting intelligent plays (some new, some unfairly forgotten, many new) without much regard for pushback—2014 saw *American Psycho,* the musical, which went on to Broadway. Almeida St. off Upper St., N1. www.almeida.co.uk. ℂ **020/7359-4404.** Tube: Angel.

Hackney Empire ★   One of London's greatest and most ornate old houses (1901) was where, once upon a time, you could catch Charlie Chaplin as a vaudeville act. The ever-changing slate still presents the best of variety, but with an urban, multicultural twist: kids' shows, opera, Christmas pantomime, hip-hop drama, and concerts. 291 Mare St., E8. www.hackneyempire.co.uk. ℂ **020/8985-2424.** Tube: Hackney Central Overground.

Lyric Hammersmith ★   Riding high after the 2014 opening of a £16.5 million expansion, this venue's core may look like a fusty Victorian jewel-box theater, but you'll find spectacular stuff—a mix of multimedia-based shows, avant-garde experiments, and an annual Christmas show to write home about. Its kids' shows are its bread and butter. Lyric Square, King St., S6. www.lyric.co.uk. ℂ **020/8741-6850.** Tube: Hammersmith.

The Print Room ★   As the Coronet, this place was built as a small variety house in 1898, but for most of the 20th century it was a cinema—this is where Hugh Grant's character wistfully attended a movie starring his estranged girlfriend (Julia Roberts) in *Notting Hill.* Now it's one of the most respected up-and-coming Fringe theatres, specializing in revitalizing ignored works by great writers. 103 Notting Hill Gate, W11. www.the-print-room.org. ℂ **020/3642-6606.** Tube: Notting Hill Gate.

Roundhouse ★★   Located in a rehabbed 1846 locomotive shed, the Roundhouse picks up on the maverick spirit of neighboring Camden with a frisky, fast-changing lineup of innovative musical dramas and spectaculars, many of them given a crowd-pleasing, dance-inflected, shock-to-the-system twist. In the 1960s, it was one of London's most important stages, particularly for counterculture concerts. In more recent seasons, you're just as likely to see one-off comedy events or concerts. Chalk Farm Rd., NW1. www.roundhouse.org.uk. ℂ **084/4482-8008.** Tube: Chalk Farm.

Soho Theatre ★   The Soho functions like a one-building arts festival; it casts a wide net in looking for the latest voices in theater, comedy, and cabaret. On weekend days, come for kids' shows. Its Theatre Bar is a fine hangout even sans tickets. 21 Dean St., W1. www.sohotheatre.com. ℂ **020/7478-0100.** Tube: Tottenham Court Rd.

The Unicorn Theatre ★   A children's theater that caters to kids without suffering from a debilitating case of preciousness, the Unicorn runs at least two productions, one for each of its theater spaces. Some are script-based and some sensory-based for younger kids and kids with autism. Many are designed to expose kids to other cultures, places, and classic stories. If only every city had a kids' facility as lush. 147 Tooley St., SE1. www.unicorntheatre.com. © 020/7645-0560. Tube: London Bridge.

Young Vic ★   Spry and in top form, this company programs a mixed bag of jarring plays, conversational touchstones, edgy musicals (in 2018, *Fun Home*), and affordable opera, then stands back and hopes for *frisson*. It often achieves it, and if it fails, it doesn't dally long, since it has three theaters (seating 500, 160, and 80) to fill. There's nearly always something high-quality to plumb here. 66 The Cut, SE1. www.youngvic.org. © 020/7922-2922. Tube: Waterloo or Southwark.

Pub Theaters

For something easy, cheap, and daring, try this option. In the early 1970s, a new form of alternative theater swept London: the pub theater. Often just a tatty back room where you can bring your beer from the scruffy front bar, your typical theater pub is where some of the city's most affordable, idiosyncratic, let's-try-this-and-see-if-it-works stuff is found—which is why they launched so many megastar actors to fame. Some of the most respected fringe venues in town are pub theaters, and they have just as much artistic power as many better-heeled West End palaces. Four fantastic ones, all charging £15 or less for most shows, are:

The Etcetera Theatre ★★   Odd, challenging fare (sometimes several different shows a night) are presented in this very small black box. 265 Camden High St., NW1. www.etceteratheatre.com. © 020/7482-4857. Tube: Camden Town.

Hen & Chickens ★   Frequent comedy bookings as well as strong writing are presented by the resident company, Unrestricted View. 109 St Paul's Rd., N1. www.henandchickens.com. © 020/7354-8246. Tube: Highbury & Islington.

The King's Head ★★★   Alums include Kenneth Branagh, Clive Owen, Joanna Lumley, Ben Kingsley, Juliet Stevenson, Hugh Grant, and John Hurt in their younger, braver, poorer days. 115 Upper St., N1. www.kingsheadtheatre.com. © 020/7226-8561. Tube: Angel.

Old Red Lion ★   The very pubby ORL hires its 60-seat space to a variety of aspiring producers and hosts the occasional comedy night. 418 St John St., EC1. www.oldredliontheatre.co.uk. © 0844/412-4307. Tube: Angel.

OPERA

Opera can be a budget-breaker. Frugal travelers should try the street singers who perform daily at the **Covent Garden Piazza** (Covent Garden tube). That's not a joke: Performers are auditioned before being awarded buskers' licenses, so the caliber is high. Also check to see if there's a touring opera putting down stakes at Sadler's Wells (p. 231). Of course, nothing compares to these institutions:

English National Opera ★★   With the Royal Opera entrenched as the country's premium company, the ENO at the gorgeous London Coliseum (built in 1904) is the progressive one that angles for younger audiences. Tightening purse strings have made it slimmer and more crowd-pleasing; its 2016 revival of Glenn Close in *Sunset Boulevard* was a particular smash. The slate consists of both progressive choices and classics: In 2018, those include an adaptation of the thriller *Marnie* by Nico Muhly, a new *La Traviata,* and Philip Glass's *Satyagraha.* Best of all, it sets aside 500 seats at every performance for £20 or less. St Martin's Lane, WC2. www.eno.org. ✆ **020/7845-9300.** Tube: Leicester Square.

Royal Opera House ★★   Opera fans don't need to be reminded of the role the ROH plays on the world scene, but outsiders might be surprised at how inviting and attractive its terrace and cafe are. The main house, which is shared by the Royal Opera (conducted by Antonio Pappano until 2020) and the equally prestigious Royal Ballet (now in its 70th year here), is supplemented with two smaller spaces for chamber opera and studio dance. Happily, 40% of the tickets cost £40 or less—if you move quickly—and surtitles

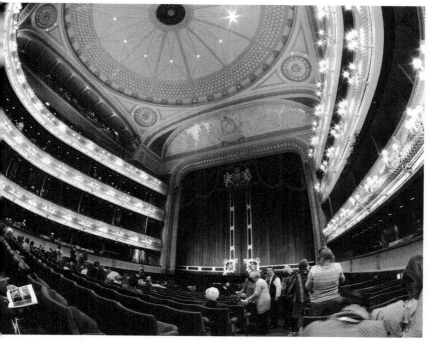

Covent Garden's Royal Opera House hosts both opera and ballet.

appear on little screens or monitors. There are three daytime tours available, too, one for backstage, one for workshops, and one for its 2,256-seat, horse-shoe-shaped auditorium (✆ **020/7304-4000;** £9–£12; 75 min.; children 7 and under not permitted; sells out 2–3 months ahead, calendar online). Bow St., Covent Garden, WC2. www.roh.org.uk. ✆ **020/7304-4000.** Tube: Covent Garden.

DANCE PERFORMANCE

London's dance scene has yet to achieve the vibrancy of New York's or Germany's, but that's not to say there's nothing to see; it's just that some of the best terpsichorean productions are put on by visiting companies, not by Londoners. The first thing to do is check the schedules at the Barbican (p. 227), Roundhouse (p. 233), Sadler's Wells (p. 231), and Southbank Centre (p. 232), which present a cornucopia of performance genres. The country's largest company, **Royal Ballet** ★★, shares space with the Royal Opera (p. 235). The adventurous **English National Ballet** ★ tours Britain much of the time but finds itself in London often (www.ballet.org.uk; ✆ **020/7581-1245**), especially for its December *Nutcracker.*

The Place ★★★ (17 Duke's Rd., WC1; www.theplace.org.uk; ✆ **020/7121-1100;** Euston tube) is known for contemporary dance—specifically, as the home of the Richard Alston Dance Company—and the host venue of some 100 companies a year from around the world. The lucky tenant of a gleaming translucent building by the same team that designed the Tate Modern, **Trinity Laban** (Creekside, Greenwich, SW8; www.trinitylaban.ac.uk; ✆ **020/8691-8600;** Cutty Sark DLR or Greenwich National Rail) puts on a mixed bill of works from around the world and by up-and-comers from its conservatory.

CLASSICAL MUSIC

Cadogan Hall ★   With 900 seats, this onetime Christian Scientist church (built 1907 in the Byzantine Revival style) is now the home of the Royal Philharmonic Orchestra and, in summer, the BBC Proms, which books it during the summer for its chamber music as a supplement to its concerts at Royal Albert Hall. 5 Sloane Terrace, SW1. www.cadoganhall.com. ✆ **020/7730-4500.** Tube: Sloane Square.

King's Place ★★   If you find yourself bored in London, it's not King's Place's fault. The relatively new development behind King's Cross has become the city's most versatile, exciting venue, with spaces for multiple galleries, chamber groups, and orchestras. It has some bright ideas to keep programming fresh; regular festivals for global music and opera and 50 great chamber concerts determined by a vote. Comedy, folk music, jazz, interviews with world notables—surprises abound. 90 York Way, N1. www.kingsplace.co.uk. ✆ **020/7520-1490.** Tube: King's Cross St Pancras.

Royal Albert Hall ★★★ Imposing, ornate, and adored by music lovers worldwide, the RAH is one of the few performance arenas on earth where, once they have performed there, artists can truly claim to have made it. During the summer, the storied BBC Promenade Concerts (the Proms) fill this historic, 5,200-seat circular hall with classical music, but the rest of the year, the space books a hodgepodge of tours, arena-style musicals, Cirque du Soleil, concerts (the house organ is 21m/69 ft. tall and has 10,000 pipes)—even tennis matches. See p. 147 to tour it. Kensington Gore, SW7. www.royalalberthall.com. ✆ **0845/401-5034.** Tube: South Kensington.

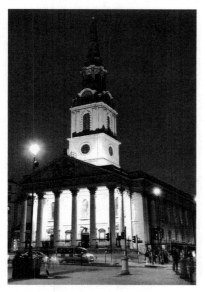

St Martin-in-the-Fields in Trafalgar Square offers candlelight concerts and lunchtime performances.

St Martin-in-the-Fields ★★★ Right in the thick of Trafalgar Square, this handsome church's evening candlelight concerts and lunchtime performances are London traditions. It's non-fussy with clean acoustics. Trafalgar Square, WC2. www.smitf.org. ✆ **020/7766-1100.** Tube: Charing Cross or Leicester Square.

Wigmore Hall ★★ Opened in 1901 as a recital hall for the Bechstein piano showroom that was next door, it was seized (along with the company) as enemy property in World War I. A nasty start, but in time performers came to include Ravel, Saint-Saëns, Britten, and Artur Rubinstein. Today the hall, notable for a bombastic Arts and Crafts cupola over the stage, is known for ideal acoustics and a roster of some 450 concerts, mostly classical, each year. Some nights, there's free music in the bar. 36 Wigmore St., W1. www.wigmore-hall.org.uk. ✆ **020/7935-2141.** Tube: Bond St.

THE MUSIC SCENE

Just as many of London's live music venues don't draw a heavy line between the genres they present, no rigid division exists between gig venues and dance venues; in fact, many spaces switch from live music to dance in a single evening. That's one of the things that makes the city's nightlife so vibrant, but it's also why it's important to check programming in advance. Students can often get discounts on entry—as if you needed any more proof that education is valued in England. Bring your ID—under 18s aren't usually admitted.

PRINCE CHARLES CINEMA: THE WORLD'S silliest MOVIE THEATER?

The family-friendly "Sing-a-Long-a" *The Sound of Music*, a silly participatory screening of the 1965 classic, was born in 1999 at the eccentric **Prince Charles Cinema** (7 Leicester Place; www. princecharlescinema.com; ℂ **020/7494-3654;** Leicester Square tube) and swept the world thereafter. Participants—some of whom arrive dressed as Nazis and nuns, without regard to gender—receive a "magic moment" bag with edelweiss, curtain swatches, and a party popper to deploy at the moment of Maria and the Captain's kiss. And it hasn't stopped with "Do-Re-Mi." On Friday nights, other Netflix favorites are given the call-and-response treatment, *Grease*, *Frozen*, *Moulin Rouge*, and *Dirty Dancing* among them. On other nights, it's an all-night Disney musical pajama party. Or a *Labyrinth* Masquerade Ball. Or a *Mean Girls* "bitch-along." Or full 70mm projections of essential cinematic masterpieces such as *Lawrence of Arabia* or, um, *Dune*.

Live Music, Including Jazz, Pop, Folk & Rock

Dozens of theaters and arenas in town book concerts by recognizable names, but it would be fruitless to list them since they're almost all rented by promoters and don't always have something going on. The better advice is to stay on top of who's playing by checking *Time Out* (www.timeout.com) or *New Musical Express* (*NME;* www.nme.com) magazines. Since big shows sell out months in advance, the best recourse is to book ahead via **See Tickets** (www. seetickets.com; ℂ **087/1220-0260**); **Stargreen** (www.stargreen.com; ℂ **020/ 7734-8932**), which has a small office at 20/21a Argyll St., outside the Oxford Circus Tube station; **Ticketweb** (www.ticketweb.co.uk; ℂ **0333/321-9990**) or its partner **Ticketmaster** (www.ticketmaster.co.uk; ℂ **0333/321-9999**), all of which levy fees but let you buy from abroad. Also visit **SouthbankLondon. com** to see what's playing in all the Southbank venues.

The 100 Club ★★   Many decades have passed since this was a prime hangout for U.S. servicemen homesick for the jazzy sounds of Glenn Miller (who died serving in the U.K., you'll remember) and his colleagues. In 1976, after passing through an R&B and jazz period that had Louis Armstrong puckering up for audiences, it sponsored the world's first punk festival, and bands like the Sex Pistols—unsigned at the time—took the stage. This battered red-walled basement room with good sightlines and expensive drinks still can't decide which era to honor, so it careens between punk, swing, R&B, jazz, and up-and-coming bands. 100 Oxford St., W1. www.the100club.co.uk. ℂ **020/7636-0933.** Cover £10–£21, 25% discounts often available in advance. Music starts around 8:30pm. Tube: Tottenham Court Rd.

The Betsey Trotwood ★★   This adorable, wood-floored Victorian pub has three levels, two with cozy performance spaces, and hosts bluegrass, comedy, and a few singer-songwriters a month—such as Jason Mraz early in his career. 56 Farringdon Rd., EC1. www.facebook.com/TheBetseyTrotwood. © **020/ 7253-4285.** Tube: Farringdon.

The Borderline ★   A Soho institution since the 1980s, this tiny basement space (which holds 275 people, uncomfortably) was recently renovated to install much-needed AC and upgrade its sound system. It books country, folk, Britpop, and blues. Cheap beer, young crowd. There are club nights, too: electro, hip-hop, R&B, pop. Orange Yard, Manette St., W1. www.theborderlinelondon. com. © **0844/847-1678.** Cover: live music around £15. Tube: Tottenham Court Rd.

Camden Assembly ★   When it was known as Barfly, this dark, intimate bar/performance space in Camden was the launch pad for a thousand indie bands, some of which actually ended up soaring (Coldplay, Blur, and the like). Today it offers a good mix of club nights and concerts for students, musicians, and old-time locals. Gentrification has tamed the overzealous moshers. When the bands wrap up, a house DJ spins for a few more hours while the audience chills. 49 Chalk Farm Rd., NW1. www.barflyclub.com. © **020/7424-0800.** Cover under £10. Tube: Chalk Farm.

Dingwalls ★   An ever-popular house of rock, folk, and acoustic guitar since 1973, this former industrial space by Camden Lock with a good sound system grants audiences the dignity of sitting at tables to enjoy the music. Performers here have included Mumford and Sons, Jello Biafra, and Foo Fighters, but now and then you'll find something like burlesque, too. Middle Yard, NW1. www.dingwalls.com. © **01920/823-098.** Cover ranges from "pay what you roll" on a die to £22. Tube: Camden Town.

Dublin Castle ★   Any bar that proclaims itself the birthplace of the '70s ditty band Madness would not, on the surface, seem to be a place you'd want to enter without prior insobriety. But it has street cred—it was the first bar in London to win a late liquor license from the government, so it became an important nightspot. Really no more than a threadbare, greenish pub with a teeny backroom stage, it hosts bands struggling to make it—and a few (Blur, for one, and Madness for two) that actually have. On weekends, late-night DJs spin. 94 Parkway, NW1. www.thedublincastle.com. © **020/7485-1773.** Cover £5–£7. Tube: Camden Town.

Electric Ballroom ★★   One of those dicey, utilitarian halls (ca. 1938) that never loses the lingering smell of old beer, the Electric Ballroom has hosted the likes of Sid Vicious, The Clash, and Garbage. Steel yourself for a steady roster of punk, goth, industrial, glam, hardcore, metal, and other genres (like British pro wrestling). Their aficionados could hardly inflict more architectural damage to the premises than what's already been done by the ravages of time and benign neglect. The divine Ultimate Power club event is all power ballads, all night long. 184 Camden High St., NW1. www.electricballroom.co.uk. © **020/7485-9006.** Cover: live music £15–£20, club nights £7–£14. Tube: Camden Town.

The Garage ★★　This 600-person concert space has so much cred as a modern choice for indie and rock that Harry Styles chose it for a surprise gig in 2017. Overpriced drinks in cans, intimate but loud; you know the drill. 20–22 Highbury Corner, N5. thegarage.london. ⓒ **020/7619-6720.** Tube and National Rail: Highbury & Islington.

Green Note ★★　This welcoming vegetarian cafe/bar books acoustic live gigs, from folk to jazz, roots to singer-songwriters. Softened by pillows and upholstered seating, it's a laid-back scene with no dancing. You can eat in the front room (tapas at sensible prices, no meat, all organic) and hear the music, or a cover charge will let you swing into the bar in the back room just for the show. 106 Parkway, NW1. www.greennote.co.uk. ⓒ **020/7485-9899.** Opens 7pm. Cover £2–£15. Tube: Camden Town.

Jazz Café ★★★　The prime Camden venue for "names" keeps the music going to 2am, usually in the form of acts (jazz, soul, bluesy vocalists, from Adele to Winehouse) seen up close. Converted from a bank and renovated with Deco touches in 2016, it has both cabaret tables and an upstairs gallery with food. In the past, there have been occasional club nights for EDM or funk dancing, so check the schedule. 5 Parkway, NW1. www.thejazzcafelondon.com. ⓒ **020/7485-6834.** Cover: live music £10–£14. Tube: Camden Town.

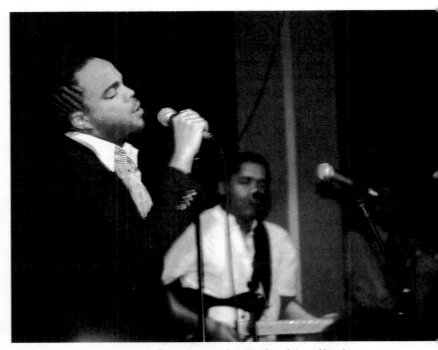

Camden's Jazz Café is a lively venue for music acts such as British soul singer Nate James.

Koko ★ Favored today by visiting indie bands, in its first life as the Camden Hippodrome this pretty 1,500-person multilevel space saw performances by Charlie Chaplin. In the '70s and '80s, it became an epicenter for pop—the Eurythmics, Boy George, and Wham! played their earliest gigs here, and it's where Madonna made her U.K. debut. The name Koko brings respect, although the setting isn't intimate and the sound can be muddy. Club nights are fun: Buttoned Down Disco is the first Saturday of the month. 1A Camden Rd., NW1. www.koko.uk.com. ✆ **087/0432-5527.** Cover under £10, student discounts before midnight. Tube: Mornington Crescent.

Pizza Express Live ★★ Unlikely as it may seem, this restaurant chain holds lunchtime and night concerts in a few on-site jazz clubs. The **Jazz Club** in Soho 10 Dean St., W1; ✆ **020/7439-4962;** Tottenham Court Rd. tube) has seen respected acts such as Jamie Cullum, Norah Jones, and Roy Haynes. Even Amy Winehouse played there. There's also an upscale supper club for live music and talks by notables at the **Pheasantry** in Chelsea (152 Kings Rd., SW3; Sloane Square tube). www.pizzaexpresslive.com. Cover free–£30.

Ronnie Scott's Jazz Club ★ Since the 1960s, when it was first recommended in Frommer's, Ronnie Scott's has been London's standard bearer for stylish, American-style jazz, and it honors a long tradition of pairing visiting U.S. greats with local acts. But the old dive got ritzy—after a £2.1-million renovation, the 255-seater began charging prices in the £45 range. Still, it's true that the club draws names, including Patti Austin, Van Morrison, Tom Waits, Cleo Laine, Chaka Khan, and Kyle Eastwood. Upstairs on Wednesdays, it hosts a loose "jazz jam" for under £10. 47 Frith St., W1. www.ronniescotts. co.uk. ✆ **020/7439-0747.** Tube: Leicester Square.

Scala ★★ When it was a cinema, Stanley Kubrick shut it down for screening *A Clockwork Orange* without permission. Good thing he did, or this 1920 theater might not have been reborn as a pleasing place to catch an acoustic or lyrical band. Its three levels give nearly everyone a good view of the stage, fostering a sense of intimacy appropriate to its capacity of around 1,000 people. A warren of rooms confuses the drunk ones and conceals the shy ones. Weekdays, it hosts gigs by indie bands, and weekends, it turns to club nights (Face Down, on Fri, is rock). 275 Pentonville Rd., N1. scala.co.uk. ✆ **020/7833-2022.** Cover £8–£15. Tube: King's Cross St Pancras.

The Water Rats ★★ If you're not a headbanger, the singer-songwriters here may appeal more than Camden's squalling sets. Once it was a pub known as the Pindar of Wakefield; Bob Dylan made his U.K. debut on its back-room stage in 1962, Oasis braved London audiences for the first time there in 1994, and Katy Perry played it before arenas—and returned for a nostalgia gig in 2017. A recent revamp gave it decent seating, but the food should be ignored. 328 Grays Inn Rd., WC1. www.thewaterratsvenue.london. ✆ **020/7209-8747.** Cover from £7 for several bands. Tube: King's Cross St Pancras.

Major Venues

If you want to get into the big-name shows, you have to book ahead, before you arrive. The most important venues post their schedules and link to ticket sellers on their websites. Grittier, midsize venues include **Bush Hall** (www. bushhallmusic.co.uk); the **O₂ Academy Brixton** (www.O2academybrixton. co.uk), good for metal and alt-rock; the **O₂ Academy Islington** (www. O2academyislington.co.uk); the recently renovated, Art Deco **Eventim Apollo** in Hammersmith (www.eventimapollo.com); the **O₂ Empire Shepherds Bush** (www.O2shepherdsbushempire.co.uk); and the **Electric Ballroom** and **Koko** (see above). The most massive venues—where your favorite artist will look like a tiny, bouncing smudge on the far side of an ocean of sweaty fans—include the **Copper Box Arena** (7,500 spectators; www. copperboxarena.org.uk) at the Queen Elizabeth Olympic Park; **London Stadium** (www.london-stadium.com), originally the main stadium at Queen Elizabeth Olympic Park, re-opened as a concert venue and the home of West Ham United FC; and **SSE Arena Wembley** (www.ssearena.co.uk). Sometimes you'll also see big gigs on the sports pitches at Arsenal football club's **Emirates Stadium** (www.arsenal.com/emiratesstadium; tours available) or **Twickenham Stadium** (www.englandrugby.com/twickenham), well outside of town.

The O₂   The £789-million boondoggle on the Thames in East London is a dome 10 times the volume of St Paul's. It's where gargantuan acts from Dolly to Gaga to Kylie to Monty Python appear, packing in their own religious followings, in a 20,000-place arena (ladies, there are 550 toilets for you, too) fringed by a mall for food and clubs. Michael Jackson was in rehearsal for a concert series for the O₂ when he died; during the 2012 Olympics, it housed gymnastics and basketball. For those not keen to squint at their favorite artist reduced to a speck on a distant arena stage, there's O₂ dome's "intimate" performance space, **IndigO₂** (⟨ **020/8463-2700**) although even that is still plenty big, with 2,800 places. An acoustically superior, contemporary room, it has four bars, and attracts major comics and talent (the late Prince, Black Eyed Peas). If you aren't carrying a ticket for a show, there's not much to do there except eat—there are no retail stores—but if you need something more jolting, you can climb above it, at the **Up at the O₂** roof-walking attraction (p. 173). One of the keys to O₂'s explosive success has been the fact the Jubilee line's sleek North Greenwich station runs beneath it. *Thames Clippers* (p. 318) docks here, too. Peninsula Square, London, SE10. www.theo2.co.uk. ⟨ **020/8463-2000.** Tube and ferry: North Greenwich.

Clubs

The city's dance scene, being embedded in the style scene, is various and shifting, and by the time you read this, the variety will have shifted again. Aside from club nights at the venues listed above in Live Music (p. 238), the best source for tips on parties you stand a chance of getting into is *Time Out* (www.timeout.com/london/clubs). The clubs around Shoreditch, Old Street, and King's Cross were until recently the markers of cool, but both gentrification and development have squeezed the scene northeast to Dalston, which makes getting home in the middle of the night expensive—freelance cabbies charge double. Covers nudge toward £20.

The king of clubs remains **Fabric** (77a Charterhouse St., EC1; www.fabric london.com; ✆ **020/7336-8898;** Farringdon or Barbican tune), a former butchery that for more than a decade has had lines around the block. Its all-weekend parties (from Sat 10pm 'til the cock crows on Mon) are engineered to drill teeth-chattering bass frequencies into the souls of those who dare to submit. The City is not lost to the nerds yet; the pedigreed managers of **XOYO** (32–37 Cowper St., EC2; www.xoyo.co.uk; ✆ **020/7729-5959;** Old St. tube) turned a former printworks into a stripped-down sound tank, and succeeded. The **Ministry of Sound** (103 Gaunt St., SE1; www.ministryof-sound.com; ✆ **020/7740-8600;** Elephant & Castle tube) is known around the planet for its top-notch sound system, upper-crust DJs, and extreme cover charges in the low £20s.

Otherwise, wander Dalston and its environs for cutting-edge venues and basement clubs. Huge windows overlooking a decommissioned gasworks make partying memorable at the vast, post-industrial **Oval Space** (29–32 The Oval, E2; www.ovalspace.co.uk; ✆ **020/7183-4422;** Cambridge Heath rail), with its eclectic programming of alternative and progressive music. **93 Feet East** (150 Brick Lane, E1; www.93feeteast.co.uk; ✆ **020/7770-6006;** Liverpool St. or Shoreditch High St. tube), was one of the first pioneers to reclaim disused industrial space in Spitalfields for the hipsters; it mounts a mix of experimental electronic music, live bands, club nights, and day parties. The **Dalston Superstore** (117 Kingsland High St., E8; www.dalstonsuperstore. com; ✆ **020/7254-2273;** Dalston Kingsland Overground) is a pansexual party mix of DJs, disco, and ravey go-go boys. **The Nest** (36–44 Stoke Newington Rd., N16; www.ilovethenest.com; ✆ **020/7354-9993;** Dalston Junction rail) is intimate, affordable, and at times sweaty, but has the quality lineup and sound system of a mini-Fabric.

COMEDY CLUBS

London's comedy scene is dominated by Edinburgh's. Each August in the Scottish capital, seemingly all of Britain attends the city's famous festival season, where sharp minds vie for awards, audiences, and perversely, that shiniest of brass rings, a major London booking. The rest of the year, it seems that half the stages in town are either helping artists groom material for Edinburgh (June and July schedules are packed with new shows) or cashing in on its past successes. The fevered competition has created a comedy scene that has less in common with the stand-and-discuss neuroses of New York clubs and more to do with the brittle high concepts of, say, Russell Brand or Ricky Gervais. You may miss a few local references, but you're sure to appreciate the wit. All comedy venues serve food and drink, and tickets are almost always under £10 unless it's a big name or a very central location. Main shows are usually at 7:30 or 8pm. The tiny **Angel Comedy Club** (2 Camden Walk, N1; www.angelcomedy.co.uk; no phone; Angel tube), even though it's in the back of the Camden Head pub, is (legit) one of the best places in town to catch smart up-and-comers, and it's (legit) free to enter; just get there by 7pm on weekends (shows start daily at 8pm) to avoid being shut out. It's on the upswing and, as a consequence, added a second space nearby, which it named The Bill Murray. A Saturday night stand-up showcase is the main event at **Amused Moose** (Sanctum Soho Hotel, 20 Warwick St., W1; www.amused-moose.com; ✆ 020/7287-3727; Piccadilly Circus tube); big-name comics like Eddie Izzard or Stephen Merchant sometimes appear here, without a peep of advance word, to test out new material. The cluttered **Canal Café Theatre** (The Bridge House, Delamere Terrace, W2; www.canalcafetheatre.com; ✆ 020/7289-6054; Warwick Ave. tube) puts on a dozen shows a week; its biggest draw is "NewsRevue" (www.newsrevue.com; runs Thurs–Sun), a weekly send-up of current events running since 1979, which gives it the Guinness world record for longest-running live comedy show. The 400-seat **Comedy Store** (1a Oxendon St., SW1; www.thecomedystore.co.uk; ✆ 0844/871-7699; Leicester Square or Piccadilly Circus tube) was created in 1979 in imitation of clubs popular in New York; it launched both Eddy Izzard and Jennifer Saunders. Today it presents improv on Wednesday and Sunday, and mainstream stand-up the other nights of the week. In a former wood warehouse 20 minutes from the center of town, **Pleasance Theatre Islington** (Carpenters Mews, North Rd., N7; www.pleasance.co.uk; ✆ 020/7609-1800; Caledonian Rd. tube) has stronger ties than most to Edinburgh; it operates the Scottish festival's chief comedy venue and it starts previewing entrants in the spring.

CINEMA

Major movie premieres attended by major movie stars are routinely held at a handful of giant cinemas around Leicester Square. Chief among them is the **Odeon** (24–26 Leicester Square, WC2; www.odeon.co.uk; ✆ 087/1224-4007; Leicester Square tube), opened in 1937; it's the largest cinema in the country, with seating for about 1,700. But tickets for Leicester Square theaters can cost over £20. For better prices—in even more historic houses—look elsewhere. Because so many handsome old cinemas have survived, moviegoing can still feel like an event. In most theaters, you even select your seats when you buy your ticket—London was doing that long before America was.

BFI Southbank ★★★ The programming of the British Film Institute (BFI) is mind-bogglingly broad and savvy, from classics to mainstream to historic—more than 1,000 titles a year. For example, on one day in a recent July, its three screens unspooled a retrospective of Indian director Satyajit Ray, Alfred Hitchcock's *Dial M for Murder* in 3D, a mid-century series from the largely forgotten Boulting Brothers, and outdoor screenings of Gothic monster schlock. As the country's preeminent archive and exhibitor, it also programs plenty of talks, special previews, and the occasional free screening. The on-premises **Mediatheque** is a free video arcade for quiet, on-demand viewing of tons of titles you'd never see abroad because of rights issues. The shop stocks an incomparable list of rare DVDs, including many treasures the BFI has personally restored and re-released, such as Charlie Chaplin's early Keystone and Mutual films, and war-era British propaganda films, which you can only find here. There are also two popular bars, one in the lobby and one on the water. Belvedere Rd., South Bank, SE1. whatson.bfi.org.uk. ℂ **020/7255-1444.** Tube: Waterloo.

The Electric Cinema ★★★ It's one of the world's great screens: Leather seats are softer and deeper than anything you have at home, and each one is equipped with a footstool, table, and a wine basket—it's a luxurious, romantic way to pass a few hours. The bar in the back of the house sells

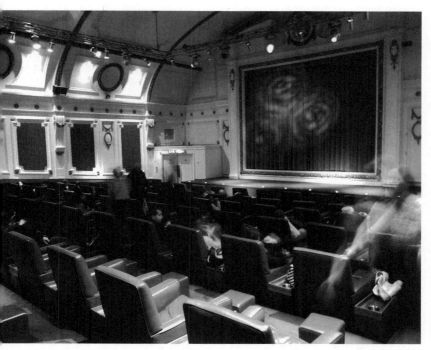

The Electric Cinema in Notting Hill offers comfortable leather seats with footstools and wine baskets.

everything from crudites to booze, and downstairs is a barrel-roofed French-American diner. Meanwhile, films, which change daily, hop between first-run and well-received art house movies—nothing too obscure. Shockingly, this place stood derelict from 1993 to 2001, and only a fierce campaign saved it. Now it's run by the exclusive Soho House, which opened a private club here. Its outpost in Shoreditch is a new build and not so richly historic. 191 Portobello Rd., W11. www.electriccinema.co.uk. © **020/7908-9696.** Tube: Ladbroke Grove or Notting Hill Gate.

Phoenix Cinema ★ Thought to be the oldest purpose-built cinema in the U.K., the Phoenix was constructed as the Premier Electric Theatre in 1910; by 1985, despite its handsome Edwardian barrel-vault ceiling, it was nose-to-nose with the wrecker's ball until fans (including director Mike Leigh) rallied. It screens an immense range of films from across eras and borders, plus frequent transmissions of live theater. It also has a liquor license. 52 High Rd., East Finchley, N2. www.phoenixcinema.co.uk. © **020/8444-6789.** Tube: East Finchley.

GAY & LESBIAN

London's gay and lesbian scene is collapsing in the face of development. The last few years saw the unthinkable closure of Camden's half-century-old drag landmark The Black Cap, and several important Soho bars including Madame Jojo's and Molly Moggs have been forced out or have been sold. Nevertheless, the city still has one of the most varied scenes in the world. The music seems to crank a few notches louder when the jolly and outrageous **Pride London** (prideinlondon.org) season rolls along, in late June or early July.

Daily gay-oriented pursuits have traditionally been centered around Soho, where the bars and clubs take on a festive, anyone-is-welcome flair, and after work, guys spill into the streets. But as a mark of a truly integrated city, now nearly every neighborhood has its own pubs and gay nights. Where you spend an evening depends on your proclivities and willingness to commute. At most places, there aren't usually cover charges unless an event or show is on, when they're about £5 at bars and £11 for clubs. Lesbians who want to go out at night must usually plan a little because most girls' events take the form of weekly scheduled nights in bars that might cater to other niches during the rest of the week.

The weekly **Boyz** (www.boyz.co.uk) and **QX Magazine** (www.qxmagazine.com) publish schedules that favor club events. *Time Out* also has a weekly "Gay and Lesbian" section that dwells more on clubbing than on well-rounded pursuits.

There are many smaller venues, but these standout venues in every flavor are welcoming to tourists and will provide a good overview of the culture.

Comptons ★★ This old two-level pub wears the tatty garb of a bygone saloon but it's one of Soho's most beloved hangouts for men who are out of their bubble-gum years. **Admiral Duncan,** across the street, and the **Duke of Wellington** ("Duke of Welly's"), where Old Compton Street T-bones into Wardour Street a few steps west, cater to the same professional age group. 51–53 Old Compton St., W1. www.centralstation.co.uk. ☎ **020/3238-0163.** Tube: Piccadilly Circus.

G-A-Y ★★ Once renowned for their literary prowess and cleverly coded hints about their sexuality, London's homosexuals have allowed their wit to become somewhat less nimble: They named one of their top clubs G-A-Y. Just G-A-Y. It's about partying, cruising, and dancing. The main event is the Saturday night club at Heaven, near Charing Cross Station. No other dance club in Europe, gay or straight, comes close to attracting such a pantheon of legendary live performances: Kylie, the Spice Girls, Cyndi Lauper, Bjork, and, of course, Madge, all performed here at the height of their fame. Increasingly, however, there's nothing more exciting than *RuPaul's Drag Race* contestants. Every night, G-A-Y also runs a light pre-show hangout, G-A-Y Bar, where a young, twink crowd steeps in cheery Europop and watches videos on the plasma screens. And you can imagine the vibe at its G-A-Y Late venue, which goes until 3am. **Club:** Heaven, Under the Arches, Villiers St., WC2. Tube: Charing Cross or Embankment. **Bar:** 30 Old Compton St., W1. www.g-a-y.co.uk. ☎ **020/7494-2756.** Tube: Leicester Square. **Late:** 5 Goslett Yard, W1. ☎ **020/7734-9858.** Tube: Tottenham Court Rd.

Ku Bar ★★ A manageably sized, young-skewing, three-level lounge is the place you go when you don't want a scene but you wouldn't mind being served by shirtless boys. It has a later license: until 3am Monday to Saturday. Tuesday is lesbian night. 30 Lisle and 25 Frith sts., WC2. www.ku-bar.co.uk. ☎ **020/7437-4303.** Tube: Leicester Square.

Royal Vauxhall Tavern ★★★ A 2013 biography revealed that Diana, Princess of Wales, once secretly attended this gay drag landmark dressed as a man. That gives you an idea of RVT's heft in British culture, as well as the fact that inside, anything goes. There are three shows a night, all transgressive, or just dancing, and when the party's thumping, this little brick building literally leaks dance-floor fog. 372 Kennington Lane, SE11. www.rvt.org.uk. ☎ **020/7820-1222.** Tube: Vauxhall.

She Soho ★ She's one of London's only 7-days-a-week lesbian bars, and given that there aren't too many part-time girl bars, either, it attracts a wide spectrum of types—even tag-along men. 23a Old Compton St., W1. www.she-soho.com. ☎ **020/7437-4303.** Tube: Piccadilly Circus.

XXL London ★★★ London's biggest dance night for "bears" (for the uninitiated, those are men who would never dream of shaving their chests like the young "twinks" do), it's colossal beyond belief. Its arched-ceilinged dance floor—actually you're in vaults beneath a railway—gets super sweaty, which must be the only reason why thousands of assembled men strip off their shirts and grind on. 1 Invicta Plaza, South Bank, Blackfriars Rd. at Southwark St., SE1. www.xxl-london.com. ℗ **020/7403-4001.** Wed and Sat. Cover £15. Tube: Southwark.

The Yard ★★   On weekends, all the cute jock types are here, cramming the courtyard-like space, or watching the action from the Loft lounge area upstairs. Weekdays, it's more subdued and a place for the after-work crowd, but it's always straight-friendly. Developers are licking their chops over the space. 57 Rupert St., W1. www.yardbar.co.uk. ℗ **020/7437-2652.** Tube: Piccadilly Circus.

WALKING TOURS OF LONDON

Paying for a bus tour seems smart in principle. You glimpse monuments, briefly, and you hear one or two eye-glazing facts about them as they whiz past. But no coach tour, no hokey sightseeing boat, goes at your speed. None convinces you that the things you're seeing are quite real, or allows you to mull what's before you, or lets you breathe in the atmosphere. Get up close to London. Don't pass it. Touch it—so that it can touch you.

WALKING TOUR 1: WESTMINSTER, WHITEHALL & TRAFALGAR SQUARE

START:	**Westminster Tube station**
FINISH:	**Trafalgar Square**
TIME:	**Allow 60 minutes, not including time spent in attractions**
BEST TIME:	**Be at the starting line just before noon to hear Big Ben deliver its longest chime of the day**
WORST TIME:	**After working hours, when energy drains out of the area**

When most people hear the word "London," this is the area they picture: the Houses of Parliament, the wash of the Thames, the gong of Big Ben, and the Georgian facade of No. 10 Downing St. Kings and queens, prime ministers and executioners, despots and assassins—this is where they converged to shape a millennium of events, at the command center for England and the British Empire. History buffs, lace up.

1 **Westminster Tube Station**
The best train to take here is the Jubilee line, which was added at great expense in 1999. The station's concrete-grey, 36m-deep (118-ft.) cavern, ascended by escalators from the Jubilee's platforms, is one of the city's finest new spaces, providing a modern-day analog to the majestic space of Westminster

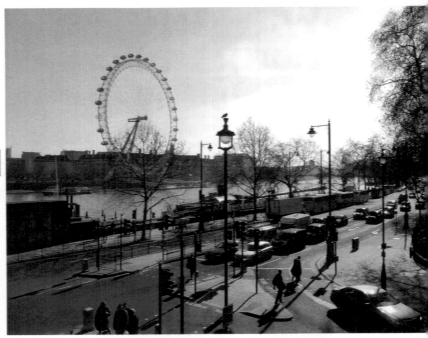

The Victoria Embankment features gardens, statues, and glorious Thames views.

Abbey nearby. Portcullis House, where many MPs (Members of Parliament) keep offices, is overhead.

Find your way to the Westminster Underground station, Exit 1, and walk outside.

2 Victoria Embankment at Westminster Bridge

Once you're outside, you'll see the River Thames. If you stood here in 1858, in the midst of what came to be known as The Great Stink, you'd have choked on the fumes rising from the fetid effluvia floating in the river below. Until then, the city had no sewers to speak of—only pipes that dumped into the water. The solution was the Victoria Embankment, a daring engineering project, completed in 1870, that saved engineers from having to dig up the whole city. They simply built a new riverbank, laid sewers along it, paired that with new Underground railway tracks, and topped the unattractive additions with a garden and a road. Destructive, but effective—how Victorian.

Today, the embankments' benches are raised to allow a good view of the water, and it's dotted with triumphant statuary like Boudicca in her bladed chariot, which you can also see from here. This tribal queen rose up against the Romans; she failed politically but, as you see, succeeded aesthetically.

Walking Tour 1: Westminster, Whitehall & Trafalgar Square

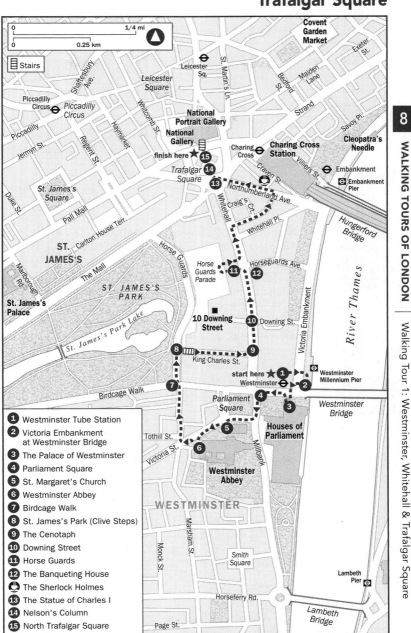

0 | 1/4 mi
0 | 0.25 km

📧 Stairs

Covent Garden Market

Leicester Sq.

Leicester Square

Piccadilly Circus — *Piccadilly Circus*

National Portrait Gallery

National Gallery

finish here ★ **15**

Trafalgar Square

14

13

Charing Cross

Charing Cross Station

Cleopatra's Needle

Embankment

Embankment Pier

Northumberland Ave.

Whitehall Pl.

Hungerford Bridge

St. James's Square

Pall Mall

ST. JAMES'S

Carlton House Terr.

The Mall

ST. JAMES'S PARK

Horse Guards

Horse Guards Parade

Horseguards Ave.

11 **12**

St. James's Palace

St. James's Park Lake

10 Downing Street

10 Downing St.

River Thames

Birdcage Walk

8 🚇
King Charles St.

7

start here ★ **1**
Westminster 🚇

Westminster Millennium Pier

2

9

4

Parliament Square

3

Westminster Bridge

Tothill St.

5

Victoria St.

6

Houses of Parliament

Westminster Abbey

WESTMINSTER

Smith Square

Lambeth Pier

Horseferry Rd.

Page St.

Lambeth Bridge

1. Westminster Tube Station
2. Victoria Embankment at Westminster Bridge
3. The Palace of Westminster
4. Parliament Square
5. St. Margaret's Church
6. Westminster Abbey
7. Birdcage Walk
8. St. James's Park (Clive Steps)
9. The Cenotaph
10. Downing Street
11. Horse Guards
12. The Banqueting House
🔵 The Sherlock Holmes
13. The Statue of Charles I
14. Nelson's Column
15. North Trafalgar Square

The London Eye, spinning on the opposite bank, had a tricky birth in 1999; it was constructed lying flat over the river, resting on pontoons, and then it was laboriously hoisted upright and into place. The mock-baroque building behind it is County Hall—it looks old, but it only dates to the early 20th century—which was once the seat of the London city government.

At the bridge's opposite landing, you can see the South Bank Lion. Weighing 14 tons, 3.6m (12 ft.) tall, and eager-eyed and floppy-pawed as a puppy, he was carved in 1837 by the Coade Stone Factory, which once stood where County Hall stands today. Made of a durable, synthetic ceramic stone formulated by a mother-daughter team, the lion stood proudly for over a century, painted red, atop the Red Lion Brewery that was located past the London Eye. Blitz bomb damage destroyed his roost, but at the request of King George VI, he was saved and placed just feet from his birthplace.

Go back into Westminster station, head down the corridor, and turn left before the set of four stairs. Leave the station via Exit 3, marked Houses of Parliament.

3 The Palace of Westminster

You're now standing under the iconic Elizabeth Tower of the Houses of Parliament, once called St Stephen's Tower but renamed in 2012 in honor of QE2's Diamond Jubilee. This is as close as you can get to it, so have a good look at the assorted crowns, kings, and crests carved into the facade. These buildings may look like they're from the Gothic period, but in fact they date to 1859, when they rose from the ashes of the old Parliament House, destroyed by a nightmarish fire in 1834. Big Ben, the name of the largest of four bells inside (2.7m/9 ft. in diameter, 13 tons), was named for the portly commissioner of works who oversaw its installation. (There's actually a bigger bell in town: Great Paul at St Paul's is 2 tons heavier.) Each side of the Clock Tower's four faces is 6.9m (23 ft.) long. Since 1923, the very earliest days of wireless, the BBC has broadcast the 16-note prelude (called "Westminster Quarters" and replicated in doorbells around the world) of Big Ben before its news summaries. Thanks to a crack that developed in the 1860s, the bell is now slightly off from its original note—E above middle C—but you'd need perfect pitch to tell.

This plot of land has been used by royals since 1050, when Edward the Confessor built a palace here, away from the hubbub of the walled city. Kings ceased living on this block as of Henry VIII, when nearby Whitehall became his main London pad, followed in later reigns by St James's and, currently, Buckingham palaces. But Parliament's land is nationally owned, so technically it meets in Westminster Palace.

Head away from the river to:

4 Parliament Square

The heavy metal bars on the spiked fence that distances you from this building are not there out of mere paranoia; as far back as the thwarted

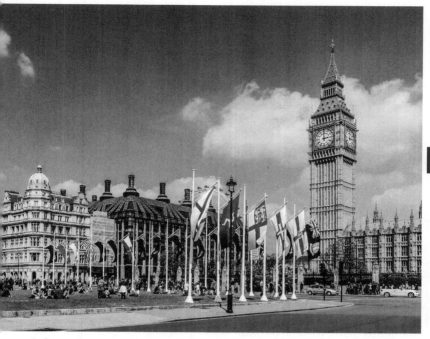

Parliament Square is an important stop on your walking tour.

Gunpowder Plot of 1605, the Houses of Parliament have been a target for would-be revolutionaries. Prime Minister Spencer Perceval was fatally shot on the steps of the House of Commons by a former convict on May 11, 1812, and in the Blitz, the buildings were smashed on more than a dozen occasions, including one (May 10, 1941) that caused the near-total destruction of the House of Commons.

The section of the Houses that juts into the yards, behind the statue of Oliver Cromwell, is Westminster Hall, from 1097, one of the only survivors from the 1834 fire. Charles I, Sir Thomas More, and Guy Fawkes were all condemned to death in the Hall.

For more on visiting the **Houses of Parliament,** see p. 130.

Turn left and walk in front of the Houses of Parliament. Use the first crosswalk to your right, heading toward the church. At the far side of the church, enter the gate to see:

5 St Margaret's Church

The little side church by Westminster Abbey (p. 134), the one with the four sundials on its tower, is the Church of Saint Margaret, dating to the early 1500s and much changed over the years. Sir Walter Raleigh, who was executed outside the Palace of Westminster, is buried inside, and both the poet Milton and Winston Churchill married their wives here.

You can see the statues of Parliament Square better from here. Probably the most famous one is that of American president Abraham Lincoln, at the western end; it's a copy of one in Chicago by Augustus Saint-Gaudens. During the anticapitalist protests of 2000, the statue of Winston Churchill that stands here received a temporary Mohawk made of grassy turf. This square has always attracted well-intentioned screw-ups: In 1868, the world's first traffic light was erected here. Gas powered, it blew up.

Follow the footpath to the front of:

6 Westminster Abbey

The lawn beside the abbey—yes, the one you just walked across—is in fact a disused graveyard. In a city this old, you simply can't avoid treading on final resting places. There are an unknown number of plague pits scattered through the city, into which thousands of victims were hastily dumped to avoid the spread of disease, and several city parks likely had the germ of their beginnings, so to speak, as potter's fields—group graves for paupers.

Although most of the Abbey is in the Early English style, the stern western towers above you now were the 18th-century work of Nicholas Hawksmoor, a protégé of Christopher Wren. Hawksmoor's designs are famous for emphasizing the forbidding, angry side of God; some critics accuse him of using architecture to frighten people into piety. Most of the time the people who use this main entrance in an official capacity do so in a crown, a gown, or a coffin. For more on visiting **Westminster Abbey,** see p. 134.

If you peer down Broad Sanctuary, which becomes Victoria Street, you can see the Italianate tower of Westminster Cathedral, the primary cathedral of England. Good news, Catholics: The English don't execute you anymore!

Cross the street to your right (Broad Sanctuary), and cross again. You should be a block west of Parliament Square on Storey's Gate now. Walk straight until you find yourself at the corner of St James's Park. You're at:

7 Birdcage Walk

You've just walked past a variety of European Union offices; the proximity to the Houses of Parliament has appealed to paper-pushers for centuries. The military has a presence here, too. The road that heads to the left, Birdcage Walk, leads to the front of Buckingham Palace. Halfway down, you'll find the Wellington Barracks, the headquarters of the Guards Division, where a battalion of one of the queen's five regiments of foot guards (Grenadier, Coldstream, Scots, Irish, and Welsh) bunks down. There's also a small, curio-packed Guards Museum (www.theguardsmuseum.com; ⓒ **020/7414-3271;** daily 10am–4pm; £6), where you learn that their tall "busby" helmets are made of Canadian brown bearskin. Who knew?

Storey's Gate, the street you just walked, was named for the keeper of Charles II's aviary. Birdcage Walk, the street you're now on, was named after a royal aviary that stood in St James's Park; until 1928, only the Hereditary Royal Falconer was permitted to drive on Birdcage Walk. The park continues its tradition of hosting bird menageries; the pond is a haven for ducks and geese, and a small flock of pelicans has been in residence since the 1600s. They are fed fresh fish daily at 2:30pm.

Cross Birdcage Walk and walk 1 block up Horse Guards Road, passing the Treasury Building on your right, until you reach Clive Steps at King Charles Street on the right. On your left, peek into:

8 St James's Park

See if you can spot the lake in the park. The body of water was originally a formal canal belonging to St James's Palace, the official royal residence from the burning of Whitehall in 1698 to the time Victoria moved into Buckingham Palace in 1837. The old canal was prim and straight in the French style and outfitted with gondolas, a gift of the Doge of Venice. In winter, as Samuel Pepys described in the 1600s, it would freeze over, and people would frolic upon it using skates made of bone. It was later sculpted into something calculated to appear more random and thus more English. St James's Palace, which is not open to the public (except for Clarence House, in summer; p. 138), is located on the north (far) side of the park. You might be able to make out a rustic-looking shack just inside the park. That's Duck Island Cottage, built in 1840 as a dwelling for the bird keeper. Not shabby for a servant's quarters.

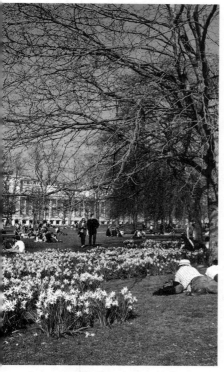

St James's Park offers pleasant strolling around a graceful pond with ducks.

You'd think that if London were under attack from flying bombers that you'd be much safer if you were a little farther from the Houses of Parliament. Yet in the basement of the sturdy 1907 Treasury Building, Britain's leaders orchestrated their country's "finest hour." Unbeknownst to the world, it was the hideout of Winston Churchill and his cabinet. Famously, but hardly wisely, that daredevil Churchill went onto the roof of the building so he could watch one of Goering's air raids slam the city. The cellar, preserved down to its typing pool and pushpins, is now the **Churchill War Rooms** (p. 129), a superlative museum paying homage to the bulldoggy prime minister.

Who is Robert Clive, the cutlass-wielding subject of this statue on the steps? He was the general who helped the East India Company conquer India and Bengal, partly through a series of underhanded bribes, thus delivering the region into the control of the British Empire for nearly 2 centuries. Don't be too hard on this hardened colonialist; the opium-addicted fellow committed suicide by stabbing himself with a penknife.

Walk down King Charles Street and through the arches at the end. You are now on Parliament Street. Look into the center of it. The somber stone column in the traffic island is:

9 The Cenotaph

The Cenotaph (from the Greek words for "empty" and "tomb") is a simple but elegiac memorial to those killed in the two World Wars. A 1919 plaster parade prop that was made permanent in stone by Edwin Lutyens the next year, it was executed with inconceivable restraint when you consider that nearly a million British subjects died in the Great War alone. Its inscription to the "Glorious Dead," coined by Rudyard Kipling, is repeated on other memorials in Commonwealth nations; the Cenotaphs in Auckland, New Zealand, and in London, Canada, are replicas. Uniformed servicemen and -women will always salute it as they pass, and on the Sunday closest to November 11, Britain's Remembrance Day, the sovereign lays the first wreath while other members of the Royal Family observe from the balcony of the Foreign Office. You may see flowers around it, or possibly silk poppies (red flowers with black centers), the national symbol of remembrance.

Walk left up Parliament Street, which becomes Whitehall. In about 30m (98 ft.) on the left, you reach a black fence with glass lanterns. Look inside the gates. This is:

10 Downing Street

On the right, by the tree and tough to make out, is No. 10, the official home of the prime minister. It's famous for its lion's head knocker—although to be frank, if you have to knock, you aren't welcome. Once, you could walk around in there, but Margaret Thatcher made many enemies, so you'll have to make do with peering down the lane through metal bars. Such security was a long time coming. In 1842, a lunatic shot and killed the secretary to the prime minister, mistaking him for the big man; and in 1912, suffragette Emmeline Pankhurst and friends pelted the house with stones, breaking four windows, in one of many acts of civil disobedience in the fight for voting rights for women. If sentries prevent you from approaching, then the prime minister might be on the move. Prepare for the black gates to burst open, spew forth an armada of cars, and watch the prime minister's Jaguar blast onto Whitehall as if fleeing a bank heist.

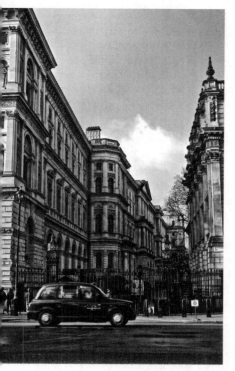

The lane was laid out by George Downing, the second man to graduate from Harvard University in America and by all accounts a shady individual, a turncoat, and a slumlord. He's one of history's great scoundrels; his underhanded dealings resulted in Dutch-held Manhattan being swiped by the British and the slave trade multiplying in the Colonies. Strange that the most important street in British politics should bear his name.

Downing built No. 10 (then, no. 5) as part of a row of terraced houses in the late 1600s, fully intending for it to fall apart after a few years (instead of actually laying bricks, he just painted on lines with mortar). Yet George II had his eye on the house, and he kicked out a man named Mr. Chicken—further information about him, tantalizingly, is lost to the mists of time—to give it as

Entrance to Downing Street is heavily secured.

a gift to the first prime minister, Robert Walpole, in 1730. Walpole insisted that the house be used by future First Lords of the Treasury, his official capacity. He also connected it to a grand home behind it on Horse Guards, now nicknamed The House at the Back—this deceptive Georgian facade actually conceals 160 rooms. No. 10 is also connected with nos. 11 and 12, and it's even linked to Buckingham Palace and Q-Whitehall, a sprawling war bunker, by long underground tunnels. Many prime ministers elected to live in their own homes, using No. 10 for meetings, but not William Pitt, who moved in upon becoming prime minister at the virtually pubescent age of 24 in 1783. He lived here for more than 20 years, longer than any other prime minister, until his death at 46. Whitehall became a slum in the mid-1800s, and the house fell out of fashion, but then it served as the nerve center for the two World Wars and became indispensable to the British spirit. You can see the original front door, now replaced by a stronger one, on display at the Churchill Museum at the Cabinet War Rooms (p. 129), two stops back.

A little up Whitehall from Downing Street, look for the bronze monument to "The Women of World War II," which depicts no women, but rather their uniforms and hats, hanging on pegs as if they'd been put away after a job well done. The implication of this 6.6m-tall (22-ft.) tableau is, of course, that the women went back to the kitchen after briefly filling a more robust societal role. This sly bit of statuary-as-commentary was unveiled by the queen in 2005. Some 80% of the cost of the memorial was raised by a Baroness who won money on ITV's *Who Wants to Be a Millionaire?*

Continue up Whitehall, past the monumental government buildings. In about 60m (200 ft.), you will reach another black gate broken by two stone guardhouses. Head inside the yard to view:

11 Horse Guards

Built in the Palladian style between 1750 and 1758 on a former jousting field of Whitehall Palace, the Horse Guards is the official (but little-used) entrance to the grounds of St James's Palace and Buckingham Palace. Two mounted cavalry troops are posted in the guardhouses every day from 10am to 4pm, and they're changed hourly. At 11am daily and 10am Sunday, the guard on duty is relieved by a dozen men who march in from The Mall behind, accompanied (when the queen is in town) by a trumpeter, a standard bearer, and an officer. Don't try to crack up guards with your shenanigans. You'll look boorish and rude—and they still won't react.

If you think the clock tower arch looks small, you're right. Its designer made it that way so that its proportions would match the rest of the building. Walk through the clock tower arch to reach the graveled Horse Guards Parade, the city's largest non-park gathering space, which you may recognize as the setting for volleyball during the Olympic Games.

Return from the yard to Whitehall. Across the street you'll see:

12 The Banqueting House

Built by Inigo Jones, this is not a home but it is the last remaining portion of the great Whitehall Palace. Inside is a bombastic ceiling by Rubens depicting the king as a god. That vainglorious posture, and the king's grabs for more power, led to the gory event that happened on this spot on January 30, 1649. If you were standing here then, you would have been in the crowd that watched King Charles I mount the scaffold (wearing two shirts so that he wouldn't shiver—he was no true god, after all), place his head on the block, and be decapitated, handing the reins of the country to a military dictatorship led by Oliver Cromwell. When the executioner held the head aloft, one witness said there was a queasy silence, followed by "such a groan by the thousands then present, as I never heard before and I desire I may never hear again." Charles I was buried privately at Windsor, not at Westminster Abbey, to avoid more unpleasant scenes. If you want to see what poor Charles looked like, hang on for the next stop. The regicide was somewhat for naught; by 1660, the country grew weary of its leadership and Charles I's son, the hedonistic spend-thrift Charles II, was back on daddy's throne. In revenge, the second Charles chose the Banqueting House as the site for his restoration party, and then had the nerve to show up late. England was royal again—and how. For more on visiting The Banqueting House, see p. 138.

Continue up Whitehall. Take the next right, Great Scotland Yard (the corner of Scotland Place was the "visitor's entrance" of the Ministry of Magic in the Harry Potter movies) and then cross Northumberland Avenue, veer slightly left, and head into Craven Passage.

The Sherlock Holmes 🍺

Time for a pint and maybe some traditional English pub grub, so head to **The Sherlock Holmes** (10–11 Northumberland St.). In 1957, a collection of Arthur Conan Doyle memorabilia was assembled as a tourist attraction for the huge Festival of Britain that gave London the Southbank Centre, and it became the centerpiece of this pub. It's nowhere near 221B Baker St., but it has a roof garden and a terrace.

Return to Northumberland Avenue and turn right. When you reach Trafalgar Square, cross the street so you're in the oval traffic island.

13 Statue of Charles I

That this bronze statue stands here is a miracle. It's of Charles I, pre-headectomy, and is a precious Carolinian original from 1633. When the king was beheaded, the Royal Family was deposed (permanently, so people thought). The owner of this statue was commanded to destroy it, but he was clever enough to bury it instead. After the Restoration, it was dug up and placed here, in about 1675. That was even before Trafalgar Square existed (the zone was, as an equestrian statue suggests, used as stables). Charles wasn't a tall man, and boosting him with a horse went some way toward making the luckless fellow seem imposing. Someone stole his sword in 1867, and he went into hiding again during the Blitz, but otherwise, this is one of the oldest things in this part of London that remains in its original place. Its pedestal, unloved and weathered, could use a restoration, too.

This is a good spot, free of traffic and obstructions, to survey your sur-roundings and take some photos. Look back down Whitehall, from where you just came, and you'll see Big Ben's tower. To the right, the vista through Admiralty Arch concludes in the distance with the grand Victoria Memorial at Buckingham Palace. Important buildings for two Common-wealth nations stand astride Trafalgar Square: Canada House to the left (west) and South Africa House to the right (east; its country's name is inscribed in Afrikaans as Suid-Afrika).

14 Nelson's Column & Trafalgar Square

Why is Lord Nelson atop that column? Money. The Admiral sacrificed his life in 1805 to defeat Napoleon Bonaparte's naval aspirations at the Battle of Trafalgar, thus securing Britain's dominance over the oceans— and pumping untold wealth into London. In the late 1800s, lightning struck Lord Nelson—or at any rate his statue—damaging his left arm. It took until 2006 for the city to finally eliminate the bronze bands that held him together, repairing him with the same Craigleith sandstone with which he was constructed in 1843. During the work, they realized that the monument is actually 4.8m (16 ft.) shorter than guidebooks had been claiming for generations—it's 51m (167 ft.) from the street to the crown of his hat. The man himself is 5.5m (18 ft.) tall. The column's base is lined with four bronze reliefs that were said to be cast using metal from French cannon captured at the battle that each one depicts. All are guarded by four reclining lions (1867), the mascots of the square. History is full of instances of public rabble-rousers climbing the lions' plinths to stand beside the cats and whip crowds into states of political agitation.

Lutyens, who did the Cenotaph (p. 256), also designed the plaza's two fountains (from 1845 originals), which were ostensibly for beautification but conveniently prevented citizens from gathering in numbers. Trafalgar Square has long been the setting for demonstrations that turned from complaint to unrestful, such as infamous riots over poll taxes and unemployment. The English gather here for happy things, too, as they did for the announcement of V-E Day (May 8, 1945), and as they still do for festivals and free summer performances. In the southeast corner, you'll see a stone booth big enough for a single person; that's the city's smallest police station, built in 1926. Once a closet for a phone that was used to summon backup, now it's used mostly to store chemicals for the fountains.

You may have heard about Trafalgar's Square's famous pigeons. So where are they? Banished for overactive excretion. Until the early 1990s, the square swarmed with them—the fluttering flock was estimated to peak at 35,000—and vendors made a living from selling bird feed to tourists. Eventually, the GLC, London's government, grew tired of shoveling streaky poo off the statues and decided to return the square to its original function as a great public space to edify its great museum, the National Gallery. They began feeding the pigeons themselves first thing in the morning, and then hired a team of hawks, tended by a leather-gloved keeper, to patrol the square. The flock learned to chow down and then clear out for the day; anyone who feeds the birds is subject to a £500 fine.

15 North Trafalgar Square

At night when landmarks are picked out by lights, the views down Whitehall are sublime. Most of the statues dotting the square are of forgotten military men and nobles: James II (1686; in front of the National Gallery) is finely crafted, but he looks ridiculous, pointing limply in those Roman robes. He was deposed in the Glorious Revolution just two years after the statue was cast. It used to stand outside the Banqueting House; for years, detractors joked he was pointing in the direction he planned to flee. (And yes, that's George Washington, who wrested the Colonies from the Crown, standing nearby. Feelings are no longer hard—he was a gift from Virginia a century ago. Urban legend has it the pedestal contains a layer of Virginia earth so he can be said to remain on American soil.) The northwestern plinth of Trafalgar Square was designed for an equestrian statue of its own, but money ran out and it stood empty from 1841. More than 150 years later, the naked spot was named The Fourth Plinth and filled by works commissioned by a subversive panel of top artists. Sculptures show for 12 to 18 months, and they get the city talking. Marc Quinn's *Alison Lapper Pregnant* (2005) depicted a snow-white, nude woman born with limb deformities and heavy with child, and *Hahn/Cock* (2013) was Katharina Fritsch's two-story, ultramarine rooster, a sly send-up of the pompous military iconography elsewhere in the square. In early 2018 it's David Shrigley's elongated thumbs-up *Really Good* (2016), followed by Michael Rakowitz's re-creation, out of Iraqi date-syrup cans, of a statue destroyed by ISIS.

Along the north terrace, by the Café on the Square, look for the Imperial Standards of Length, which were set into the wall in 1876 and moved in 2003 when the central stairs were installed. They are the literal yardsticks against which all other British yardsticks are measured, showing inches, feet, and yards, plus mostly obsolete measures such as links, chains, perches, and poles.

And now, reward yourself with a visit to the loo, left of the stairs, and a spot of tea in the cafe. Or, if you crave some more substantial victuals, head over to the street east of the square to St Martin-in-the-Fields church, finished in 1724. Its combination of spire and classical portico was controversial at the time, but today, it pleases people of all persuasions with its excellent Café in the Crypt (p. 84). And, of course, two of the city's greatest museums, the National Gallery (p. 122) and the National Portrait Gallery (p. 124), share the same block and tower above you now.

8

WALKING TOURS OF LONDON | Walking Tour 1: Westminster, Whitehall & Trafalgar Square

START:	St Paul's Tube station
FINISH:	The George Inn, near London Bridge Tube station
TIME:	2 hours, not including restaurant breaks or attractions
BEST TIMES:	Weekend days in good weather, when the area is abuzz; Borough Market is most vital from Thursday to Saturday
WORST TIMES:	After dark, when cobbled streets are too dark to see well

It was the best of advertisements, it was the worst of advertisements. Charles Dickens' novels, largely social protests wearing the cloak of entertainment, made readers feel as if they'd traveled to London when they never left their own armchairs. Trouble is, the city that Dickens has primed visitors to expect—the foggy, coal-smudged metropolis teeming with pickpockets and virtuous orphans—is nowhere to be found. Partly thanks to Dickens' work, London reformed itself. On this tour, you'll explore what's left of its darker side—from the libertine London of Shakespeare's day to the desperate one Dickens sought to solve with his pen. Along the way, you'll enjoy gourmet food and a beer on the Thames, which conceals a body count of its own.

1 St Paul's Tube Station

If you just took the Central Line here, you rode what was once called the Central Railway. In the first 75 years of the Underground, train lines were independently owned, and separate tickets were required each time a passenger changed trains. Fares were cumbersome, calculated according to the distance traveled and the class of carriage chosen. When the Central Railway held its grand opening in 1900, in the presence of American wit Mark Twain (who lived in London at the time), it soared above its competitors by dint of several innovations, the most important of which was that anyone could ride as far as they wanted on a flat fare. The so-called "Twopenny Tube," which had one class of carriage like today's Tube trains, was a sensation. Gilbert and Sullivan, swept along, amended a line in their operetta *Patience* from a reference to the threepenny bus to "the very delectable, highly respectable Twopenny Tube." The Central Railway helped democratize public transit and accelerated expansion into the suburbs—even if authorities eventually went back to the old format of charging passengers by distance. The St Paul's station opened on July 30, 1900, as Post Office station—the city's main Post Office was then across the street (hence the name of Postman's Park just north; p. 160).

Exit the St Paul's Underground station and turn left, toward:

2 Panyer Alley

Panyer Alley, where you're standing, was named for the basketmakers, or panyers, who once traded here. Look for a plaque on the wall depicting a child sitting on a basket. This plaque, the so-called Panyer Stone, is

Walking Tour 2: St Paul's & Southwark

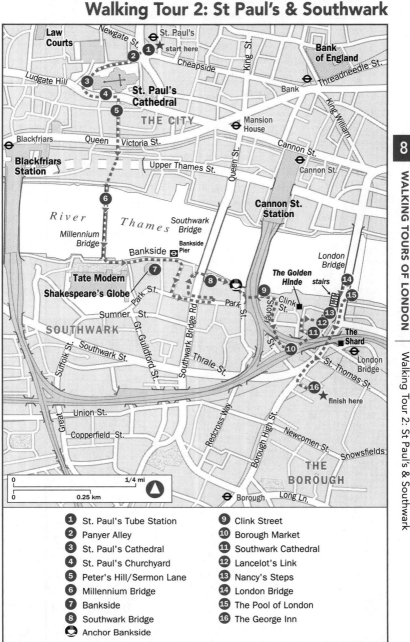

1. St. Paul's Tube Station
2. Panyer Alley
3. St. Paul's Cathedral
4. St. Paul's Churchyard
5. Peter's Hill/Sermon Lane
6. Millennium Bridge
7. Bankside
8. Southwark Bridge
   Anchor Bankside
9. Clink Street
10. Borough Market
11. Southwark Cathedral
12. Lancelot's Link
13. Nancy's Steps
14. London Bridge
15. The Pool of London
16. The George Inn

dated "August the 27, 1688," and reads, "When you have sought / the citty round / yet still this is / the highest ground." The artists behind this stone surely knew that Ludgate is not the highest point in The City; that's Cornhill, which is about 30cm (12 in.) higher. But the sign has been here so long that it would quite literally be a crime to take it down.

Head left, toward St Paul's, and make a right through the pedestrian alley, Paternoster Row, to Paternoster Square. Go through the ornate arch at the far left:

3 St Paul's Cathedral

The area you've just walked through, Paternoster Row, ranks among the most sacred in London. There have been major houses of worship on the plot of St Paul's as far back as 604, and for centuries these narrow surrounding streets have teemed with ecclesiastical scribes and clergy, as well as untold hordes of supplicants desperate for a handout from the merciful church. Paternoster Row was later known as the center of literary London, first for its publishers—who replaced the scribes—and later for its book market. This is where Shakespeare bought the historical texts that inspired him to write his plays. Yet what you'll see today is modern; even the 23m-tall (75-ft.) column in Paternoster Square was created only a few years ago to appear older than it is. Why would planners permit the wholesale demolition of such a rich heritage? They didn't. This was

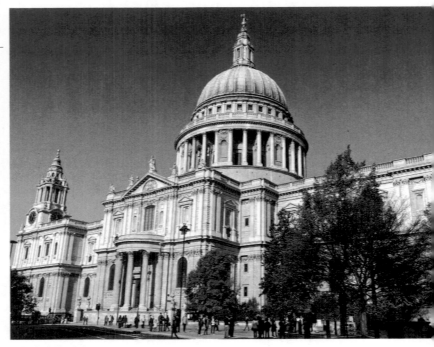

St Paul's Cathedral.

Ground Zero of the Blitz in 1940. The Germans, recognizing that the destruction of St Paul's would demoralize the nation, focused their power on it, and the spillover devastated everything around it. Every firefighter was called to the cathedral, saving it at the expense of just about everything else.

The ornate stone archway that you pass through, however, is a true antique. It's Temple Gate, one of eight ancient gateways to The City of London, which originally stood where Strand becomes Fleet Street from 1672. Charles Dickens described it in *Bleak House* as "a leaden-headed old obstruction." It was dismantled in 1878 and was destined for a dump somewhere when a visionary stepped in and brought the stones home. After spending more than a century in the hinterland of his family's Hertfordshire estate (and being spared the Blitz), the gate, possibly designed by Christopher Wren, was restored and re-erected here in November 2004. The seven other gates, including Aldgate and Moorgate, were all lost over time.

In front of the cathedral, a statue of Queen Anne, who ruled England when St Paul's was completed, looks down Ludgate Hill. In attendance are ladies symbolizing England, France, Ireland, and North America, which she considered her subjects. The statue is an 1886 copy of the 1712 original, which (like Temple Gate once did) now resides, in scabby condition, in the countryside.

Herbert Mason's iconic photograph of St Paul's dome, snapped during the mighty conflagration that engulfed London after air raids on December 29 and 30, 1940, was taken from Ludgate Hill. Next time you see that picture, note that it's lit by firelight. For more on visiting St Paul's, see p. 161.

Skirt the cathedral along the busy street called:

4 St Paul's Churchyard

At the crossing, go over the street. Now's a good time to duck into The City of London Information Centre (Mon–Sat 9:30am–5:30pm, Sun 10am–4pm), located inside the origami-style, wing-roofed building, and stock up on free tourist brochures and timetables. It also runs daily guided walks in the afternoon.

If you don't need information, turn left. If you do use the office, when you come out again, turn right. After the patch of grass, turn right again. You can see down Peter's Hill to a white pedestrian bridge over the river. Stroll down:

5 Peter's Hill/Sermon Lane

On the right is the Firefighters National Memorial, which depicts a young man gesturing wildly toward St Paul's as two others grapple desperately with a hose. It's impossible to exaggerate the devastation caused by the Blitz, both in property and in lives. The superheated firestorms created damage greater in area than those of the Great Fire of 1666. More than

20,000 people were killed, and 1.4 million left homeless. The names of some 1,000 victims, all volunteer firefighters defeated by the wild blaze and collapsing buildings, are inscribed on the octagonal base. Winston Churchill dubbed this monument "The Heroes with Grimy Faces." For their families, the survival of St Paul's Cathedral amidst utter devastation remains a testament to their sacrifice. Keep going toward the river.

Go onto the:

6 Millennium Bridge

You're now on the steel Millennium Bridge, the central city's first new crossing over the Thames since the Tower Bridge in 1894. Its design, which features side-located suspension cables that sag about six times shallower than a conventional suspension bridge's supports do, was a little too advanced for its own good. When the bridge opened in 2000, it was discovered that the shifting weight of pedestrians caused it to sway, and people had to grasp the rails for support. (At the start of *Harry Potter and the Half-Blood Prince,* Death Eaters attack the bridge and make it wobble—that was an inside joke for Londoners.) Engineers closed the 325m (1,066-ft.) span, poured in another £5.2 million to solve the issue, and reopened it in 2002. Now locals love it because it has transformed accessibility to the river's southern bank, and they're planning more foot crossings. It's still not perfect—it's plagued by joggers with little regard for idle strollers—but crossing the river here, in view of many of the city's landmarks, young and old, makes for some stirring photos.

Straight ahead is the monumental Tate Modern (p. 155), signaled by its factory-like "campanile" smokestack, which from 1952 to 1981 belched exhaust from the Bankside Power Station. Energy has been a fundamental part of the district's character for generations. The power station replaced an earlier one that dusted everything near it with a coating of soot, and that plant, too, supplanted a foul gasworks. Before that, the district was the domain of a legion of coal merchants who shuttled their filthy wares around town in shallow boats. These "lightermen" worked from docks that lined the entire southern shore, where land was cheaper than it was in The City on the northern side. The building you see before you is a direct descendant of the way of life that prevailed on the bank in the 1700s.

How deep is the Thames? The river fluctuates greatly with tides (so it's dangerous for swimming—in fact, that's illegal between Putney and the Thames Barrier), but depending on when you measure around here, it's generally 8.9m (29 ft.) deep at highest tide and 1.8m (6 ft.) at low tide. The Thames' moodiness is the main reason Southwark, the side of the river where the Tate Modern sits, was written off for so many centuries. Until medieval times, the low-lying southern bank was boggy and mostly uninhabitable, so was instead thought of as part of Surrey, the county south of London. Londoners made use of the waterlogged land by turning it into gardens for secret trysts and fish farms (the Pike Garden, or Pye Garden, stood pretty much in front of you around the Tate's eastern flank). It wasn't until the latter part of the 1700s that people figured out how to drain the water and settle the area fully. Southwark was where you went for a rowdy time—that is, until the Puritans quashed the fun in 1642.

Before you completely cross the river, look down at the debris near the river wall. Turn back for a stupendous view of St Paul's dome symmetrically rising from the center of the bridge.

Once you're on the opposite bank, with the river in front of you, turn right. Stand midway between the cluster of houses and the building with the thatched roof. You're on:

7 Bankside

This river promenade also continues west, past the Tate Modern, to the London Eye and the Houses of Parliament. In *Four Weddings and a Funeral,* when Hugh Grant told Andie MacDowell he loved her (in the words of David Cassidy), he did it farther along this walkway by the National Film Theatre. There's no better place to stroll, people-watch, and appreciate the sweep of the city.

As late as the 1960s, the path you're on, which at this place is called Bankside, was a vehicular street bearing two-way traffic, as it had been since the 1600s. Each building on the street owned rights to the docks or water-stairs on the river opposite it, so tenants were usually people who needed access to the water, such as ferrymen or sailors. The four-story white house at the left of the blind Cardinal Cap Alley, no. 49, was built around 1710 on the foundations of a pub, the Cardinal's Cap, which itself was built in 1547 to entertain the people who came to Southwark to carouse. No. 49 was home to successive generations of coal merchants, but not, as its plaque purports, to Sir Christopher Wren as he built St Paul's. Wren did live nearby, but in a building that was torn down when the power station needed land. This plaque hung on that vanished home, but was appropriated by a D.I.Y. revisionist in the mid–20th century. No. 49 has received its own biography, *The House by the Thames* by Gillian Tindall.

To the left is Shakespeare's Globe Theatre (p. 155), which made a premature exit in its own era, only to be rebuilt in ours. The circular Globe's stage is even at the same compass point as the 1599 original's. Interestingly, the city's theatrical life was centered here from about 1587 to 1642, when it was illegal to operate a theater in The City proper. Once the laws relaxed, the entertainment venues moved back into town, where they've been ever since.

Southwark was the Tudor version of a multiplex, and the biggest blockbuster was bear-baiting—the spectacle of vicious dogs let loose upon tethered bears. Even Henry VIII and Elizabeth I were huge fans; he had a bear pit installed at Whitehall Palace, and she barred Parliament from banning the pursuit on Sundays. One short block past the Globe, turn down a lane called Bear Gardens to find a small courtyard, three-quarters of the way down the street. That's the former location of the Davies Amphitheatre, one of the most popular bear pits. Samuel Pepys wrote in his diary in 1666 of attending one such slaughter where he "saw some good sport of the bull's tossing the dogs—one into the very boxes. But it is a very rude and nasty pleasure."

Under a modern office building in the next street, Rose Alley, lie the foundations of another theater known to have premiered plays by Shakespeare, the Rose (p. 155). It lasted from 1587 to about 1606. The Swan stood nearby, too, although we may never find the footprint. The Rose's footprint gave us vital clues about what Elizabethan theaters looked like—architects also studied sketches made of it by a Dutch tourist in 1596. (Are you sketching your trip?)

Historians think they know where the original Globe stood. If you'd like to see it, head down Bear Gardens (between two modern buildings) one block to Park Street, turn left and go under the bridge, and just after it, past the buildings on the right, you'll find slightly red cobbles showing locations of fragments archeologists found in 1989. Not very suggestive, is it? In 1949, it was even drearier. It lay behind the gate of the decrepit Anchor Brewery, and when American actor Sam Wanamaker (father of Zoë, who played Madam Hooch in the Harry Potter movies) dropped by to pay pilgrimage, the indignity of the meager plaque (still there) so enraged him that he resolved to rebuild the Globe as a living home for England's great theatrical tradition—which is what came to pass, albeit 4 years after his 1993 death. Oscar-winning actor Mark Rylance was its first artistic director, serving for a decade.

Continue along the river, keeping it to your left. You'll go through a pedestrian tunnel under:

8 Southwark Bridge

On the wall of the tunnel, you'll see illustrations of skaters and revelers at the bygone "Frost Fairs" that, starting in 1564, were regularly held on the icy Thames. No matter how many winters you spend in London, you'll never see the Thames freeze over. But back then, they had the London Bridge, a few hundred yards downstream. Its 19 arches were so narrow, and its supports so thick, that the river's flow became sluggish, allowing water (and the outhouse filth that churned within it) to freeze. By contrast, during outgoing tides the rush was so fierce that boats capsized and passengers (few of whom knew how to swim, given the filth) drowned. When the bridge was dismantled in 1814, the Frost Fairs melted into history.

Take a look underneath Southwark Bridge where it meets the shore. You can still discern the remains of some water-stairs, dating to before the construction of the first bridge here in 1819. Back then, getting across the river usually required boatmen, the taxi drivers of their day. Ferrymen would court business by shouting destinations to theatergoers after their plays: "Eastward ho!" or "Westward ho!"

In 1912, this bridge's central 72m (236-ft.) span was the largest ever attempted in cast iron. The drab hunk of a building to your right is the headquarters of the *Financial Times*.

The Anchor 🍺

Few pubs are more idyllic than the **Anchor** (p. 102), situated where Bankside meets the railway viaduct. The riverside patio is open in good weather; otherwise, the interior is charming. This pub was once controlled, as nearly all pubs once were, by a brewery; it was Barclay Perkins, located just behind it from 1790 until about 1980. Even before that, it was a fixture; in 1666, Samuel Pepys watched the Great Fire rage from here before coming to his senses and hurrying across the river to rescue his possessions from his home in Seething Lane, near the Tower of London. In the 1950s, the Anchor was considered a slum and nearly was demolished.

After the Anchor, the path jogs inland. Take the first left onto:

9 Clink Street

Pass under the railway arch. In a few moments, you've gone from Elizabethan Southwark (theaters, bear-baiting) to Georgian Southwark (coal merchants, breweries). Now you're in Victorian Southwark, a claustrophobic underworld teeming with fetid-smelling industry and river rats. You can almost hear distant reverberations on this narrow wharfside street. You might even call the sensation Dickensian, and you wouldn't be wrong, since when the writer was 12 years old, his father was thrown into a debtor's prison near where you're standing, off the Borough High Street.

Prisons were something of a cottage industry for the area; the Clink Street Prison stood here from 1127, when the Bishop of Winchester built it as a lockup for his Winchester Palace, until 1780, when the anti-Catholic Gordon riots saw the dismal hole destroyed. Although the Clink gave its name as slang to all prisons that came after it, no one knows for sure how it got the name itself—Flemish or Middle English words for latch are likely

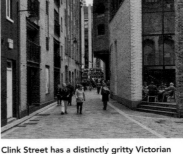

Clink Street has a distinctly gritty Victorian vibe.

the origin. Suffice to say it was awful—and so is the museum here that purports to tell its story. Avoid it.

In the 1800s, warehousing goods instead of people became this street's stock-in-trade. You'll still see hints of the street's past maritime uses, from wooden loft doors to cranes used to hoist crates into upper floors, but in recent years even the original cobbles were removed. Today, these spaces house media companies and architects. During the week, you'll see them in their fashionable clothes, strutting in their Italian shoes to mid-afternoon cocktails.

The latter Bishops of Winchester were not nice guys. Henry II (1133–89) gave them control of this neighborhood, and because it was outside the jurisdiction of the city, they could pretty much get away with whatever they wanted to. Principally, they cultivated countless brothels and skimmed the profits for themselves—which is how Southwark got its rep as a den of vice. Anyone who annoyed them (heretics, troublemakers) wound up in the Clink, where no one was likely to find them again. As you continue down Clink Street, past the modern building with the rounded grid of windows, on your right you'll see all that's left of the Bishops' palace: a fragment of old stone wall, dating to the 1300s, with a round panel of stone tracery at the top. That tracery once held a rose window, which lit the palace's great hall. This fragment was forgotten behind a wall until a warehouse fire exposed it again. Double back to Stoney Street.

Turn down Stoney Street and walk under the railway. On your left, you'll see:

10 Borough Market

Stop at the frilly grey portico.

The mood of the neighborhood has changed drastically again. To your left, behind the portico, is Borough Market, a fantasy for the tongue (described in gastronomic detail on p. 95) and the oldest fruit and vegetable market in the city. A market has been held around here since A.D. 43, when Roman soldiers noted passing a market on their way to sack The City. More reliable records date it to 1014, when it served the denizens on the old London Bridge, the city's only river crossing. The cream-grey portico is not original to this place; it's the cast-iron Flower Hall of Covent Garden, rescued when the Royal Opera House was renovated in 2003. If it seems to blend seamlessly, it's because it was made around the same time as the rest of the Borough Market structure (1859–60). You are standing very near the spot, by the Wheatsheaf pub, where police swiftly put an end to a ghastly Saturday night terrorist attack by knife-wielding attackers in June 2017.

The Market is best known for gourmet supplies. Park Street, which runs into Stoney Street, looks as quaint as a movie-set version of old England; in fact, it was used in *Harry Potter and the Prisoner of Azkaban*, and no. 7A was the entrance of The Leaky Cauldron. The Market itself has appeared in films including *Howard's End* and *Bridget Jones's Diary.* The city's first railway, a 6.4km (4-mile) run to Greenwich, plowed its route .8km (½ mile) east of here in 1836. Even after tunneling technology improved, railway tycoons thought nothing of barricading thriving neighborhoods with massive brick viaducts, cutting them off from each other and creating slums. On your tour, you have crossed under a number of railway viaducts built that way, and shortly, you'll see how narrowly one of England's most historic churches averted its own destruction.

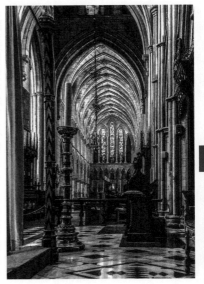

Southwark Cathedral.

Enter the market to the right of the portico and walk straight. Cross the next street and enter the brick arch marked Green Market. Before you is:

11 Southwark Cathedral

(If for some reason the Green Market arch is closed, turn left down Bedale St.—it's not marked—until you see a church appear on your right.)

Before you stands the oldest Gothic church in the city, and the oldest building in Southwark. You'll see its tower appear in every old drawing of the city. In Roman times, it was the site of a villa. Its Christian chapter was begun by the daughter of a ferryman in the 7th century; it was rebuilt in the 850s and again 300 years later. There was once a monastery and a chapel in this yard, where office workers now lunch on gourmet items from Borough Market, but those came and went, too. Southwark teemed with the poor, with factory workers, and with grubby river men. One such blue-collar child was John Harvard, one of nine kids of a man who owned a tavern and butcher shop just northeast of here. John was baptized in this church in the early 1600s, but when he grew up, he fled this slum for the Massachusetts Bay Colony, where Harvard University was later named for him. In time the place was limping along as a humble parish church called St Saviour's and dissolving into dilapidation. The rerouting of London Bridge Road sheared away several small chapels, and in 1863, the rumbling railway forced its way alongside the yard. But by 1905, its fortunes reversed when it was elevated to a cathedral, and now it's so well cared for that it's hard to discern its true age and sordid past.

The cathedral has some beautiful painted monuments, including one of England's oldest wooden effigies (1280). Shakespeare's brother Edmond was buried here in 1607, as was Philip Henslowe, who built the Rose, in an unmarked grave. Other worthwhile sights include Edwardian stained-glass tributes to the Bard's plays, the Harvard Chapel with masonry from the Norman period, and some of the original ceiling bosses, carved in 1469 and saved when things got bad. How bad? During Elizabeth I's reign, the retro-choir (the part behind the altar) was walled off and rented to a baker. Later on, vestrymen discovered the baker was also raising swine in there.

Just north of the cathedral, running parallel to its nave, a separate entrance leads into a glass-roofed corridor, which traces the line of an alley that was called:

12 Lancelot's Link

Nelson Mandela opened this addition in 2001. Have a look at the display inside, which preserves surprising discoveries made in this small area during a 1999 renovation. Look down into the well on the far right, and you'll see the original paving stones from the Roman road that cut through this space in the 1st century. You crossed over this same road several times already today; you were standing above it when you entered Borough Market. Other relics, piled on top of each other, include a stone coffin, probably from the 1200s, with a carved slot for the head, and a kiln from the 1600s, soot marks intact—bits of the Delftware made here have been found as far away as Williamsburg, Virginia.

Back down the corridor, exit. Go through the yard into the lane (it's Montague Close; the Thames is in front of you). Turn right, and just before the overpass, look left for:

13 Nancy's Steps

These are popularly held to be the location, in the Dickens novel *Oliver Twist,* where Noah Claypool eavesdrops on a conversation that leads to Nancy's murder by Bill Sykes. In the book, those steps faced the Thames, but these steps are in fact a rare surviving remnant of the New London Bridge, built here in 1821 as a replacement for the 600-year-old, over-crowded London Bridge. (The steps that Dickens wrote about were sold in 1968 to an American oilman. Locals superciliously quip he was duped, but, in fact, he knew exactly what he was doing and preserved what the English wouldn't. He had most of the New London Bridge shipped, stone by stone, to Lake Havasu, Arizona, to form a tourist attraction, and there it remains today, standing near a marina on a desert lake.) These steps were left behind and attached to the existing London Bridge, a featureless 1973 replacement.

Just so you know, the modern London Bridge was not the source of the nursery rhyme "London Bridge Is Falling Down"—that either referred to the burning of a wooden version in 1013, during a skirmish between Danes and Norwegians; or to Henry III's "fair lady" Queen Eleanor, who skimmed the tolls of the medieval bridge for her own purse, leaving its maintenance in a parlous state.

Climb the stairs to the road above. You're now on:

14 London Bridge

At the top of the stairs, you'll see a pedestal topped by a dragon, the symbol of the city, holding London's crest. You'll see these dragons at several of the city's medieval borders. About 30m (98 ft.) east of here, under modern buildings, is where you would have entered the Stone Gateway, the entry to the disaster-prone medieval London Bridge. For more than 3 centuries, tar-dipped heads of executed criminals were impaled on pikes and stuck atop the Gateway as a vivid warning to would-be ne'er-do-wells.

Turn to the right to use the crosswalk. Go to the opposite side of the street and walk onto London Bridge, over the river. Don't cross the river—just enjoy the view of the:

15 Pool of London

This section of the Thames between London Bridge and the Tower Bridge is known as the Pool of London. It may be quiet now, but for nearly 2,000 years, it was the heart of international trade. So many goods passed through here that warehouses along the southern bank became known as "London's Larder." Ships finally became so large that they had to unload downstream, closer to the sea. The section of river in front of you, parallel to this bridge, is where the medieval London Bridge stood.

Across the river from the Tower, you'll just make out an egg-shaped glass building. That's City Hall (2002), designed by Norman Foster (who also did the Millennium Bridge) to be ergonomic, with a huge spiral staircase curling around its atrium and "smart" windows that open on hot days. Just like a politician, it has no edge and you can't tell if it's coming or going. Former London mayor Ken Livingstone, a man not known for tact or restraint, called it "a glass testicle." Anyone can have a ball in its public spaces from 8:30am to 5:30pm on weekdays (www.london.gov.uk).

Turn around and follow London Bridge inland, keeping on the left side of the road. This street becomes Borough High Street. You will pass under a railway arch. Just after you pass Southwark Street forking off to the right, look for "The George" sign. It marks:

16 The George Inn

Because the London Bridge was the only crossing to the city from the south for so many centuries, this area became the equivalent of a train depot, and it was dotted with inns, stables, coach yards, and pubs. Everyone going to or coming from southern England or Europe stopped here, often spending the night before pushing into the shoulder-to-shoulder crowds of London Bridge. If you've ever read *The Canterbury Tales,* you'll recall that in 1386, the pilgrims began their journey to the shrine of Thomas à Becket from the Tabard Inn. Until 1873, that was located a short walk farther down Borough High Street, on the left. The George, described on p. 103, is the last survivor from this bustling coaching era. Although the wooden building, which once encircled the entire yard, dates to 1677, the inn was here for at least another 130 years before that, if not longer. We know it was typical of the time because John Stow, in *A Survey of London* (1598), termed it "a common hostelry for travelers." A drink here makes a fitting end to your journey through time. Look up and you'll see the jagged glass spire of The Shard (p. 157), Europe's tallest building, peering down as you sit where people have lifted beer for nearly half a millennium.

WALKING TOUR 3: **SHOPPING, SOHO & GIMME SHELTER**

START:	**Oxford Circus Tube station**
FINISH:	**Goodge Street Tube station**
TIME:	**2 hours, not including shopping or restaurant breaks**
BEST TIMES:	**Weekdays, when Berwick Street's market is on and Oxford Street is slightly less crowded**
WORST TIMES:	**Evening rush hour, when Oxford Circus Tube stop is positively rammed, and after dark, when stores and markets close**

All churched out? London is more than stories about dead queens and bloody uprisings. It's always been cosmopolitan, too, and the flash point for trends that ripple out to the rest of the world. Songs first sung at the clubs of Soho soon caused toes to tap on the other side of the planet, and fashion trends born on Carnaby Street remain internationally iconic 40 years later. Bring along your credit cards as we roam some of the city's best shopping streets and touch upon a few leftovers from London's recent past, including forgotten air-raid shelters and the settings for some good, old-fashioned sex scandals. This is the London you found out about from the radio and the runways, not from your social studies teacher.

1 Oxford Circus

Leave the Tube station using Exit 2. Position yourself out of the fray.

You are in the thick of mile-long **Regent Street,** which to the right is punctuated by the witches-hat steeple of All Souls Church and to the left curves toward Piccadilly Circus. When the Prince Regent, later George IV, was planning his new pet project, Regent's Park, he decided he also wanted a road to connect his house to it. He chose this particular location because, in his mind, it would provide a suitable demarcation line

Walking Tour 3: Shopping, Soho & Gimme Shelter

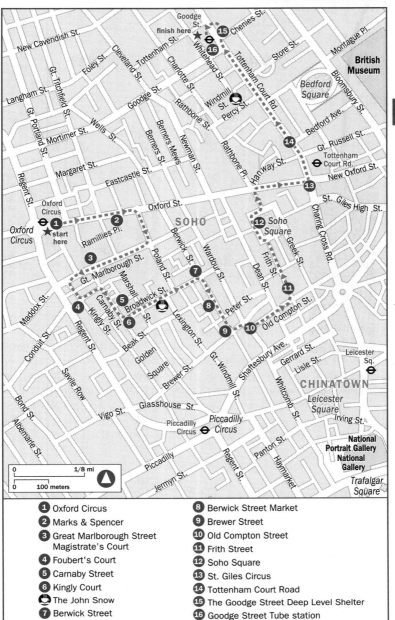

1. Oxford Circus
2. Marks & Spencer
3. Great Marlborough Street Magistrate's Court
4. Foubert's Court
5. Carnaby Street
6. Kingly Court
7. The John Snow
8. Berwick Street
9. Berwick Street Market
10. Brewer Street
11. Old Compton Street
12. Frith Street
13. Soho Square
14. St. Giles Circus
15. Tottenham Court Road
16. The Goodge Street Deep Level Shelter
17. Goodge Street Tube station

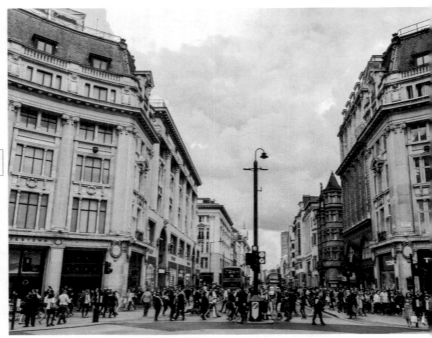

The bustling intersection known as Oxford Circus.

between the gentry of Mayfair, to the west, and the rabble of the traders who lived in Soho, to the east. George tapped John Nash to do the job, completed in 1825. Originally, the sidewalks were covered by stone colonnades, but when those attracted prostitutes, they were removed, and most of the original buildings were later rebuilt—the only Nash original is now All Souls. Even if most of the facades you see now mask more modern buildings, few streets in London impart such a sweeping, uplifting feeling, though few are also as congested with the hoi polloi George would have spurned.

The other avenue intersecting before you is Oxford Street, following the same line as a Roman road. George's class-centered definition of the landscape has more or less held: The exclusive shops of Oxford Street still lie west of Regent Street, and the downmarket stores tend to be east of it. Having a presence on Oxford Street is considered crucial for brands with mass appeal.

Head right, east on Oxford Street. You will pass Argyll Street on the right. When you pass Ramillies Street, prepare to stop in front of:

2 Marks & Spencer

London has a love-hate relationship with Oxford Street. People come here to shop by the thousands, but they often despair of the crush of the experience. Charles Dickens, Jr., described the street thusly in 1888: "It ought to be the finest thoroughfare in the world. As a matter of fact it is not by any means, and though it is, like all the other thoroughfares, improving, it still contains many houses which even in a third-rate street would be considered mean." We're only going to walk down a sample of Oxford Street. It's usually so crowded, that's as much as you can probably handle if you're keeping one eye on this book.

Marks & Spencer (p. 205), or M&S, dates to 1894 and is the favored British department store for staples. Perhaps proof of its appeal is that the chain can afford to run two giant frontages on Oxford Street; its flagship store is remarkably near here, between Bond Street and Marble Arch Tube stations. Its Food Halls (at this store, in the cellar) are well known as an ideal place to pick up prepared foods, sandwiches, and inexpensive but well-selected wines.

Turn right at Poland Street, walk 1 block, and turn right again onto Great Marlborough Street. Soon on your right, at nos. 19–21, you'll see a stout white building. That's the:

3 Great Marlborough Street Magistrate's Court

Charles Dickens worked here as a reporter just before hitting it big as a novelist, and a variety of other big names appeared before the judges here, including the Marquess of Queensbury (defending himself from Oscar Wilde's libel charge). When this neighborhood turned bohemian in the Swinging '60s, the court began trying a string of drug charges against the likes of Mick Jagger, Johnny Rotten, Keith Richards, Francis Bacon, and, curiously (and coming full circle), the guy who wrote the musical *Oliver!*, Lionel Bart. It's now a hotel, but I suggest you go inside briefly, because much of the old judicial fittings were left intact. You can have a cocktail in one of the old jail cells—now converted into private booths— or even peek into a restaurant slotted into the authoritative Number One court, which still has its witness stand, bench, wood paneling, and vaulted glass ceiling.

Beyond the Courthouse Hotel on the left, you'll see a Tudor-style building of black beams and white plaster. This is Liberty (p. 205), famous for its haute fabrics. It's also famous for its building—it was made in 1924 using wood recycled from junked ships.

Great Marlborough Street runs into Regent Street. Turn left there and walk the short distance to:

4 Foubert's Court

Times have been better on Regent Street. Walmart-style box stores in the suburbs have put the screws on the destination shops of the city, and this avenue has seen long-termers lose their sizzle. Dickins & Jones, a department store at the corner you just turned, closed its doors in early 2006 after nearly 170 years, and the same old shopping mall brands are moving in.

Two doors farther from Foubert's Court, though, at nos. 188–196, is a well-loved holdover from the street's glory days. It's Hamleys (p. 219), one of the largest toy stores in the world. Some 5 million customers pour through its doors every year, but since the sales force is famous for putting on a nonstop show on every floor, it's understandable if many of those customers come to gawp and not to buy. If you go into Hamleys, when and if you come out again, turn right and go back to Foubert's Court.

Walk down the very short Foubert's Court for 1 block; you'll see "Carnaby" on a metal arch. Go under it and head 1 block. Go right, and now you'll see a larger arch on:

5 Carnaby Street

Yes, those obnoxious arches proclaim your location with a self-promotion that proves this street is no longer the super-cool, forward-trending street of the kids in the know. It's more of a mall with an edge. The days of Swinging London, when men could cruise from store to store trying on hip-hugging black trousers and frilly shirts, are behind it. *Time* magazine spilled the secret of Carnaby Street in 1966, and by the 1970s, it was pedestrianized as a shopping street, making hipness a matter of retrospect.

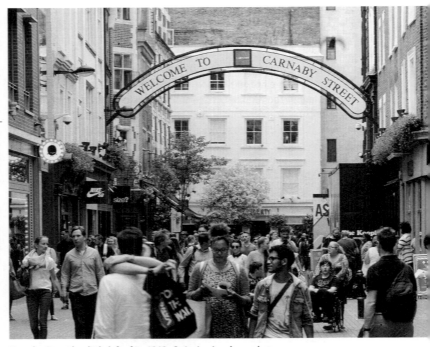

Carnaby Street has little left of its 1960s Swinging London cachet.

Just after you cross Ganton Street, where Broadwick Street hits Carnaby Street, duck into the passageway on the right:

6 Kingly Court

Clever entrepreneurs capitalized on Carnaby Street's rep with this development, a retail experiment in a former timber warehouse. The stores here are mostly boutiques pushing young designers.

Slip out the back door of Kingly Court, opposite its front door, and hang a left on Kingly Street. No. 9 is the Bag 'O Nails pub, where future Wings-mates Paul McCartney and Linda Eastman first clapped eyes on each other—and also where in 1961 John Profumo met Christine Keeler, kicking off the notorious Profumo Affair. It's also where Fleetwood Mac's John McVie proposed to Christine.

Return to Kingly Court. Retrace your steps out of it, cross Carnaby Street, and head down Broadwick Street. You'll stop around:

John Snow Pub 🍺

So grateful were Dr. Snow's neighbors that they renamed their pub for him, albeit a century later. It stands at no. 39, at Lexington Street, on the site of his practice. Raise a pint in his honor here, as we read the words of Dr. Snow himself: "I feel it my duty to endeavor to convince you of the physical evils sustained to your health by using intoxicating liquors even in the greatest moderation." (Oops.)

Continue on Broadwick Street to:

7 Berwick Street

About 160 years ago, this block was a foul slum. French, Greek, and Italian immigrants fled hard times and revolutions by cramming into these tight streets, and by the 1850s, cholera was storming through the overstuffed city. An 1854 outbreak killed 500 people in barely 10 days. Common wisdom at the time held that the disease was spread through the air—a reasonable conclusion, given how terrible the sewage-smeared city smelled—but a local anesthetist, John Snow (for whom the pub you just visited was named) had a different theory. Suspecting polluted water was the cause, he got permission to inspect the public pump at Broad Street, now Broadwick Street (in the block before Berwick St.) and found that it was being contaminated with sewage leaking from no. 40 nearby. The saga was recently retold in the book *The Ghost Map* by Steven Johnson, and in 2015 the site of no. 40 was dug up to build a giant new development.

When you reach Berwick Street, look left. Think of this location as the modern-day Abbey Road. It's where, in 1995, Oasis photographed the cover of *(What's the Story) Morning Glory?,* one of the seminal CDs of the age. The photographer shot from farther down the street, aiming south, toward where you're standing. (Noel Gallagher, with characteristic tact, said he thought the album cover was "s**t.")

And here's another slice of rock history: One miniblock farther down Broadwick Street at no. 7, the corner shop covered in striking rust-colored tiles (now Sounds of the Universe record store, a local landmark for world music) was the Bricklayers Arms pub. Brian Jones auditioned the Rolling Stones here in 1962, and they held formative rehearsals upstairs. Across the road at no. 6 is Agent Provocateur, a noted lingerie shop, a hint of how unsavory the area once was. The word "Soho" is probably derived from a hunting cry used when this area was parkland—it's nice to see that some folks around here are still on the hunt.

Turn south on Berwick Street. Walk down it to:

8 Berwick Street Market

This is the vestige of the last great market in the center of the city,—it's been in operation at least since the 1840s (vestry records indicate some illicit trading was going on as far back as 1778). London's first publicly available grapefruit was sold here in 1890. Now that the Cockney produce sellers have been mostly elbowed aside for gourmet nibbles, the market again caters to those with exotic, expensive tastes.

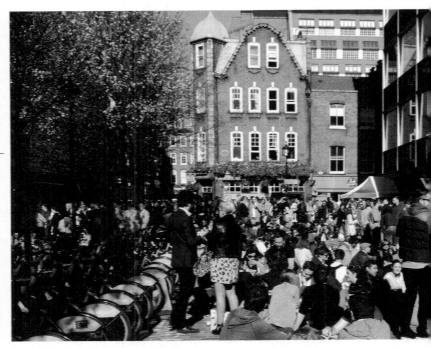

Berwick Street Market.

Pass over Peter Street and under Maurice House, going under the crossover and winding up on:

9 Brewer Street

From the late 1700s to the 1950s, it was impossible for a single gentleman to pass unpropositioned through Soho. A 1959 act chased the open salesmanship indoors, to be replaced by drinking joints where men could buy lap time with a lady, and by the 1970s, even those were forced to seek a lower profile. By law, today's displays are not permitted to titillate, complying with the British reputation (inaccurate in my book) for sexual modesty.

It was in this fleshy carnival that Laura Henderson bought a theater at Great Windmill and Archer streets and got around indecency laws by ensuring that the performers in her naughty entertainment, the Revudeville, never moved a muscle. Famously, the Windmill never closed, not even during the Blitz. You might have seen it in the film *Mrs Henderson Presents.* By the 1950s, Soho was a den of gang warfare and prostitution, full of craftsmen of every sort—costumers, ostrich feather trimmers, gun makers—until the Conservative government re-zoned the neighborhoods to admit offices, and the old ways were priced out.

Go left to Wardour Street, make a right and then a quick left. You'll be at the head of:

10 Old Compton Street

First, note the church of St Anne's, a few yards down Wardour Street, on the left. It was built in 1685, possibly by Wren (which ones weren't?), 2.5m (8 ft.) higher than the street because it went on top of a graveyard for 60,000 bodies (until 1853, when burials stopped, the neighborhood reeked from it). Everything save the church's tower was creamed by the Nazis.

Walk down Old Compton Street, Soho's de facto main street, which is busy round the clock and a center of gay life. No. 54 is the Admiral Duncan, where Dylan Thomas once drank (then again, where didn't he?). It was here, in 1999, that Nazi sympathizer David Copeland planted a bomb stuffed with 500 nails, which killed three people and injured many more. Copeland, an obvious madman, also bombed the South Asian population of Brick Lane and blacks in Brixton, but his only fatalities were here.

On the corner of Dean Street, look right. Down the block on the left, at no. 49, is the French House, more commonly called the French Pub. During World War II, it was the drinking haunt of Charles de Gaulle; here the exiled leader formed the Free French government and army. The street beyond the French House is Shaftesbury Avenue, the famous theatrical thoroughfare; many of the side streets between Old Compton and Shaftesbury contain the stage doors for the major playhouses, where famous actors report to work. Now look left, north up Dean Street. In the attic of no. 28, Karl Marx dwelled in abject poverty with his wife and several kids, but no running water or toilet. Three of his kids died while he was in residence in Soho in the early 1850s. No wonder he thought communism would be better.

Turn left at:

11 Frith Street

Bar Italia, the stylish cafe at no. 22, is a nightlife landmark of its own (p. 84). Upstairs is where, in 1925, John Logie Baird privately tested a homemade invention he called "noctovision," using his grocer's delivery boy as a test subject. The next year, he unveiled an improved model for the science nerds of the Royal Institution upstairs in this building. (Unsatisfied, he made another attempt in 1928 that involved hooking up a fresh human eyeball he'd rushed by taxicab from Charing Cross Ophthalmic Hospital. It created a mess.) Baird's system, which used a spinning disc, was eventually discarded, but it debuted ahead of American Philo T. Farnsworth's more famous electronic version. Within a decade, the BBC was broadcasting "television"—its new name—regularly. In the 1940s, Baird invented the first color picture tube.

Walk up three doors. For 10 months starting in September 1764, the 8-year-old Mozart lived with his father and sister at a house at no. 20 (the building was replaced in 1858). While he was in London, the prodigy amused King George III, wrote his first two symphonies, and befriended fellow composer J.C. Bach, who mentored him. By the 1800s, Soho's Wardour Street was the violin-making center of Europe. Music history of another kind happened at no. 47, which in 1969 hosted the first public performance of The Who's *Tommy,* and then Jimi Hendrix's last performance, in 1970.

Use the gate to head into:

12 Soho Square

Laid out in 1681, Soho Square was, early on, fashionable and mansion-lined. Later it became the center of the ambassadorial and scientific cliques. Sir Joseph Banks, who made his name collecting exotic specimens as a tagalong on Captain Cook's voyages, moved here in 1777. These days, Soho is a center for the music and film industries.

In the center of the square, which is technically a private garden even though it's been open to the public for half a century, is a cottage you'd swear was Tudor in origin. In fact, it's an 1895 imitation made to hide an electrical transformer. Beneath the lawns lie empty air-raid shelters.

Exit the opposite side of the square and go straight down Soho Street. You'll soon hit Oxford Street again. Turn right and head for the next major intersection, officially called:

13 St Giles Circus

Look across the next major street, and you'll see the 35-story Centre Point development. Built in 1964 with heavy government concessions, it

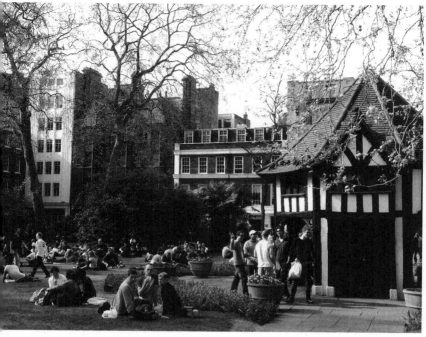

Soho Square.

was kept empty for years by its unscrupulous owner, partly to hold out for astronomical rents and partly because doing so would get him off the tax hook, even as the city struggled through a homeless crisis. The charity Centrepoint, which started in the basement of St Anne's church in Soho and grew into a force in housing issues, derisively took its name from the waste. Still, it's indisputably one of the landmarks of the skyline.

The area around the Tube station is under major redevelopment as part of the mammoth Crossrail project (opening in late 2018), a train line that will connect Canary Wharf in Docklands with West London.

Turn left and head up:

14 Tottenham Court Road

Fans of Andrew Lloyd Webber (anyone?), or at least of T. S. Eliot, will recall that this is the "grimy road" roamed by Grizabella in *Cats,* who sings "Memory." On the first corner, the Dominion Theatre was one of London's biggest cinemas, then a major concert venue (Judy Garland played here more than in any other London house, and Dolly Parton shot a TV special here). Now it's one of the largest West End theaters. Just 5 minutes ahead, on your left, you will see Goodge Street, with pubs frequented by students who attend the several universities in this area.

Duck into Chenies Street, on your right. At the curving side alley of North Circle, look for the striped, rounded buildings. That's:

15 The Goodge Street Deep Level Shelter

In 1939, planners decided to build an express train line beneath the existing Northern line platforms of Goodge Street. War intervened. In 1942, the unfinished tunnel was allocated to the Americans, and it was under the ground here where General (later President) Dwight D. Eisenhower orchestrated D-Day and announced it to the world, in 1944. There were eight deep-level shelters around town, five of which were open to bomb-shocked civilians; this is one of the most central and best kept. It retains its ground-level entry blocks, one pillbox and one octagonal, connected by a brick building—thousands of Londoners pass them daily but don't know their original purpose. Since the Cold War, the shelters have been used for storage.

Double back onto Tottenham Court Road. Across the street will be:

16 Goodge Street Tube Station

Before you end your tour at the Tube station opposite, turn right. The Goodge Street Deep Level Shelter could originally be accessed from a second point on the west of Tottenham Court Road opposite Torrington Place; some brick-and-concrete structures and vents linger. Back on Tottenham Court Road, notice how no. 79 stands alone—its neighborhood was blasted away by the final V2 rocket attacks in 1945. Nine people died here; 2,700 perished this way citywide. The site remains undeveloped. Goodge Street Underground station, opened in 1907 and still sporting much of its original tile work, uses elevators, not escalators. You can always take the 136 steps—that is, if you have the juice after your walking tour.

DAY TRIPS FROM LONDON

You've flown all the way to England. It would be a shame to miss seeing some of the sights that make it special—the rolling countryside, the stately mansions cradled by ancient trees, the ageless villages built on slow-flowing rivers. An excursion enriches you with two experiences for the price of one: You'll taste everyday English life while you immerse yourself in world-famous landmarks.

Britain has comprehensive transport, but it's not quick as mercury. Because of traffic and a dearth of superhighways, you can expect a 48km (30-mile) trip to take an hour, so a spot that's 129 to 161km (80–100 miles) each way, such as Stonehenge or Bath, will require you to rise at dawn if you want to buy yourself much touring time at all. Going by bus is often less expensive than by rail, but the inefficient journey will involve narrow roads.

The tourist offices listed will be able, for a fee (£4–£5, plus 10% of the room rate), to hook you up with a bed for the night, should you decide that you'd rather not trek back to London right away. You can find lots more information at **Visit England** (www.visit england.com) and **Visit Britain** (www.visitbritain.com).

For in-depth coverage of everything outside of London, get a copy of *Frommer's England & Scotland*. For casual day-trippers, though, here's what you need to know to dash out of the city and see the best of these destinations.

WINDSOR & ETON

Buckingham Palace is a mere *pied-à-terre*. The queen actually prefers this great castle, which dominates the skyline of town like a cloud of stone. Windsor Castle (32km/20 miles west of London) has been the home of the Royal Family for some 900 years, far longer than anything in London. Queen Victoria is buried in the backyard (although they don't phrase it quite that way). Despite the inevitable crowds, this is unmissable.

Essentials

GETTING THERE The price difference between transport options is negligible. Riding the rails is quicker, so it's got the edge.

Trains (www.nationalrail.co.uk; ✆ **08457/48-49-50**; 38–56 min.; £10–£12) go directly from Waterloo station to Windsor & Eton Riverside or from Paddington to Windsor & Eton Central with a change at Slough. Both Windsor stations are a 3-minute walk from the Castle. Trains requiring no changes leave twice an hour, and trains requiring a change leave a little more frequently. Or take a coach by **Green Line** (www.greenline.co.uk; ✆ **0871/200-2233**; 1 hr. 45 min.; £10 single, £15 return, 40% less after noon). Nos. 700, 701, or 702 leave from Hyde Park Corner or Victoria Coach Station, south of Victoria Station.

VISITOR INFORMATION   Stop by **Royal Windsor** (Old Booking Hall, Windsor Royal Station, Thames St.; www.windsor.gov.uk; ✆ **01753/743-900**; windsor.tic@rbwm.gov.uk). From there, you can be referred to Blue Badge guides for **town walks.**

TOURS   The most appealing way to see the area is by **boat,** departing from Windsor Promenade, Barry Avenue, for a 40-minute round-trip with fine views of the castle. Tours are operated by **French Brothers,** Clewer Boathouse, Clewer Court Rd., Windsor (www.frenchbrothers.co.uk; ✆ **01753/851-900**; 40-min. trip £8.50 adults, £7.80 seniors, £5.65 children 3–13, cheaper online; 2-hr. trip £15 adults, £13 seniors, £9.65 children 3–13).

Exploring Windsor

Legoland Windsor (www.legoland.co.uk; ✆ **0871/222-2001**; Mar–Oct; £35–£60 seniors and children 3–15, cheaper online), 2 miles from town, has top-notch rides catering to small children and some impressive Lego constructions. The Green line from London goes there, as do shuttles from Windsor's Theatre Royal. The tourist office sells discounted tickets for late-afternoon entry.

Windsor Castle ★   You may have had your fill of palaces in London proper, but you haven't seen the best. A fortress and a royal home for more than 900 years, it was expanded by each successive monarch who dwelled in it—more battlements for the warlike ones, more finery for the aesthetes. The resulting sprawl, which dominates the town from nearly every angle, is the queen's favorite residence—she spends lots of time here—and its history is richer than that of Buckingham Palace.

The castle's **State Apartments** are sumptuous enough to be daunting, and a tour through them—available unless there's a state visit—includes entrance to some mind-bogglingly historic rooms. Around a million people file through every year, so sharpen your elbows. *Warning:* There are no cafes (they're building one for 2018), so eat first.

The palace has a cache of priceless furniture (some of it solid silver), paintings, ephemera (look for the bullet that killed Lord Nelson, sealed in a locket) and weaponry, all of which, frustratingly, the audio guide, signage, and £5 souvenir book do little to describe, so the only recourse is to pepper staff with questions. In 1992, one-fifth of the castle area was engulfed by an accidental

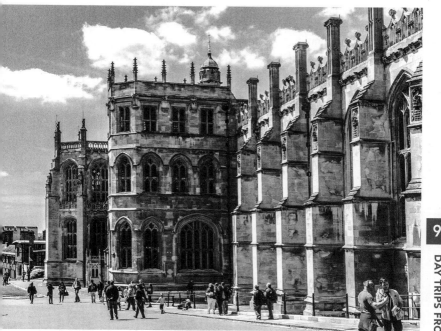

St George's Chapel at Windsor Castle.

fire; the queen recounted her despair over that, plus the breakup of two of her children's marriages, in her now-famous "annus horribilus" Christmas speech to the nation, and much effort and funding went into returning everything to the way it was before. In fact, the queen originally opened Buckingham Palace to visitors to fund the restoration.

St George's Hall, one of the repaired areas, is the queen's chosen room for banquets. Kids love **Queen Mary's Doll's House,** a preposterously extravagant toy built for the allegedly grown-up Queen Mary in the 1920s with working electricity, elevators, plumbing, specially written library books, and other details so extravagant they're borderline offensive. From October to March, the tour also includes the **Semi-State Rooms,** George IV's private area, considered by many to be among the best-preserved Georgian interiors in England. In August and September, you can climb the **Round Tower** for views, and sometimes in January and midsummer, the castle's ancient **Great Kitchen** is open. There's also a **Changing the Guard** ceremony at 11am (Mon–Sat, but alternate days Aug–Mar; check the website). **St George's Chapel** (closed Sun), a delicately vaulted Gothic spectacle opened by Henry VIII, is his final resting place and that of nine other monarchs, including Elizabeth II's father (George VI). Elizabeth II's mother (the Queen Mum) and sister (Princess Margaret) are with him in a side chapel; it's safe to assume that this is where she will wind up one day, too.

The Castle is the superstar here, but supporting roles are played by the succinctly named **Great Park** adjoining it, and the 4.8km (3-mile) pin-straight **Long Walk** that culminates with an equestrian statue of George III. **Frogmore,** open a pitiful few days in the summer, is the house where Victoria and Albert share their mausoleum. Just south of the castle is the **Guildhall,** where Prince Charles and Camilla Parker-Bowles had a quiet civil marriage in April 2005; it's no St Paul's, where in 1981 Charles wed his first wife, what's-her-name, but it is also the work of Christopher Wren (note its delicate arches). The building was apparently designed without the center columns, which made councilors nervous; Wren threw up some columns but left them an inch shy of the ceiling, just to prove that his architecture was sound.

Castle Hill. www.royalcollection.org.uk. ✆ **020/7766-7304.** Admission £21 adults, £19 students and seniors, £12 children 5–16, free for children 4 and under, £53 family of 5 (2 adults and 3 children 16 and under), cheaper if the State Apartments are closed. Mar–Oct daily 9:30am–5:30pm, last admission 4pm; Nov–Feb daily 9:45am–4:15pm, last admission 3pm. Closed for periods in Apr, June, and Dec, when the royal family is in residence. National rail: Windsor Central or Windsor & Eton Riverside.

Eton College ★ A 15-minute walk over a footbridge on the Thames (narrow at this western remove), you're in a world served by snooty stationers and haberdashers. Eton is probably the most exclusive boys' school on Earth. Princes Harry and William are alums, known as Old Etonians, as are kings and princes from around the world. There's a museum in its wine cellars—and the fact this school has a wine cellar tells you what kind of rich these kids are. Be nice to them. They're tomorrow's dictators. Public access is restricted; small tours tend to go Friday afternoons at 2pm, May to September.

Keats Lane, Eton, Windsor. www.eton college.com. ✆ **01753/370-603.** Admission £12. 2-hr. tours May–Sept. Fri at 2pm. Reservations required.

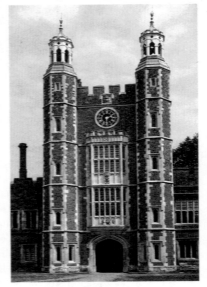

Clocktower and entrance to Eton College.

BATH

Easily roamed on foot, Bath, about 161km (100 miles) west of London, is revered as a splendid example of Georgian architecture—to tourists, Bath is resolutely stuck in that past. The pleasing sandstone hue of its buildings set against the slate-grey British sky, the assiduously planned symmetry of its streets, the illusion that Jane Austen (who lived here in 1800–05) is taking tea

Train fares listed in this section are provided as a guideline; National Rail pricing schemes are complicated and unpredictable. The good news is that for all of the destinations served by trains, if you return to London on the same day that you leave it, you can pay just a little more than the price of the usual one-way (single) ticket. Rail clerks call this a "day return." More tips:

o Tickets tend to be most costly on Fridays, when Londoners head out of town.

o You can find incredible deals (up to 70% off) if you happen to be among the first customers to get tickets for a given departure. Book starting 12 weeks out.

o Prices are highest for "open" tickets with no restrictions, so opt for the restricted fare since you probably won't need to change your plans.

within one of its 18th-century Palladian town houses—Bath's magic comes from its consistent and regal design. No wonder the upper crust of the 1700s found it so fashionable, and no wonder their descendants have not dared to alter it. And no wonder UNESCO inscribed it as a World Heritage Site—a rarity for an entire city.

Essentials

GETTING THERE The fastest **trains** (www.nationalrail.co.uk; ℂ **08457/ 48-49-50;** 90 min., twice an hour; £18 with advance purchase) leave from Paddington and let off in Bath Spa, an ugly section of town about 5 minutes' walk from the good stuff. Because buses take twice as long, I don't recommend National Express (www.nationalexpress.com; ℂ **08705/80-80-80;** 3 hr.; £12 single). Most of the major tour bus companies (see box on p. 318) come here, combining with Stonehenge (p. 302) for about £70.

VISITOR INFORMATION Visit Bath/Bath Tourist Information Centre (Abbey Chambers, Abbey Churchyard; www.visitbath.co.uk; ℂ **090/6711-2000** [50p/min.], from overseas ℂ **011-44-844-847-5257;** tourism@bath tourism.co.uk).

TOURS The Mayor's office provides professionally guided, free 2-hour **Walking Tours of Bath** (www.bathguides.org.uk; Sun–Fri 10:30am and 2pm, Sat 10:30am; May–Aug also Tues and Fri 7pm). Meet by the Abbey Churchyard entrance to the Pump Room. Download the free **Official Bath App** for orientation. You can also purchase 50-minute walking tours on downloadable MP3s from **Tourist Tracks** (www.tourist-tracks.com; £5 for two).

Exploring Bath

Begin your tour of Georgian Bath at **Queen Square** for some of the famous streets laid out by John Wood the Elder (1704–54). Walk up to the **Circus,** three Palladian crescents arranged in a circle, with 524 different carved emblems above the doors. His son designed the **Royal Crescent,** an elegant half-moon row of town houses. Robert Adam put up **Pulteney Bridge,** a shop-lined crossing of the River Avon, in 1773, just as a similar bridge in the same medieval style, London Bridge, was crumbling.

Roman Baths ★   The Romans (ca. A.D. 60) were the first to recognize the tourism potential of the natural hot springs, which bubble at a rate of 250,000 gallons a day. Springs were re-developed or re-bored every few centuries; the current buildings are mostly from the 1800s, but Roman artifacts are occasionally found, and the restoration and accompanying museum are excellent. The Victorians mounted a proud colonnade around the excavation, and water has long been drawn in the adjoining Pump Room; you can drink a glass of the sulfuric stuff if you like, or settle down for a pricey lunch in neoclassical style. It's been the done thing in Bath since your great-great-great-grandma was in bloomers.

Bath Abbey Church Yard, Stall St. www.romanbaths.co.uk. ⓒ **01225/477785.** Admission £16–£17 adults, £14–£16 seniors and students, £9.80–£14 children 6–16 (higher prices are July–Aug). July–Aug daily 9am–9pm; Sept–Oct and Mar–June daily 9am–5pm; Nov–Feb daily 9:30am–5pm; last exit 1 hr. after closing.

No. 1 Royal Crescent ★   First-time visitors are blown away by the sweep and elegance of the Royal Crescent, a dazzling 30-house development that took some 8 years to complete, from 1767 to 1775. Its first house, which recently absorbed the old servants' quarters in a massive restoration that religiously presents daily life in those days, is worth a swing-by if you want the full Regency effect.

1 Royal Crescent. www.no1royalcrescent.org.uk. ⓒ **01225/428126.** Admission £10 adults, £7 students and seniors, £4 children 6–16, family ticket £22. Tues–Sun 10:30am–5:30pm; Mon noon–5:30pm; last admission 1 hr. before closing. May be closed late Dec to Jan.

Fashion Museum & Assembly Rooms ★   The grand **Assembly Rooms,** designed by the younger John Wood and completed in 1771, once played host to dances, recitals, and tea parties. Damaged in World War II, the elegant rooms have been restored and look much as they did when Jane Austen and Thomas Gainsborough attended events here. Housed in the same building, the **Fashion Museum** offers audio tours through the history of fashion from the 16th century to the present day through some 165 dressed mannequins. Exhibits change every 6 months. There's also a "Corsets and Crinolines" display where enthusiastic visitors can experience the masochism of period garments.

Bennett St. www.fashionmuseum.co.uk. ⓒ **01225/477-789.** Assembly Rooms: free admission. Fashion Museum admission (includes audio tour) £9 adults, £8 students and seniors, £7 children 6–16, £29 family ticket, free for children 5 and under. Mar–Oct daily 10:30am–5pm, Nov–Feb daily 10:30am–4pm; last exit 1 hr. after closing.

Jane Austen Centre ★   This small homage to Britain's favorite 19th-century writer isn't in her house, but Miss Austen did live up the hill (at no.

Yes, it's super-touristy—just go with it. The Regency stiffness of Bath is bound to give you a craving for that quintessentially English tradition of afternoon tea served with jam, clotted cream, and scones. Try the **Pump Room** at the Roman Baths (p. 290), which serves "Bath buns" (sweet buns sprinkled with sugar), or **Sally Lunn's** at 4 North Parade Passage (www.sallylunns.co.uk; ✆ **01225/461634**), which makes such a big deal of its light Sally Lunn buns you'd swear you'd even heard of them before, which you haven't. The latter's building itself is one of the oldest in Bath, dating from 1482, and shows little hint of any changes with its crooked floors and low ceilings. For £8 to £13, you can sample a range of cream teas, which include toasted and buttered buns served with strawberry jam and clotted cream. The **Regency Tea Rooms** at the Jane Austen Centre offer "Tea with Mr. Darcy" sets (yes, I know . . .) for £18 to £56 for two, and basic cream tea from £9.

25) for a few months in 1805. Exhibits and a video convey a sense of what life was like when Austen lived in Bath between 1801 and 1806. Ladies can also learn the esoteric skill of using a fan to attract an admirer. Wholesome, corny fun. Allow at least 45 minutes. The tearoom is worth a visit (see "Taking Tea in Bath," below).

40 Gay St. www.janeausten.co.uk. ✆ **01225/443-000.** Admission £11 adults, £9.50 seniors, £8.50 students, £5.50 children 6–16, £23 family ticket. Apr–Oct daily 9:45am–5:30pm; Nov–Mar Sun–Fri 10am–4pm, Sat 9:45am–5:30pm.

OXFORD

Whereas the face of London, 92km (57 miles) east, has been forcibly reshaped by the pressures of war, disaster, and commerce, Oxford was made stronger by them. When plague killed townspeople, the colleges snapped up their houses, and when the Reformation cleaned out the churches, the colleges took their land, too. Academies used the extra space to carve out some of the most beautiful college buildings in the world. Here, the reverence for education borders on the ecclesiastical. Yet Oxford is no cloister; it's a decidedly modern city—thriving, sophisticated, and busy.

Essentials

GETTING THERE   The least expensive, easiest method is by coach, since companies compete for students with regular buses rolling round the clock. The so-called **Oxford Tube** bus (www.oxfordtube.com; ✆ **01865/772250;** 100 min. with no traffic; £15 single or £18 same-day return) leaves every 10 to 20 minutes at all hours. It picks passengers up near the Tube stations at Marble Arch, Victoria, Notting Hill Gate, and Shepherd's Bush. Give rush hours wide berth. **Trains** (www.nationalrail.co.uk; ✆ **08457/48-49-50;** 1 hr.; £15–£25 single with advance purchase) go from Paddington station to Oxford, sometimes via Reading.

VISITOR INFORMATION In addition to selling (yes, selling—not giving) maps and guides, the **Oxford Information Centre** (15–16 Broad St.; www.experienceoxfordshire.org; ℭ **01865/686430**) offers daily walking tours using accredited guides. You can download free maps of the city from Visit Britain (www.visitbritain.com).

TOURS The Information Centre offers excellent **theme tours** such as "Harry Potter and Alice in Wonderland," "C.S. Lewis and J.R.R. Tolkien," and ghost trails; book ahead. **Oxford River Cruises** (www.oxfordrivercruises. com; ℭ **0845/226-9396**) runs several boat tours along the River Thames; the tranquil 50-minute Oxford Experience (cheaper online: £12 adults, £6 children 15 and under) is popular. You can also purchase various walking tours on downloadable MP3s from **Tourist Tracks** (www.tourist-tracks.com; £3, or £7.50 for three).

Exploring Oxford

Wandering Oxford's cobbled streets and ducking into its colleges to soak up their hidden loveliness makes for a happy afternoon, particularly for fans of architecture. Many of the most iconic building clusters in this city of 140,000 (30,000 of whom are students) are collected together in the center of town. Oxford, like Cambridge (p. 296), is comprised of individual colleges that feed off a central university system. Each of the 39 colleges has its own campus, tradition, character, and disciplines. Unfortunately, many close their grassy inner sanctums to visitors. During the school terms (mid-Jan to mid-Mar, late Apr to mid-June, Oct to early Dec), some university buildings required for study (libraries, residence halls) are closed to the public, or only open on Saturdays. At all times of year, watch out for zooming bicyclists; an unwritten law appears to grant them ownership of the city.

To get the most out of Oxford, poke around, looking inside cloisters and above rooftops. The doors between the inner and outer quadrangles of **Balliol College** (Broad St. and St Giles; www.balliol.ox.ac.uk; ℭ **01865/27-77-77;** £3 adults, £1 seniors and students; daily 10am–5pm) still bear scorch marks from where Bloody Mary burned two Protestants alive for refusing to recant. Viewpoints are popular attractions here: The 22m (72-ft.) rectangular **Carfax Tower** (Carfax; ℭ **01865/790522;** £2.30 adults, £1.20 children 15 and under; Apr–Sept daily 10am–5:30pm, Oct–Mar daily 10am–4:30pm) is the last remaining chunk of the 13th-century St Martin's Church; it has only 99 steps so it's not too taxing, which may be why it's a well-known suicide spot. It's located by the crossroads of the city center. Other popular panoramas are from the octagonal cupola above Sir Christopher Wren's **Sheldonian Theatre** (Broad St.; www.sheldon.ox.ac.uk; ℭ **01865/277-299;** £3.50, £8 with guided tour; Mon–Sat 10am–4:30pm, also Sun in July–Aug; closes at 3pm Dec–Jan). Perhaps the top view is from the **University Church of St Mary the Virgin** (www.university-church.ox.ac.uk; ℭ **01865/279113;** free admission; daily 9am–5pm, closes 6pm July–Aug).

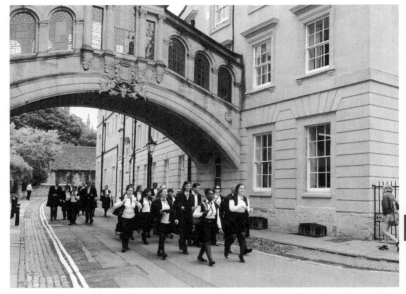
Oxford students, in their academic gowns, stroll under Hertford Bridge, aka the Bridge of Sighs.

The Ashmolean Museum ★ Offering more than just a pretty facade, the Ashmolean was founded way back in 1683, literally before anyone knew what the word "museum" meant. It houses an important hodgepodge of antiquities and art on par with (but on a smaller scale than) the British Museum, including a lantern carried by Guy Fawkes during the foiled Gunpowder Plot; the Anglo-Saxon Alfred Jewel of gold, enamel, and rock crystal; a Stradivarius violin; and assorted Old Masters paintings. Oh, and you know, minor stuff by Raphael and Michelangelo.

Beaumont St. at St Giles. www.ashmolean.org. ℭ **01865/278-000.** Free admission. Tues–Sun 10am–5pm. Closed Dec 24–26.

Bodleian Library ★ The main research library in a town that made its name in research, "the Bod" opened in 1602 and has been burrowing under the streets of Oxford, trying to find new places to store its multiplying collection (11 million tomes and counting), ever since. The round **Radcliffe Camera** ("Rad Cam"; open via guided tours at the Bodleian) was built in the 1740s to house scientific books. It stands on the north side of Radcliffe Square.

Catte St. www.bodleian.ox.ac.uk. ℭ **01865/287-400.** Admission £1, Divinity School only; £14 for 90-min "Extended tour" including reading rooms, £8 for standard 60-min tour, or £6 for 30-min "Mini tour"; check current tour times online. Mon–Fri 9am–5pm; Sat 9am–4:30pm; Sun 11am–5pm. Closed for week around Christmas and New Year's.

Christ Church ★ The largest, most beautiful, and most popular college to visit looms large in children's literature; it was copied for Hogwarts School in the Harry Potter films, and it was where Lewis Carroll (aka mathematician Charles Dodgson) befriended the little girl for whom he wrote *Alice in Wonderland*. The college chapel, which dates from the 12th century, also serves as Oxford Cathedral for the local diocese. Bowler-hatted "custodians" still patrol the pristine lawns, and Christ Church Meadow, still grazed by cattle, is a delightful place to watch punters on the rivers Isis and Cherwell. Just being here makes you feel smarter.

St Aldate's. www.chch.ox.ac.uk. ℗ **01865/ 276-150.** Tours £7–9 adults, £6–8 seniors, students, and children 5–17, free for children 4 and under. Mon–Sat 9am–5pm; Sun 2–5pm. Last admission 4:30pm. Closed for week around Christmas and New Year's.

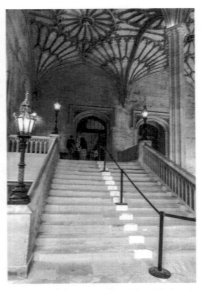

The stairway leading to Christ Church College's dining hall may look familiar from the Harry Potter movies.

Magdalen College ★ Pronounced "*Maud*-lin," it is one of the largest and most peaceful colleges here; its tower is the city's highest point, and its chapel is carved with breathtaking detail. Its site has a virtual tour to prep you on your explorations. U.S. Supreme Court justice Stephen Breyer attended.

High St. www.magd.ox.ac.uk. ℗ **01865/276-000.** Admission £6 adults; £5 seniors, students, and children. July–Sept daily noon–7pm; Oct–June daily 1–6pm or dusk (whichever is earlier). Closed for a week around Christmas and New Year's.

The Pitt Rivers Museum ★ An imposing 1886 cast-iron cathedral-like building, not unlike a railway station, houses an oft-freakish blend of folk art and anthropology—think shrunken heads and bundles of poisoned arrows

---

Punting the River Cherwell

Punting on the River Cherwell is an essential if slightly eccentric Oxford pastime. From mid-March to October at the **Cherwell Boathouse,** Bardwell Road (www.cherwellboathouse.co.uk; ℗ **01865/515-978**), you can rent a punt (a flat-bottomed boat for up to five people, maneuvered by a long pole and a small oar) for £16 (Mon–Fri) to £18 (Sat–Sun) per hour. **Magdalen Bridge Boathouse,** the Old Horse Ford, High Street (www.oxfordpunting.co.uk; ℗ **01865/202-643**), charges £22 per hour, daily 10am until dusk. Both outfits will give you some basic training.

BLETCHLEY PARK: ENIGMA no more

For decades, it was top secret. Few people realized what had happened during World War II in these rotting temporary wooden huts, which were nearly bulldozed for a housing development. But in time, we learned what codebreaker Alan Turing and his brilliant team accomplished at **Bletchley Park** (www.bletchleypark.org.uk; ✆ **01908/640-404**), hidden from the world on a former estate 88km (55 miles) northwest of London. Here they cracked the Enigma machine code, breaking the German blockade that threatened to starve an entire country. In 2014, the year their story, *The Imitation Game*, was released, the fully restored Bletchley Park campus was opened as a fascinating day out. It's like a spy novel set in a park, suffused in the urgency, intrigue, and excitement of those terrifying years when computers were born and Nazis were a few chess moves away from storming England. You can tour more than a dozen buildings around its soothing central pond, exploring the methods, experiments, and lucky breaks that enabled round-the-clock workers—including many gifted women—to translate a jumble of meaningless letters into life-saving intercepted secrets. The cramped, rudimentary Huts 3, 6, and 8, dressed to look like they probably did then (no one is sure—photographs were forbidden), were the heart of the operation, but you can also tour the ground floor of the mansion that served as its command post and outbuildings that housed the computers,

which were later dismantled down to the rivets to prevent anyone from duplicating them. Head to the basement of Block B, where modern fans have rebuilt one. The number of Enigma-related artifacts and the level of codebreaking detail can be head-spinning, so children may tire quickly, but interested adults could spend 3 or 4 absorbed hours wrapping their heads around it, a pursuit made easier by the three cafes spread around its grassy acres. Admission costs £18 adults, £16 seniors, £11 students 12–17, and is free for children 11 and under. It's open daily, 9:30am–5pm from March to October (the rest of the year it's 9:30am–4pm). Last admission is 1 hour before closing

Next door, you'll find the **National Museum of Computing** (www.tnmoc.org; ✆ **01908/374708;** admission £7.50 adults, £5 seniors, students, and children), where volunteers are rebuilding historic systems that were lost to time, including Bletchley's own Colossus. That exhibit is open daily, but the rest of the museum, including the world's largest collection of historic computers, is only open Thursday, Saturday, and Sunday from noon to 4pm. The level of computing detail there isn't for everyone.

Trains to Bletchley leave Euston a few times an hour (50 min.; £16 single) and the gates are only 182m (200 yards) from the station; sit on the left of the carriage for good views of the Grand Union Canal as you go. If you fancy a country drive, Avis, Enterprise, and Budget are clustered near the Bletchley train station.

brought back by British explorers over hundreds of years. It is, to use an academic term, totally gnarly.

Parks Rd. www.prm.ox.ac.uk. ✆ **01865/270-927.** Free admission. Tues–Sun 10am–4:30pm; Mon noon–4:30pm.

OUTSIDE OXFORD
Blenheim Palace ★   Within 30 minutes, the half-hourly S3 bus from the Oxford train station or Gloucester Green whisks visitors to Hensington Road,

Woodstock, and the gates of the birthplace of Winston Churchill, now a UNESCO World Heritage Site. The British rarely remind you that their oh-so-English savior was, in fact, half American; his mom Jennie, who was from Brooklyn, married an English lord, and Winston was born here in 1874, several hundred years into the palace's history. A few decades later, the home was saved from financial ruin when the Duke of Marlborough married another American, a Vanderbilt; their descendants still live here for part of the year. Tours of the grounds, landscaped by Capability Brown, and the state rooms, which are in excellent nick, take about 3 hours.

Hensington Rd., Woodstock, Oxfordshire. www.blenheimpalace.com. ℰ **01993/810-530.** Admission palace and grounds £25 adults, £21 seniors and students, £14 children 5–16. Daily 10:30am–5:30pm, last admission 4:45pm.

CAMBRIDGE

Oxford is a city in its own right, but Cambridge, in the marshes 79km (49 miles) northeast of London, would barely have a pulse without its university. That makes Cambridge manageable—it's also cheaper to visit. It feels in some ways like a typical English town, with a daily market for crafts and food on its central square, Market Hill. Its best rewards come when you wander through randomly chosen iron gates or along a river path—that's when the inviting little town really opens up.

Essentials

GETTING THERE   Nonstop **coaches** from National Express (www.national express.com; ℰ **08705/80-80-80;** 2½ hr.; £7–£8 single) leave hourly from Victoria Coach station; don't get off at Trumpington, but wait for the city center stop. There are **trains** from Liverpool Street or King's Cross, but be warned that Cambridge's station is several miles from the city center, so you will need to bike or call a taxi; coaches are the smarter way to travel. If you insist, though, note that some trains take about 45 minutes and some take twice that, so ask about journey times (www.nationalrail.co.uk; ℰ **08457/48-49-50;** 45–90 min.; £10–£23).

VISITOR INFORMATION   Cambridge Visitor Information Centre (Peas Hill; www.visitcambridge.org; ℰ **0871/226-8006** in U.K. or 011-44-1223/464-732 overseas) sells maps and guides but won't dispense them for free. You can download free maps of the city from Visit Britain (www.visit britain.com).

TOURS   The **Cambridge Visitor Information Centre** (see "Visitor Information," above) has several types of walking tours of the city, from £6 to £19 for adults, and up to £7 for children 11 and under. Book tours at www.visit-cambridge.org/official-tours (ℰ **01223/457-574**). You can also purchase hour-long walking tours on downloadable MP3s from **Tourist Tracks** (www. tourist-tracks.com; £5 for two).

Exploring Cambridge

Like Oxford, Cambridge's glory is the elaborate and ancient architecture of its colleges. However, unlike in Oxford, it's easy to venture into the cloistered grounds of many of Cambridge's colleges, though doing so usually requires a few quid. (Cambridge took shape in the early 13th c., after a squabble in Oxford drove several scholars to leave there and establish a second educational capital. The oldest Cambridge College, Peterhouse, was founded in 1284.) Mill Lane leads to the River Cam, where you can rent a punting boat for £6 or sit at The Mill pub overlooking the water. (If you want to seem savvy to Cambridge traditions, punt from the back of the boat. In Oxford, they punt from the front.) The meadows along the Cam, known as the **Backs,** make for idyllic walks.

The head of Oliver Cromwell, which was impaled outside Westminster Hall in London as a warning against regicide (albeit 3 years after the man died of natural causes), was finally buried within an antechapel (not open to visitors) at Sidney Sussex College in 1960. It's in an unmarked grave to keep pranksters from pinching the much-abused thing. That's Cambridge in a nutshell: It has many secrets, but since it's still a working university town, marvels won't be handed to you. You have to wander, wonder, and ask questions. Outside of term (terms run mid-Jan to mid-Mar, late Apr to mid-June, and Oct to early Dec), colleges aren't open, and street life is at a minimum.

Fitzwilliam Museum ★   Cambridge's most storied attraction is a first-rate neoclassical building full of applied arts and Old Masters that a city 10 times Cambridge's size (population 108,000) would covet. If a colonial Englishman could carry it home on a ship, it's here: precious antiquities from Rome, Greece, Egypt, Asia, and paintings by every famous name under the European sun.

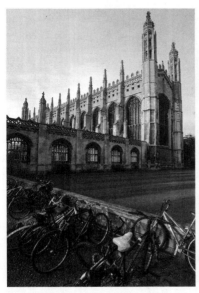

King's College, Cambridge, is known for its magnificent chapel.

Trumpington St., near Peterhouse. www.fitzmuseum.cam.ac.uk. ⓒ **01223/332-900.** Free admission; donations appreciated. Tues–Sat 10am–5pm; Sun noon–5pm. Closed Mon, Good Friday, Dec 24–26 and 31, and Jan 1. Sat guided tours at 2:30pm (£6).

King's College Chapel ★   For some reason, the marauding Puritans neglected to smash the 16th-century stained-glass windows of this chapel—they probably thought they were too divine to destroy, just as you will. The chapel's fanned and vaulted ceiling, a work of craftsmanship that stuns even those who care little for such things, was completed at the behest of Henry VII. Its famous choristers sing at services during term time.

King's Parade. www.kings.cam.ac.uk. © **01223/331-212.** Admission £9 adults, £6 students and seniors, free for children 11 and under. Mon–Fri 9:45am–3:30pm; Sat 9:30am–3:15pm; Sun 1:15–2:30pm; check website ahead for changes.

Pembroke College ★ The third-oldest college in town is one of the best, distinguished by the oldest gatehouse in Cambridge and by a chapel with an ornate plaster ceiling, which was the first completed work by Christopher Wren (after finishing this, the man seemed never to rest again). Unlike many of the colleges, Pembroke never charges visitors to poke around its common areas.

Trumpington St. www.pem.cam.ac.uk. © **01223/33-81-00.** Free admission. Daily 2–5pm, except mid-May to mid-June when closed for exams.

Queen's College ★ Founded in 1448 by the wife of Henry VI and the wife of Edward IV, Queen's is regarded as the most beautiful of Cambridge's colleges. Entry and exit are by the old porter's lodge in Queens' Lane. Tourists are often told that the wooden **Mathematical Bridge** (1749) spanning the Cam behind it (see it from Silver St.) was constructed using no nails, and when curious students disassembled it to figure out how, they couldn't put it back together without using screws. The college is curiously defensive about the tale, saying that anyone who believes this "cannot have a serious grasp on reality."

Silver St. www.quns.cam.ac.uk. © **01223/335-511.** Admission £3 adults (including guide booklet), free for children 9 and under. Mid-Jun–Sept and Nov–mid-May daily 10am–4:30pm; Oct Mon–Fri 2–4:30pm and Sat–Sun 10am–4:30pm. Closed late May to late June.

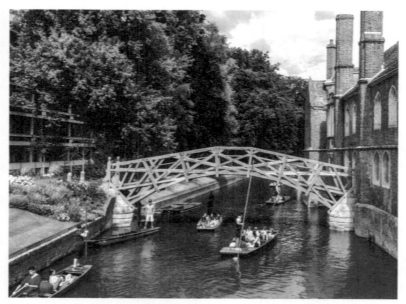

Punting under the Mathematical Bridge on the River Cam.

THE TRADE-OFF WITH escorted tours

Arranging your own day trips using public transportation will almost always be the most cost-effective method, but there are cogent reasons for choosing a guided coach tour. It's simply quicker to allow someone else to drive you around, making sure you cram a laundry list of major sites into a short time span, and consuming spoon-fed nuggets of information about each place. What you learn won't have much depth, but at least you'll have been there.

You'll pay a pretty penny to be sealed on that bus: Most tours cost at least £70 a day, not including food. You get a richer experience (and one that doesn't have you idling in traffic or waiting for other tour members to catch up), when you do it yourself. But some people desperately want to soak up as many sights as they can, even if it means viewing sights as a blur from the motorway. For them, here are the major players in the coach-tour biz, sold aggressively through concierges at expensive hotels (who love getting the commissions):

- **Evan Evans Tours** (www.evanevans tours.co.uk; in the U.K. ℂ **020/7950-1777,** in the U.S. 866/382-6868)
- **Gray Line's Golden Tours** (www. goldentours.co.uk; in the U.K. ℂ **020/7233-7030,** in the U.S. 800/509-2507)
- **Premium Tours** (www.premiumtours. co.uk; in the U.K. ℂ **020/7713-1311,** in the U.S. 800/250-5775)

Better yet are the more affordable **London Walks** (www.walks.com; ℂ **020/7624-3978**), which run frequent day trips (p. 195). These use public transportation and don't include admission fees, but you'll have a guide every step of the way to show you how it's all done.

Trinity College ★   Trinity is the largest and most endowed of Cambridge's 31 colleges. Sir Isaac Newton first calculated the speed of sound here, at Neville's Court, and Lord Byron used to bathe naked in the Great Court's fountain with his pet bear. (The University forbade students from having dogs, but there was no rule against bears.) In *Chariots of Fire,* sprinters tried to get around the .8-hectare (2-acre) yard in the time it took for its clock to strike 12. Your attempts will not be appreciated.

Trinity St. www.trin.cam.ac.uk. ℂ **01223/338-400.** Free admission. The Wren Library: Mon–Fri noon–2pm; Sat 10:30am–12:30pm. Various other areas open at different times and may incur a £2 charge; inquire at the porter's lodge.

STONEHENGE & SALISBURY

Stonehenge is a circle of rocks. If it's raining, it's a damned circle of rocks. But people still ask to go, and if that's their dream, then they should do it. Just understand that it may not blow you away.

Most coach tours offer an itinerary that combines Stonehenge with Bath (p. 288); bus and train connections make it difficult to do that if you're traveling independently. However, it's quite doable to combine Stonehenge with a visit to Salisbury, a lovely and relatively well-preserved cathedral town.

Essentials

GETTING THERE This one's a pain. Trains don't go directly to Stonehenge; the nearest station is in Salisbury, nearly 16km (10 miles) south. So the easiest way to get here is to drive. The rocks are located 3.2km (2 miles) west of Amesbury in Wiltshire on the junction of A303 and A344/360. If you must do public transportation, take a half-hourly **train** (www.nationalrail.co.uk; ℂ **08457/ 48-49-50;** 90 min.; £38 single with advance purchase) from Waterloo station to Salisbury station. There used to be a cheap public bus to the rocks from there, but it says a lot about the values of local tourism authorities that they replaced that route entirely with the expensive but convenient Stonehenge Tour Bus by **Wilts & Dorset Buses** (www.thestonehengetour.info; ℂ **0845/0727-093;** 30 min.; round-trip £14 adults, £9 children 5–15, buy from driver), which leaves from Salisbury station seven times a day between 10am and 4pm. A few extra buses are tossed in during the summer; check its website for updated schedules. Many tour companies offer round-trip all-day coach tours from London that take 10 or 11 hours. One of them is **Premium Tours** (see above) for £49 adults, £46 seniors, and £39 children 3 to 16. Versions that also include Bath cost about £30 more.

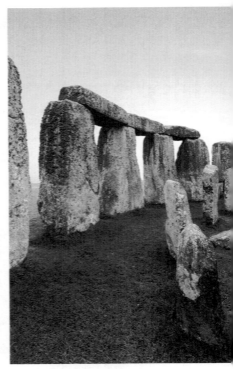

Mysterious Stonehenge has drawn visitors since before 1562.

VISITOR INFORMATION Salisbury and Stonehenge (Fish Row, Salisbury; www.visitwiltshire.co.uk; ℂ **01722/342-860**). Visit Wiltshire produces a free app (called Visit Wiltshire) that rounds up the area's offerings.

TOURS You can easily see Salisbury on foot, either on your own or by taking a guided daytime or evening walk run by **Salisbury City Guides** (www. salisburycityguides.co.uk; ℂ **07873/212941**). Tickets are £6 for adults, £3 for students, and free for kids.

HIGHCLERE CASTLE, THE real DOWNTON ABBEY

The 8th Earl and Countess of Carnarvon still dwell under the sandstone turrets of **Highclere Castle** (Highclere Park, Newbury; www.highclerecastle.co.uk; ✆ **01635/253-204;** admission £22 adults, £20 students and seniors, £14 children 4–16; last admission at 4pm, grounds close at 6pm), known to TV viewers as the idyllic and stately *Downton Abbey*. Time and spendthrift earls took their toll on this historic home, and as recently as 2009, more than 50 rooms were uninhabitable due to mold and leaks. The current Earl faces repair bills running around £12 million, so he welcomes visitors to spend the day exploring the 1,000 acres of private rolling Berkshire countryside. He also rents out to film production: The upstairs scenes of the ITV/PBS show were shot on the ground floor and first floor using the house's actual furniture, though downstairs scenes were shot on a soundstage in Ealing, west London. That's partly because at Highclere, the basement is full not of kitchens but of mummy stuff: The fifth Earl was the guy who bankrolled Howard Carter's 1923 emptying of King Tut's tomb in Luxor, so unseen beneath Lord Grantham's feet lie items taken from the tombs of Egypt. Highclere is only open 60 to 70 days a year, and they're scattered all over the calendar—typically Easter Week, bank holiday weekends, and from July to mid-September. Taking a group tour guarantees a ticket, but those sell out months ahead and herd you along. If you show up independently (download the Highclere Castle guide app, $3, first) at 10am or by 2pm at the latest, you can usually get a walk-up ticket even though advance tickets are sold out. Only once you have a ticket can you also sign up for the £30 afternoon tea in its Coach House (no children for that). Getting here on your own involves taking a 52-minute train from Paddington (from £24) or a National Express bus (1¾ hr.; from £10) to the adorable town of Newbury (stop to admire the longboats on the Kennet and Avon canal and peruse the century-old village department store, Camp Hopson) and then a £15 taxi (try www.cabco 33333.com, ✆ **01635/33333;** or www.newburytaxi.co.uk, ✆ **01635/44444**).

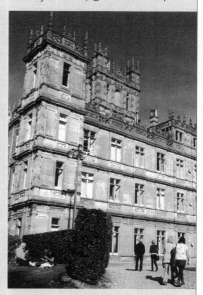

Highclere Castle, better known as Downton Abbey.

Exploring Stonehenge & Salisbury

Stonehenge ★   Construction on this bucket-list sight began about 5,000 years ago; the first recorded day trips to the megalith were in 1562. Arranged in such a way that it aligns with the rising of the sun during the midsummer solstice, this Neolithic circle of stones is certainly Britain's most important ancient wonder, and it's a UNESCO World Heritage Site (together with Avebury, a far less interesting, but still important, line of rocks 39km/24 miles north). Whether its builders, who remain anonymous, worshiped the sun or merely appreciated astronomy is only the beginning of the mystery. We also can only make educated guesses as to how these prehistoric people, using only rudimentary tools, managed to hoist these slabs from Wales to here, and then into place. Even if you don't salivate over such long-ago feats of ingenuity, the distinctive profile of the stones, surrounded by empty plains, "henge" earthworks, and hundreds of lumpen burial mounds, will surely feel iconic.

You're not allowed to walk amongst the rocks the way visitors once were; you have to stick to a footpath that curves near the circle but keeps the formation at a safe distance, good for pretty photographs but bad for curiosity. Most tourists like you and me are kept at arm's length (exception: Clark Griswold, who managed to topple them like dominoes in *National Lampoon's European Vacation*), but you can apply in advance for a 1-hour "Circle Access" pass to stroll with about 29 others among the rocks—no touching—timed in the very early morning or after it closes for the day. The application is at the English Heritage website (see below). Otherwise, you'll have a limited experience—a disappointment for many who trudge 129km/80 miles west of London to have it. Alternatively, climb **Amesbury Hill,** clearly visible 2.4km (1½ miles) up the A303. From here, you'll get a free panoramic view. Check opening times before heading out; closings are occasional.

At the junction of A303 and A344. www.english-heritage.org.uk/stonehenge. ℂ **08703/ 331181.** Admission £17 adults, £15 students and seniors, £9.90 children 5–15, £40 family ticket (higher posted prices include a "voluntary donation"). June–Aug daily 9am–8pm; Apr–May and Sept to mid-Oct daily 9:30am–7pm; mid-Oct to Mar daily 9:30am–5pm; last admission 2 hr. before closing. Train: Salisbury, then Stonehenge Tour Bus.

Old Sarum ★   Believed to have been an Iron Age fortification, Old Sarum was used again by the Saxons and flourished as a walled town into the Middle Ages. The Normans built a cathedral; parts of that were taken down to build the city of "New Sarum," later known as Salisbury, leaving behind dramatically sited remains with unforgettable views of Salisbury and rolling green hills, not to mention the opportunity to commune with grazing sheep.

2 mi N of Salisbury off A345. Castle Rd. www.english-heritage.org.uk/oldsarum. ℂ **01722/335398.** Admission £4.80 adults, £4.30 seniors and students, £2.90 children 5–15 higher posted prices include a "voluntary donation"). Apr–Sept daily 10am–6pm; Mar and Oct daily 10am–5pm; Nov–Mar daily 10am–4pm. Bus: 5, 6, 7, 8, or 9, every 30 min. during the day, from Salisbury bus station.

Salisbury Cathedral ★ Built with uncommon efficiency between 1220 and 1258 and barely touched since, this early English Gothic masterpiece is considered by many to be the most breathtaking church in the world. After you've seen it, and lost yourself in gazing at it and sighing, the rest of your time in Salisbury will be contentedly spent walking medieval streets, which were laid in a loose grid and give the city an airy character. The cathedral complex's octagonal Chapter House holds one of four surviving copies of the Magna Carta signed by King John in 1215. (Two more are in London at the British Library; p. 109.)

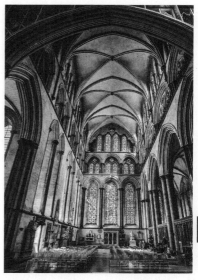

Salisbury Cathedral is an early English Gothic masterpiece.

The Close. www.salisburycathedral. uk. ℂ **01722/555120.** Admission voluntary donation £8 adults, £7 seniors, £5 students, free for children 7–17, £15 family. Mon–Sat 9am–5pm; Sun noon–4pm. Chapter House closes 5:45pm (4:30pm Nov–Mar) and all morning Sun.

CANTERBURY

The ecclesiastical capital of England, Canterbury (62 miles southeast of London) feels like a seat of English charm itself, with the squared spire of its great Gothic Cathedral rising from the cobbled cluster of its village. You can still find traces of the original city walls and punt on the calm water that meanders through town. It's also easy to explore on foot; starting your explorations at The Goods Shed, a market for luscious English dairy, meat, and alcohol (with its own gourmet restaurant; www.thegoodsshed.co.uk), conveniently beside the Canterbury West railway station.

Essentials

GETTING THERE Two National Rail stations, Canterbury East and Canterbury West, are both conveniently just outside the city walls. High-speed trains from Charing Cross, St Pancras, and Victoria take 60–90 minutes (www.nationalrail.co.uk; ℂ **08457/48-49-50;** £14–38 single). Buses are not recommended for a day trip; trains are quick and deliver you right to the town.

VISITOR INFORMATION Canterbury Visitor Information (the Beaney House of Art and Knowledge, 18 High St.; www.canterbury.co.uk; ℂ **01227/862-162**).

TOURS The popular **Canterbury Punting Company** (Water Lane; www. canterburypunting.co.uk; *☎* **07786/332-666**; £12 adults, £10 seniors and students, £6 kids) lets you ply the river, past medieval buildings in an ancient channel that weaves through town, on a wide, flat boat that crawls oh-so-slowly under the hanging bowers.

Exploring Canterbury

Canterbury Cathedral ★★
The original modern tourist attraction, it's where the pilgrims were headed in Chaucer's *The Canterbury Tales* (1478). They were going to pay their respects to archbishop Thomas Becket, who was murdered in the northwest transept, next to what is now the Chapel of Our Lady Martyrdom. Henry VIII tore down that shrine in a typical fit of pique, but this transporting place is still one of the most visited sites in Britain. The cathedral, along with **St Augustine's Abbey** and **St Martin's Church** (the oldest still-functioning church in the English-speaking world; both were founded around 597), form a World Heritage Site. Look for the medieval tombs of King Henry IV and Edward the Black Prince; Becket lies in the Trinity Chapel, near the high altar. The stained glass depicting his reported miracles is regarded as some of England's finest; fortunately, the cathedral's windows survived Hitler's bombs by being removed and hidden away.

The Precincts. www.canterbury-cathedral.org. *☎* **01227/762-862.** Admission £12 adults, £11 seniors and students, £8 children under 18. Mon–Sat 9am–5:30pm, Sun 12:30pm–2:30pm.

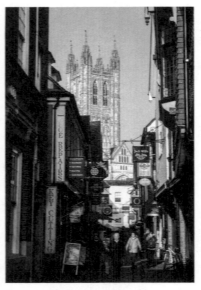

The square Gothic tower of Canterbury Cathedral rises above the town's cobbled medieval lanes.

PLANNING YOUR TRIP TO LONDON

First of all, relax. Getting to London isn't as tricky as it used to be. Some 31.5 million international visitors journeyed to London in 2015, a 20% increase over 2010—making it the most popular destination for travelers from abroad. The London hospitality and tourist industries know a thing or two about helping foreigners. Finding airfare isn't much harder than finding a cross-country flight. Being ready for the rest (money, electricity) is simply a matter of having the facts.

GETTING THERE

By Plane

10

Transatlantic flights almost always land at **Heathrow,** Europe's busiest international airport (LHR; 17 miles west), or **Gatwick,** perhaps the most disliked (LGW; 31 miles south). With a few minor exceptions, the other four airports, **Stansted** (STN; 37 miles northeast), **Luton** (LTN; 34 miles northwest), **London City** (LCY; in London's Docklands area), and **Southend** (SEN; 42 miles east) serve flights from Europe; they're where cut-rate flyers and executive jets tend to go.

FINDING THE LOWEST AIRFARE

The central question is *when* are they? London is such a popular destination (it's served by more flights from the United States than any other European city) that plenty of airlines vie to carry you across—although the ones that are not American-run are usually of higher quality. If you're not redeeming frequent-flier miles (book very far ahead if you are), there are five rules to finding bargains:

1. **Fly on days when traffic is lightest.** Some airlines post calendars that show you when their best prices are, or test fare trends on a site such as **Hopper.com**.
2. **Depart after dinner.** This saves you from paying another hotel night, since you'll arrive in the morning. You're also likely to find lower fares, because business travelers like day flights.

3. **Go off-season.** London's weather isn't extreme, so there's really not a no-go month. November through March yield the lowest airfares and hotel rates, although the late-December holidays and the last week of November (Thanksgiving in U.S.) can be busy, too. Summer prices (June–Sept) soar over a grand.

4. **Search for fares for or on a weekend.** Many major airlines post lower prices to fly then. You might also save money by booking your seat at 3am. That's because unpaid-for reservations are flushed out of the system at midnight, and prices often sink when the system becomes aware of an increase in supply.

5. **Try a bargain airline.** Norwegian Air Shuttle (www.norwegian.com) and WOW Air (www.wowair.com) are reliable.

6. **Don't buy last-minute.** Desperation has a price.

Monitor airline newsletters, sale pages, Twitter accounts, and sites for sales. Both **Airfarewatchdog.com** and **Yapta.com** spit out emails when airfare drops.

Primary websites that collect quotes from a variety of sources (whether they be airlines or other websites) include **Ebookers.com, Expedia.com, Kayak. com, Lessno.com, Mobissimo.com, Momondo.com,** and **Orbitz.com.** Always canvas multiple sites, because each has odd gaps in coverage because of how they obtain quotes. Always compare your best price with what the airline is offering, because that price might be lowest of all. Some sites have small booking fees of $5 to $10, and many force you to accept nonrefundable tickets for the cheapest prices. If you're hitting a wall, search for transatlantic itineraries that allow for one or two stops, since routes that include stops in Reykjavik or Frankfurt (on Icelandair or Lufthansa, respectively) can produce hidden bargains. No matter which airline you go with, prepare yourself for added taxes and fees, which are usually $500 or higher round-trip from the USA—London's airport fees are truly noxious.

Most times of the year, the least expensive way to reach London is with an **air-hotel package** (p. 60), which combines discounted airfare with discounted nights in a hotel. Most air-hotel deals will allow you to fly back days after your hotel allotment runs out, and at no extra charge. Keep in mind that solo travelers always pay a little more, typically $200.

AIRPORT TRANSPORTATION OPTIONS

Fares and trip duration can be found in the chart, p. 308.

BY TRAIN   Every airport offers some kind of rail connection to the central city, and that's the smart option to take. Tickets can be bought at windows in the arrivals halls, at machines, or online, where you get a discount. You'll rarely have to wait more than 20 minutes for the next train, and it's not necessary to pre-book any of them.

Heathrow Express trains (www.heathrowexpress.com; ✆ **08456/00-15-15**) zoom to Paddington every quarter-hour. First Class is a waste of money; Express Saver, the cheapest option (purchase online, on its app, or at vending machines), is plenty plush. Weekend one-way tickets are just £5.50 if you book at least 90 days ahead. The **Heathrow Connect** train service (www. heathrowconnect.com; ✆ **084/5678-6975**) is designed to give access to local stations, so it takes twice as long (still not long at all). It uses commuter-style carriages and leaves half-hourly. Both trains arrive at Paddington, where you can hop the Tube system or a taxi (above Platform 12). The cheapest way to go is via **London Underground** (£6 cash or £5.10 Oyster; 75 min.) using the Piccadilly line. If you need to go in the middle of the night and the Tube isn't running, Night Bus N9 goes to and from Trafalgar Square and Heathrow, taking about 75 minutes.

Gatwick Express trains (www.gatwickexpress.com; ✆ **084/5850-530**) run from Victoria. On **Thameslink & Great Northern** (www.thameslinkrailway. com; ✆ **0345/026-4700**), you can get to Gatwick via Blackfriars, Farringdon, St Pancras, or London Bridge stations four times an hour—service usually ends around 11:45pm, but check ahead, since timings change.

Stansted Express (www.stanstedexpress.com; ✆ **0845/600-7245**) runs from Liverpool Street station. **Luton** has rail service from St Pancras station, Blackfriars, London Bridge stations by **Thameslink & Great Northern** (www.thameslinkrailway.com; ✆ **0345/026-4700**). The correct stop is Luton Airport Parkway Station, linked by a 10-minute shuttle (5am–midnight) to the terminals.

City Airport is linked so expediently and affordably by the Docklands Light Railway that it doesn't support commuter rail or coach service. **London Southend** (www.southendairport.com) is so well-connected to a shiny new station by **Greater Anglia** rail from Liverpool Street that buses don't bother to go there, so the train is the sole option.

BY BUS **National Express** (www.nationalexpress.com; ✆ **0871/781-8181**) buses will take you from all airports (except Southend or City) for around £10 each. With extreme advance purchase, **EasyBus** (www.easybus.com) can be a few pounds cheaper (from Gatwick, Stansted, and Luton).

BY TAXI OR CAR SERVICE Because of traffic and price, taking a **taxi** (£46–£100) to the city does not have our hearty recommendation. **Uber** drivers aren't allowed to wait on airport premises, which makes rendezvousing difficult. Door-to-door **car service** (£50–£60) can take 45 minutes to 2 hours, so the train-taxi or train-Tube combo is often faster (although on trains you'll have to contend with your luggage). You can book cars ahead, which often saves about 25% off the price of a taxi: Check each airport's website for a current list of the latest approved companies. **Addison Lee** (www.addisonlee. com; ✆ **020/7407-9000**) is an established minicab company, the website

AIRPORT	COST/AVG. TIME USING NATIONAL RAIL	HOURS OF RAIL SERVICE
Heathrow (LHR), HeathrowAirport.com	Heathrow Express (www.heathrow express.com): £22 single, £37 return, kids under 15 free*/ 15 minutes OR Heathrow Connect: £10.30 single/30–45 minutes	Four times hourly 5:10am to 11:33pm
London Southend (SEN), www.southend airport.com	Greater Anglia: About £17 single/53 minutes	4am to midnight
Gatwick (LGW), GatwickAirport.com	Gatwick Express (www.gatwick express.com): £20 single/£36 return (in person), £18/£32 (online), kids £10/£17.50 and £9/£15.50/30 minutes OR Thameslink & Great Northern: £11 single/30 to 50 minutes	Four times hourly 5am to 12:30am
Luton (LTN), www.London-Luton.co.uk	Thameslink & Great Northern: £16 single including 5-min. shuttle bus, 45 minutes	Six times hourly 5am to midnight; hourly midnight to 5am
Stansted (STN), StanstedAirport.com	From £17 single, £28 return/ 47 minutes	Four times hourly 4:40am to 12:30am (also a 3:40am train on Monday, Friday, and Saturday)
London City (LCY), LondonCityAirport.com	N/A	DLR: 5:30am to midnight

*Ticket machine or online fare. Tickets £5 more if you wait to pay on board. Advance purchase more than a month ahead is lower.

Minicabit.com surveys companies for the best prices, and Heathrow has a partnership with **Green Tomato Cars** (www.greentomatocars.com; ℭ **020/ 8568-0022**). Also try **Airport Cars UK** (www.airportcars-uk.com; ℭ **0330/ 088-2222**) and **Carrot Cars** (www.carrotcars.co.uk; ℭ **020/7005-0557**), which serve all airports. Also look into the app **Splitcab** (www.splitcab.co.uk), which matchmakers you with other people going in the same direction to cut costs; prices start at around £12 from Heathrow to Central London.

By Train

For trips from northwestern Europe, the train is the dignified way to go. Unlike taking a flight, you won't need to set aside extra hours and pounds to

RAIL SERVICE TO	COST/TIME USING TUBE OR DLR	COST/AVG. TIME FOR NATIONAL EXPRESS SHUTTLE SERVICE TO CENTRAL LONDON	COST/AVG. TIME TO AIRPORT BY TAXI
Paddington	£5.70 cash or £5.10 Oyster/ 75 minutes on Piccadilly Line	£8.50 single, kids 3 to 15 £4.25, under 3 free (www.nationalexpress. com)/50–70 minutes	£65–£85/ 70 minutes
Gatwick Express: Victoria; T&GN: St Pancras, Farringdon, Blackfriars, or London Bridge	N/A	£5–8 each way, kids 3 to 15 £5 under 3 free (www.national express.com)/90 minutes	£100/70 minutes
St Pancras, Blackfriars, or London Bridge	N/A	From £11 (www.national express.com)/90 minutes (runs 24 hr.)	£100/ 80 minutes**
Liverpool Street	N/A	From £12 single (www. nationalexpress.com)/ 60–100 minutes	£99/ 80 minutes**
N/A	£4.90 cash, £3.30 Oyster/ 25 minutes on Docklands Light Railway	N/A	£25–£40/20–40 minutes
Liverpool Street	N/A	N/A	£80–£100/60 to 80 minutes**

** As if you'd be daft enough to want a taxi after seeing those prices and times, you're more likely to find one by booking ahead. Check www.london-luton.co.uk, www.stanstedairport.com, and www.southendairport.com for list of the latest approved companies. Addison Lee (www.addisonlee.com) is an established minicab company, and Heathrow has a partnership with Green Tomato Cars (U.K.: ℂ 0800/599-9099; www.greentomatocars.com). All services offer discounted prices for children.

get to and from airports; train stations are in the middle of town. We're living in marvelous times: The Channel Tunnel opened 2 decades ago (although they *still* seem to be working out the kinks), so you can reach the heart of London in an incredible 2 hours and 15 minutes from Paris. You can literally ride both the Tube and the Métro before lunch. In fact, you can ride both a black taxi and Space Mountain before lunch, since one Eurostar route alights in the middle of Disneyland Resort. Eurostar links London's St Pancras station with Paris, Brussels, Lille, and Calais, and from there, you can go just about anywhere using other trains.

Book via **Eurostar** (www.eurostar.co.uk; ℂ 03432/186-186 in the U.K. or 44-1233/61-75-75 outside of it; phone bookings are US$7 more) itself or the

driving IN LONDON?

Don't! Roads are clogged. In bad traffic, a trip from Heathrow to the western fringe of London can take 2 hours. And once you're in the city, just about every technology is deployed against you. There's a hefty fee just to drive to the city center. Roads are confusingly one-way. Cameras catch and ticket your honest driving errors. Parking is a fantasy. Many North Americans think of cars as the default transportation mode, but in London, trains are the thing. The only time to *maybe* drive a car is if you're on a cross-country tour—but in cities, it won't be easy for you.

The cheapest coach and van services for each airport are listed in the chart, and they all drop you off at standardized stops such as major train stations. For Gatwick, Stansted, and Luton, in addition to the usual National Express coach options, there's the no-frills **easyBus** (www.easybus.co.uk). Unless you book far in advance, it may not beat the National Express prices.

If you insist upon wheels (don't), reserving ahead from home yields the best prices. Try to return your car outside the congestion-charge zone to avoid charges and aggravation. You will find similar rates among **Nova Car Hire** (www.novacarhire.com), **Auto Europe** (www.autoeurope.com), **Europe By Car** (www.ebctravel.com), **Europcar** (www.europcar.com), and **Holiday Autos** (www.holidayautos.com). Also check the major names like Avis, Hertz, and Budget, in case they can do better. Air-conditioning, something you won't need, adds about £5 to the daily bill. Fuel, or *petrol*, is even more expensive than at home, and although most rentals include unlimited mileage, not all do. Also: Many rental cars are stick-shift models, which means you'll be driving on the left in a foreign land with a stick shift. Don't.

U.S.-based **Rail Europe** (www.raileurope.com; ☏ **800/361-7245** in North America), which also sells European rail passes. Check both sites, since prices can differ, but do it early, because rates boom as availability decreases. Advance-purchase deals regularly go as low as £29 each way.

By Bus

A few coach companies also travel between the U.K. and the Continent, usually crossing the Channel with a ferry. Because of the pressure put on the market by mushrooming no-frills airlines, rates are extremely low. You'll pay as little as £21 one-way to Paris via **Eurolines** (www.eurolines.co.uk; ☏ **08717/81-81-77**; 8–10 hr. each way). Brussels or Amsterdam are £15 with a 7-day advance purchase. Also look at **Flixbus** (www.flixbus.com), which goes from Victoria to multiple destinations around Europe (say, Antwerp from 17€, or five cities for 99€). The trade-off: It can take all day, sunrise to sunset, to reach Paris by this method.

Some other companies arrange full-on organized tours of Europe's greatest hits—but never for less than you could do independently; choose one only because you'd enjoy having company: **Contiki** (www.contiki.com; ☏ **866/266-8454**) is geared toward a party-hearty under-35 crowd, **Tucan Travel**

Adventure Tours (www.tucantravel.com; ℂ 855/444-9110) is for social scrimpers, and **Fanatics** (www.thefanatics.com; ℂ 020/7240-3233) is for followers of organized sports.

By Boat

Ferry travel is obsolete, mostly used by people who need to transfer cars. No ferry to Europe or Ireland sails directly to London. You'll have to get down to the southern coast (for France), Portsmouth (for Spain), or Liverpool or Wales (Ireland). Advance purchase can be from £39 each way with a car and including taxes (150 min.) on **P&O Ferries** (www.poferries.com; ℂ 08716/64-64-64) or **DFDS** (www.dfdsseaways.com; ℂ 0208/127-8303), both of which do Dover–Calais. Ferries to and from Ireland are also operated by **Irish Ferries** (www.irishferries.ie; ℂ 0818/300-400 in the Republic of Ireland, or ℂ 353/818-300-400 in Northern Ireland/U.K.) and **Stena Line** (www.stena-line.com; ℂ 01/204-7777). The aggregator **DirectFerries.co.uk** sells European routes from a rapidly diminishing roster of companies.

If you despise flying, one ocean liner still makes the storied 7-day trip between New York City and Southampton, which connects by rail to London in an hour. That's the *Queen Mary 2* (www.cunard.com; ℂ 800/728-6273), intermittently scheduled. Fares start around $900 per person one-way, including all your meals. Pack your tuxedos and gowns.

GETTING AROUND LONDON

There are three practical methods for taming London's sprawl: by Tube (historic and enchanting, but expensive); by bus (less expensive and less glamorous, but more edifying and often quicker); and by foot (the best method, but not always possible). Taxis are overpriced, Ubers require mobile data usage, and driving a car is lunacy.

A significant savings strategy is to choose a hotel that's within walking distance of lots of the things you want to do. Fortunately, the city's extremely walkable. Tube trains go shockingly slowly (34kmph/21 mph is the *average* and has been for more than 100 years); and in the center of town, stops are remarkably close together and the stairs can wear you out. In fact, if your journey is only two or three stations, you'll often find it less strenuous to simply walk.

The Underground

Londoners call their 402km (249-mile) metro system the Underground, its official name, or just as commonly, "the Tube." Its elegant, distinctive logo—a red "roundel" bisected by a blue bar—debuted in 1913 as one of the world's first corporate symbols, and it remains one of the city's most ubiquitous sights. The Tube is much more dignified than most American systems. In fact, seats are upholstered—that's because the British know how to take care of nice things. And yet there's no older subway system on earth—the first section opened in 1863 while America was fighting its Civil War—and it often acts its age, with frequent delays and shutdowns. Check posters and whiteboards in the ticket hall to see what "engineering works" are scheduled.

The Tube is an attraction unto itself. It's fun to seek out vestiges of the early system (1907 tilework on the Piccadilly Line; the fake house facades built at 23–24 Leinster Gardens to hide exposed tracks; abandoned stations like the one at Strand and Surrey Street). If such "urban archaeology" fascinates you, visit the **London Transport Museum** in Covent Garden (p. 120), one of the city's family-friendly highlights.

There are 13 named lines, plus the Docklands Light Railway (DLR), which serves East London, and a tram line in South London. Together they serve nearly 300 stations. Lines are color-coded: The Piccadilly is a peacock purple, the Bakerloo could be considered Sherlock Holmes brown, and so on. The newest line, the Elizabeth Line, is scheduled to begin cross-city service in December 2018.

The Tube shuts down nightly from Sunday to Thursday. Exact times for first and final trains are posted in each station (using the 24-hr. clock), but the Tube generally operates from 5:30am (0530) to just after midnight (0000), and Sundays 7am (0700) to 11:30pm (2330). On Friday and Saturday nights, many lines in Central London run every 10 minutes all night long: **"Night Tube"** trains are the Piccadilly, Victoria, Central, and Jubilee lines, plus the Charing Cross branch of the Northern line. Still, if you plan to take the train after midnight, always check the Night Tube map and schedule beforehand. The TfL offers 24-hour information at *C* **0343/222-1234.**

What happens if you miss the last train? Don't worry—you're not stranded, although your trip may take longer or cost more. Just turn to the city's network of 24-hour and Night Bus routes (p. 316).

HOW TO FIND YOUR WAY ON THE TUBE

Navigating is mostly foolproof. Look for signs pointing to the color and name of the line you want. Pretty soon, more signs separate you according to the direction you want to go in, based on the Tube map. If you know the name/color of the line you want, as well as the direction of your destination, the signs will march you, anthill-like, to the platform you need. Nearly every station is combed with staircases. You'll shuffle through warrens of cylindrical tunnels, many of them faced in custard-yellow tiles and overly full of commuters, and you'll scale alpine escalators lined with ads. Stand to the right so "climbers" can pass you.

On the DLR (the Overground) and commuter trains, the carriage may not automatically open. Push the illuminated button and it will.

One of the groovier things about the Underground is the electronic displays on platforms that tell you how long it'll be until the next train. A 24-hour information service is also available at *C* **0343/222-1234.** The best resource is the TfL Journey Planner, online at **www.tfl.gov.uk/gettingaround**. For specific journey information using a mobile device, you can text your start-point and end-point—as full postcodes (what tourist knows those?), or station or stop names, in the format "A to B"—to ✆ **60835.** TfL will fire off a text with the quickest route and scheduled times. The best resource is the free app **Citymapper,** which tells you which Tube, bus, or train to use, how long it takes, and includes mapped walking directions to the nearest stop. The **UK Bus Checker** app shows 3-D maps of routes go and where the next bus is.

The most confusing lines for tourists are the Northern line (black on the maps) and the District line (green). Owing mostly to the petty backbiting of the Victorians who built these lines as individual businesses, they split and take several paths. You can handle it. Platform displays and signs on the front of the trains tell you its route before you board, and you won't get too far off course if you mess up. If you ride the DLR (and you should—it provides a lovely rooftop-level glide through the brickwork of the old East End and the monolithic towers of Canary Wharf), those lines split variously, too, but there are lots of chances to rectify mistakes.

Search the **Underground's website** (www.tfl.gov.uk) for the "London's Rail and Tube Services Map." It's a truer picture than the Tube map alone because it shows all the places Oyster will take you by rail. (Buses are on separate maps.) The site also has terrific simplified bus maps that show you routes from any neighborhood. Plug in your hotel's address, access Citymapper via Wi-Fi, and you'll have your options.

FARES, PASSES & TICKETS

London Underground (**tfl.gov.uk/tickets**) gives 1.1 billion rides a year—and seemingly every passenger pays a different fare. Rates go up every January (these rates were current at press time and will give you a sense of proportion). Britain's system is so complicated that it's accused of having been engineered to bewilder travelers into paying more than they have to. But it can be boiled down to this: **You want to get an Oyster card and load it with money.** I'll explain.

How much you pay: The center of town—basically everything the Circle line envelops, plus a wee bit of padding—is zone 1. Heading outside of town, in a concentric pattern, come zones 2 through 6. Most tourists stick to zones 1 and 2; very few popular sights are outside those (Wimbledon, Hampton Court, and Kew being the main exceptions). Your fare is calculated by how many zones you go through, and the lower the zone number, the less you pay. If a station appears to straddle zones, you'll pay the cheaper zone's rate. One-way tickets are called "singles" and round-trips are "return."

Astonishingly, **kids 10 and under travel for free** when accompanied by an adult. Adults must buy their own ticket and then ask the staff to wave Junior through the entry gate. Ask an agent about the going discounts for kids.

There are essentially three ticket types for visiting adults.

frustrations OF THE TUBE

The Tube lists everything about itself in exhaustive detail at **www.tfl.gov.uk**, which contains more maps, planners, and FAQs than a normal person can use. As endearing as the Tube is, it is not perfect. In fact, it can be so dehumanizing that it has had to put up signs begging people not to abuse its staff (sad but true). Be prepared for a few things:

1. **Stairs.** Most stations are as intricate as anthills. Passengers are sadistically corralled up staircases, around platforms, down more staircases, and through still more staircases. Even stations equipped with extremely long escalators (Angel has the longest one in the system—59m/194 ft.) perversely require passengers to climb a final flight to reach the street. So if you bring luggage into the Tube, be able to hoist your stuff for at least 15 stairs at a time. (This is where backpacks make sense—but don't be the person who leaves it on while on a crowded carriage.) For a list of which stations are step-free (there are only 66 so far), contact **Transport for London Access & Mobility** (www.tfl.gov.uk; ✆ **020/7941-4600**).

2. **Delays.** When you enter a station, look for a sign with the names and colors of the Tube lines on it. Beside each line, you'll see a status bar reading "Good service," "Severe delays," or the like. Trust this sign—it's updated every 10 minutes and lines close without warning. If you note "Minor delays," don't worry. Do worry about labor strikes—they're unpleasantly common.

3. **Heat.** The network can be stuffy. In summer, health advisories are issued to passengers. The worst lines: Bakerloo, Central, and Northern. The best: Circle and District. AC is being added—slowly.

4. **Hellish rush hours.** Shoulder-to-shoulder, silently shuffling through airless underground cylinders. It's memorable in the wrong way.

5. **Tough weekends.** Unlike modern systems, which generally have two sets of rails in each direction, London's ancient system has one set, so entire lines have to shut down when maintenance is required. Weekends are when this happens. This is a major reason why it's smart to stay in central London, where you don't depend on a single Tube line. Check in the ticket hall to see what "engineering works" are scheduled.

1. **Via Oyster Pay As You Go (PAYG).** This is the best option, and it's what locals use. Rub this credit card–size pass on yellow dots at the turnstiles and you get the lowest fares. You load it with cash and it debits as you go, no tickets required, on all forms of in-city public transit. No matter how many times you ride the Tube (debited at £2.40 in zone 1—that's a lot better than the £4.90 cash fare!) and bus (debited as £1.50—you can't pay cash on a bus), the maximum taken off your card in a single day will **always be less** than what an equivalent Day Travelcard (see below) would cost. Nonstop Oyster use will always peak at £6.60 for anytime travel in zones 1 and 2 (£4.50 if you only took buses), versus the flat rate of £12.30 you'd have paid if you'd bought an equivalent Travelcard. It's called "price capping," and it resets daily at 4:30am. Getting an Oyster usually

requires a £5 deposit, but you can get that back before you skip town at any Tube ticket office (there's even one at Heathrow; ID may be requested). The card won't get erased if you keep it beside your mobile phone. And if you don't use up all the money you put on it, you can get a refund as long as there's less than £10 value left on your card. (Travelcards offer no refunds for unused monies.) **Buy an Oyster card.** They're sold at vending machines when you enter the Tube and then you can use it on buses, too.

2. **Via Travelcard.** Aimed at tourists, this is an unlimited pass for 1 or 7 days on the Tube, rail, and bus. "Day Anytime" Travelcards for zones 1 through 3 with no timing restrictions are £12.30. If you find you have to pop into a zone that isn't covered by your card, buy an extension from the ticket window before starting your journey; it's usually £1.50 to £2 more. 7-Day Travelcards cost adults £33 for travel in zones 1 and 2. For Travelcard prices that include more zones, visit **www.tfl.gov.uk/tickets**. You can load a Travelcard purchase onto an Oyster. Downside: Unlike PAYG, you may end up paying for rides you never use.

3. **In cash, per ride.** You could, but don't. To travel a mile in zone 1 on the Underground, the cash fare is £4.90 (more than US$7). I did the math: It costs 3½ times more to pay cash to go a mile on the Tube than to go a mile in transatlantic First Class. What's more, bus drivers don't even take cash anymore. They *do* take Oyster.

The Tube does offer **contactless payment** on turnstiles' yellow dots—charges are exactly the same as with Oyster—but there's no telling if your card issuer or bank supports it. Apple Pay and American Express with contactless payment should work. Visit **tfl.gov.uk/fares-and-payments/contactless** and confer with your own issuer to make an educated guess whether you can use contactless payment. If you do use Apple Pay, have your phone recognize your fingerprint and be ready for the transaction before you approach the turnstiles or you'll hold everyone else up.

How to use tickets: Since pricing depends on how far you've gone, you must touch your Oyster card to the big yellow reader dot both before you board *and* after your trip—even if there are no turnstiles (that's the part people always forget). The same goes if you have a paper ticket for any train, even trains that aren't part of the Tube system; keep it handy because you'll need it to get back out at the end. If you can't find it, you'll have to fork over the maximum rate. Inspectors regularly check passengers' tickets and they won't hesitate to fine you.

> ### From *Europe on $5 a Day,* 1969–1970
>
> "For those who have played the sardine in New York's subway, the London "underground" is a revelation. Quiet, clean, comfortable; the normal fare ranges from 6 to 18¢, depending on the length of the ride, but your average trip should cost no more than around 9¢."

How to pay at a vending machine: If you are using a swipe credit card to buy tickets from a vending machine, don't pull your card out of the vending machine too quickly, or it will falsely tell you it's declined. Vending machines usually accept cash and coins. If your credit card issuer offers a version of your card embedded with a SIM chip, order one ahead of your trip—it makes a lot of transactions a lot easier in London, where chip cards are the norm.

Buy ahead?: Although TfL will mail you tickets ahead of time, that's a waste of money; you can just as easily purchase them without shipping costs at any Tube stop.

Buses

The Tube and buses are seen as one piece, so the same payment systems work on both. Buses are what smart Londoners use. The buses in your city may not come often, but London's are frequent (every 5 min. or so on weekdays), plentiful (some 100 routes in central London and 700 in the wider city), and surprisingly fast (many operate in dedicated lanes). Sitting on the second level of a candy-apple red double-decker, watching the big landmarks roll past, is one of London's priceless pleasures. Best of all, the bus is cheaper than the Tube. The 1-day Oyster PAYG price cap for bus-only travel is £4.50, no matter the zone. Travelcards and Oysters (per trip £1.50; buy in Tube stations) are the best way to pay. The only **free transfers** are between two buses within a one-hour window, and be warned that surprise ticket inspections are common nowadays. Note that bus passes and Travelcards expire at 4:30am the day after you buy them. The TfL offers 24-hour information at ℂ **0343/222-1234.**

Drivers do not accept money, and very few bus shelters have automated ticket machines (cash only, and don't expect change), so you'll need to go into a Tube stop to get your Oyster card or Travelcard. All stations have easy-to-read maps that tell you where to catch the buses going to your destination. Major intersections have multiple stops named with letters, and each stop services different routes; check the map in the bus shelter to find the letter stop you need. Many shelters even have electronic boards that approximate the arrival time of the next bus.

Board the bus in front, by the driver, and get off via the door at the middle. Newer buses have reinstated a rear-door design with its own conductor, and you can leap off that back entrance whenever you want, but of course that comes with hazards. An automated voice announces stops with plenty of warning. Press a button on a handrail to request a halt at the next one.

Routes that start with N are Night Buses, which tote clubbers home after the Tube stops around midnight; many connect tediously in Trafalgar Square, so pee before setting off. London has trams, too, charged like buses, but they're in areas where tourists are unlikely to go.

National Rail

These are the rail lines that aren't operated by the Underground. These comfortable, standard-sized trains go to suburbs, distant cities, and to neighborhoods the Victorians didn't tunnel the Tube to, and they operate on a regular, reliable, published timetable—on maps, they are denoted by two red parallel lines with a zig-zag line connecting them. These lines, which for comfort are actually preferably to the Underground, are covered by Travelcards and Oyster PAYG for roughly the same price as the Tube as long as you stay in the zone system. (The major stations have information desks if you're unsure about Oyster's validity on any journey.) You must tap Oyster at the start *and* at the completion of each journey or you'll be charged as if you took the train to the end of the line. If you accidentally tap in for a wrong or missed train, alert staff. They can ensure you aren't penalized.

There are many termini, but you don't have to hunt by trial and error. Call the 24-hour operators at **National Rail Enquiries** (www.nationalrail.co.uk; *☎* **08457/48-49-50**), check **TheTrainLine.com** or its app, or plug your journey into your favorite map app such as the free **Citymapper.** Alternatively, each station posts timetables. Schedules are listed by destination; find the place you're going, and the departures will be listed in 24-hour time.

National Rail stations (not Eurostar or the Underground) accept discount cards for certain folks. Each card requires proof of eligibility (passport, ISIC student ID), but since they can be used for trips to distant cities, they pay for themselves quickly if you're doing lots of rail-riding. Get them at rail stations:

- The **Senior Railcard** (www.senior-railcard.co.uk, £30 a year): Discounts of about 33% for those 60 or over.
- The **16–25 Railcard** (www.16-25railcard.co.uk, £30 a year): Discounts of 33% for those 16 to 25, plus full-time students of any age. It requires a passport-size photo, which may be uploaded from a computer. If you're applying in the U.K., bring a passport photo for that purpose.
- The **Family & Friends Railcard** (www.family-railcard.co.uk, £30 a year) is for at least one adult and one child age 5 to 15, with a maximum of three adults and four kids on one ticket; at least one child must travel at all times. It awards adults 33% off and kids 60% off. But know that two kids age 4 and under can travel with an adult for free at all times, even without this card.

Ferries

Partly thanks to the dedication of a series of mayors, London's river ferry services are now one of the most pleasurable ways to get around. The boats, nicknamed River Bus, cover a surprising amount of terrain quickly. Some of their most useful stops include right outside the London Eye, the Tate

RED-LETTER double-deckers

A few routes are truly world-class, linking legendary sights. With routes like these, you won't need to splurge on those tedious hop-on, hop-off tour buses:

- The **15 bus,** which crosses the city northwest to southeast, takes in Paddington, Oxford Street, Piccadilly Circus, Trafalgar Square, Fleet Street, St Paul's, and the Tower of London. And it has antique Routemaster vehicles.
- The **10** passes Royal Albert Hall, Kensington Gardens, Knightsbridge (a block north of Harrods), Hyde Park Corner, Marble Arch, Oxford Street, Goodge Street (for the British Museum), and King's Cross Station.
- The **159** links Paddington, Oxford Circus, Trafalgar Square, and Westminster.
- The **RV1** hits Covent Garden, Waterloo, the Tate Modern, and as a bonus, you get to ride over the Tower Bridge to the Tower of London.

Modern, the Tower of London, Greenwich, and the O_2. Getting from Greenwich to Embankment takes all of 45 idyllic minutes (but on weekends, you may have to wait 30 min. for a boat back). You can go right under the famous Tower Bridge—and because it's intended for commuters, it's at a fraction of the price of a tourist boat.

Fares depend on how far you're going, but for a trip from Westminster to Greenwich, expect a one-way fare around £8.10 (£6.30 with Oyster). You will always save money if you buy a return trip instead of two one-ways, and always ask if your Oyster card or Travelcard grants a discount. The fast catamarans of *Thames Clippers* (www.thamesclippers.com; ✆ **020/7930-2062;** generally 6:30am–10:30pm; bookable via its app) go every 20 minutes during the day. River Roamer passes, which allow you to take as many trips as you want on a single day, cost £18.50 for adults, £37 for a family of two adults and up to three kids. You can buy at the piers or buy ahead via the Thames Clippers Tickets app, downloadable via thamesclippers.com/app. **Thames River Services** (www.thamesriverservices.com; ✆ **020/7930-4097**) offers a £12.50 single/£16.50 ride to Greenwich or the Thames Barrier. It calls these "sightseeing" trips, but note that, despite the elevated price, it's not fully guided.

Bikes

Scattered throughout town, you'll see racks of identical red bikes in racks. They're yours to borrow, day or night! They are called **Santander Cycles** (www.tfl.gov.uk/modes/cycling/santander-cycles), but Londoners call them **Boris Bikes,** after the blowsy former mayor who brought them here (or **Barclays Bikes** after a previous sponsor), and they provide more than 10.3 million rides a year. Interestingly, it's been reported this is the only part of Transport for London that makes a profit.

It works like this: You choose one and pull it out of the rack by lifting the seat. You ride it to any other docking station in the city with a free space, and you park it by slotting the front wheel in until a green light appears on the dock. When you're ready to ride somewhere else, just get another bike. You buy the right to borrow bikes for £2 for 30 minutes (payments are on your credit card) every time you pull a bike out of the rack. Go past that, and you pay the same rate: £2 per extra 30 minutes. The idea is for you to use a bike as you need it, not to keep it with you all day. You are required to follow the same traffic rules that cars do, which won't be easy, although the city's huge parks are safer places to cycle. Locations of nearby docks are listed on every pylon. Use the free apps **Santander Cycles, Spotcycle,** or **Citymapper** to find nearby stations with space.

Taxis

Even Londoners think taxis are crazy expensive. It's not the fault of the cabbies. They're the best in the world. Before they're given their wheels, every London taxi driver (there are some 24,000 of them) must go through a grueling training period so comprehensive that it's dubbed, simply, "The Knowledge." On Sundays, you'll see trainees zipping around on mopeds with clipboards affixed above their dashboards. Cabbies arrive inculcated with directions to every alley, mews, avenue, shortcut, and square in the city, and if they don't know, they'll find the answer so discreetly you won't catch the gaffe. And then there are those adorable vehicles: bulbous as Depression Era jalopies, roomy as a studio apartment, yet able to do complete U-turns within a single lane of traffic.

But for this admittedly peerless carriage, you'll pay a £2.60 minimum. Trips of up to 1.6km (1 mile) cost £5.80 to £9 during working hours; 3.2km (2-mile) trips are £8.80 to £14; 6.4km (4-mile) trips are £15 to £22; and trips of around 9.6km (6 miles) hit you for a painful £23 to £30. Rates rise when you're most likely to need a taxi: by about 10% from 8pm to 10pm or all day on weekends, and roughly another 20% from 10pm until dawn. Trips that start at Heathrow cost an extra £2.80. Mercifully, there is no charge for extra passengers or for luggage. It has become customary to tip 10%, but most people just round up to the nearest pound. Some taxis accept credit cards (don't count on it), but mostly they are a cash-only concern.

Taxis are often called "black cabs," although in fact 12 colors are registered, including "thistle blue" and "nightfire red." If you need to call a cab, **One-Number** (✆ **087/1871-8710**) pools all the companies, with a surcharge of £2.

Minicabs, which are hire cars that operate separately from the traditional black cab system, are easy to find using apps. Don't accept a ride from an unsolicited one. Among the top free apps that can hail the nearest ride: **Splitcab** (www.splitcab.co.uk), which finds people going your way to share the cost (and gives women the option of female-driven cars); **Kabbee** (www.

CAN I do that?

Some things that are considered sins back home may lead to legal pleasures in London. Which means they're not sinful as long as you're on British soil! To wit:

- The drinking age is 18. But if you're having your first legit night out, take it easy, because beers here have higher alcohol content than in many countries.

- There are no open container laws. That means you can drink beer in public. The one exception is on public transportation, where you need a drink the most.

- You may smoke Cuban cigars. Get them at any tobacconist and puff away. If you're American, though, don't try smuggling them home.

- Absinthe, the brutal quaff nicknamed "The Green Fairy," is available here. Drink up because American Customs frowns on many versions of it.

- The age of consent is 16 no matter the sexual preference.

kabbee.com; © **0203/515-1111**), which canvasses cab fleets for the best fixed price; **Minicabit** (www.minicabit.com); **Cabwise** (www.tfl.gov.uk/cabwise); taxi-calling app **Hailo** (hailoapp.com/locations/london/; minimum charges of £10 outside of 10am–5pm weekdays), which failed in the U.S. but thrives here and to which about half the city's black cabs subscribe; independent share ride app **Uber** (www.uber.com); **Gett.com** (cashless app with no minimum fare or surge pricing); and London's reigning power minicab operator, **Addison Lee** (www.addisonlee.com), which makes more than £100 million in bookings a year from its free app alone.

Renting a Car

Are you insane? Rare is the local who drives in central London, where there's a mandatory daily "congestion charge" of £11.50–£14 (don't believe me? see **www.cclondon.com**), and where parking rates look like your rent back home. Streets were cramped enough when people rode horses, and now they're dogged with one-way rules and police cameras that will ticket you for even honest errors, which you'll definitely make since you're just visiting. You'll go crazy and broke, so why do it? If you're driving out of the city for a tour of the country, fine, but *do not* rent a car for a London vacation.

GETTING AROUND THE U.K.
By Train

The original railway builders plowed their stations into every town of size, making it easy to see the highlights of the United Kingdom without getting near a car. The British whine about the declining quality of the service, but Americans, Canadians, and Australians will be blown away by the speed (and the cost, if they don't book ahead) of the system. Find tickets to all destinations through **National Rail** (www.nationalrail.co.uk; ✆ **08457/48-49-50**) or the indispensable **TrainLine.com**. Seats are sold 12 weeks ahead, and early-bird bookings can yield some marvelous deals, such as £26 for a 4-hour trip to Scotland (£125 last-minute is common). When hunting for tickets, always search for "off-peak" (non-rush hour) trips going or coming from London in general, not a specific London station, because each London terminal serves various cities. The free app **TicketySplit** (download in the U.K.) also searches the rail companies' byzantine fare schedules to tell you journey configurations that can save you many pounds. Unfortunately, not every train company website accepts international credit cards; TheTrainLine does.

Tickets bought reasonably well in advance will still be cheaper than what you'd pay for the same trips on a **BritRail pass** (www.britrail.com; must purchase outside the U.K.), good on long-distance trains but not on local London transport. Few tourists ride rails with the near-daily regularity that would make a timed pass pay for itself. Check prices against the U.S. seller **Rail Europe** (www.raileurope.com; ✆ **800/622-8600**), as quotes vary.

By Bus

National Express (www.nationalexpress.com; ✆ **0871/781-8181**) is the least expensive way to get from city to city in Britain (but not the fastest—that's usually the train). Because the country is not very big, it rarely takes more than a few hours to reach anyplace by bus. Even Scotland is only 5 hours away. A major carrier with scads of departures, **Megabus** (uk.megabus.com; ✆ **090/0160-0900** or 44-141-352-4444), which serves more than 100 cities across Europe, charges as little as £1.50 for early bookings, although £19 to £45 for Edinburgh is a more typical rate. It accepts bookings 2 months ahead; book online to avoid phone fees. Both coach services depart from the miserable Victoria Coach Station, located behind Victoria railway station (www.tfl.gov.uk/coaches).

What's the best place to hear about inexpensive ground tours? Hostels. Drop into one; most of their lobbies are papered with brochures. Don't neglect their bulletin boards, either, since you may catch wind of a shared-ride situation that'll often cost you no more than your share of the gasoline (in Britain, *petrol*).

If You Need to Fake a British Postcode

When you're online in the U.K., such as when you sign up for free Wi-Fi, you may be asked for a mobile number and a postcode before you access a signal. Of course you don't have those things— you're visiting! Bulldoze through this shortsightedness by giving a fake number you can invent at http://fakenumber. org/generator/mobile. As for a postcode, use your hotel's. Better yet, use the following code: EH2 2AN. After all, if that postcode is good enough for the queen, it's good enough for you!

By Car

Okay, *now* is when you might want to rent a car (see "Driving in London?" on p. 310 for car rental tips).

WHEN TO GO

CLIMATE   It's always time to visit London. It doesn't rain as much as they say and it hasn't been foggy since they got rid of coal. Even though it's approximately at the same latitude of Edmonton, Alberta, weather patterns keep the environment from being extreme. It gets cold in the winter, but rarely snowed in. It gets warm in the summer, but rarely blisteringly so (in fact, most buildings don't even have air-conditioning). The winter months are generally more humid than the summer ones, but experience only slightly more rain. Locals use the free, reliable **Met Office Weather app,** by the U.K.'s national weather service, to pinpoint forecasts by GPS.

London's Average Daytime Temperatures & Rainfall

	JAN	FEB	MAR	APR	MAY	JUNE	JULY	AUG	SEPT	OCT	NOV	DEC
TEMP. (°F)	39	39	43	46	52	58	62	62	57	51	44	42
TEMP. (°C)	3	3	6	7	11	14	16	16	13	10	6	5
RAINFALL (in.)	3.1	2	2.4	2.1	2.2	2.2	1.8	2.2	2.7	2.9	3.1	3.1
RAINFALL (mm)	49	39	40	43	47	52	59	57	56	62	59	53

SEASONAL CONSIDERATIONS   The principal art season (for theater, concerts, art shows) falls between September and May, leaving the summer months for festivals and park-going. A few royal attractions, such as the state rooms of Buckingham Palace, are only open in the summer when the queen decamps to Scotland. In summer, when the weather is warmest, the sun sets after 10pm, and half of Europe takes its annual holiday, airfares are higher, as are hotel rates. Summertime queues for most tourist attractions, such as the London Eye and the Tower of London, might make you wish you'd come in March. For decent prices and lighter crowds, go in spring or fall—April and October seem to have the best confluence of mild weather, pretty plantings, and tolerable crowds. Prices are lowest in mid-winter, but a number of minor sights, such as historic houses, sometimes close from November to March, and the biggest annual events take place during the warmer months.

London's Public Holidays

England observes **eight public holidays** (also known as "bank holidays"): New Year's Day (Jan 1); Good Friday and Easter Monday (usually Apr); May Bank Holiday (first Mon in May); Spring Bank Holiday (usually last Mon in May, but occasionally the first in June); August Bank Holiday (last Mon in Aug); Christmas Day (Dec 25); Boxing Day (Dec 26). If a date falls on a weekend, the holiday rolls over to the following Monday.

London's Calendar of Events

Special events are an integral part of London's calendar, and many regular happenings draw tourists from around the world. Find even more events at London's **city website** (www.london.gov.uk/events), at the **official tourism site** (www.visitlondon.com), the blog **Londonist** (www.londonist.com), and *Time Out* **magazine** (www.timeout.com/london).

JANUARY

London New Year's Day Parade. As many as 10,000 dancers, acrobats, musicians, and performers (heavy on the marching bands) promenade from Parliament Square to Piccadilly for 500,000 spectators and TV audiences. www.lnydp.com, ✆ **020/3275-0190.** January 1.

Chinese New Year Festival. In conjunction with the Chinese New Year, the streets around Leicester Square come alive with dragon and lion dances, children's parades, performances, screenings, and fireworks displays. www.chinatownlondon.org.

Get into London Theatre. Theatre gets a jolt of new audiences during this promotional period during which producers cooperate to sell some 75,000 tickets at big discounts. www.getintolondontheatre.co.uk. Early January to February.

London International Mime Festival. Not just for silent clowns, but also for funky puppets and ingenious physical tomfoolery, it's held at venues around town. www.mimelondon.com, ✆ **020/7637-5661.** Mid-January.

FEBRUARY

London Fashion Week. Collections are unveiled for press and buyers at a biannual fashion festival also held in September. It's tough to get a runway show ticket, but there's a raft of slick events and parties across the city. www.londonfashionweek.co.uk. Mid-February and mid-September.

MARCH

St Patrick's Day Festival. When you're this close to Dublin and you consider England's long rivalry with the Emerald Isle, you can expect three days of raging Irish pride—parades, music, and food stalls around Trafalgar Square, where the fountains gush green. The city also sponsors concerts and craft fairs promoting Irish culture and heritage. It's not just about drinking—it just looks that way. www.london.gov.uk, ✆ **020/7983-4000.** March 17.

BADA Antiques & Fine Art Fair. Sponsored by the British Antique Dealers' Association, it's considered to be the best in Britain for such collectors. Some 100 exhibitors move into a mighty tent in Duke of York's Square, in Chelsea, for the 7-day sales event. Don't expect a bargain. www.badafair.com, ✆ **020/7589-6108.** Mid- to late March.

Oxford and Cambridge Boat Race. This popular annual event (since 1829), held on the Thames in Hammersmith, takes less than a half-hour, but the after-party rollicks into the night and the good-natured rivalry is undying. www.theboatrace.org. Late March or early April.

APRIL

London Marathon. Although it draws some 35,000 runners, the Marathon is also a kick for spectators, so hotels tend to fill up ahead of it. The starter pistol fires in Blackheath; the home stretch is along Birdcage Walk near Buckingham Palace. If you want to run, apply by the previous October. www.virginmoneylondonmarathon.com. Sunday in mid-April.

Udderbelly Festival. Famously mounted in a giant inflatable purple cow's udder by the riverbank (really), this 410-seat offshoot of Edinburgh Fringe Festival's variety venue the Underbelly sells well over a million tickets. Dozens of acts range from comedy to musicals to circus, plus there's food, a beer garden, and other amusements. In 2017, it merged with the similar Wonderground festival to extend from 3 months to 5 months. www.udderbelly.co.uk, ✆ **0844/545-8282.** April to mid-July.

Regent's Park Open Air Theatre. Forget stuffy auditoriums. There's little shelter from sudden downpours, but in good weather the repertoire of high drama, musicals, and Shakespeare sparkles under a canopy of blue skies, towering trees, and natural beauty. www.openairtheatre.org, ☎ **0844/826-4242.** Mid-May to September.

Chelsea Flower Show. The Royal Horticultural Society, which calls itself a "leading gardening charity dedicated to advancing horticulture and promoting good gardening" (don't you just love the English?), mounts this esteemed show for 5 days on the grounds of the Royal Hospital in Chelsea. The plants, all raised by champion green thumbs, are sold to attendees on the final day, but sadly, foreigners aren't usually able to get their plants past Customs. Tickets go on sale in November for this lily-palooza, and they're snapped up quickly. The event is so celebrated that it is covered on nightly prime-time TV. Really. www.rhs.org.uk, ☎ **020/3176-5800.** Late May

JUNE

Beating Retreat. Drum corps, pipes, and plenty of bugle calls: This anachronistic twilight ceremony, held for two evenings at Horse Guards Parade by St James's Park, involves the salute of the queen (or another member of the royal family) and the appearance of many red-clad marchers. Scholars trace its origins to 1554—so for tradition's sake, it's deeply meaningful. It's the nearest relative to the better-known Trooping the Colour, but without the crowds. Reserve ahead (£15) in mid-December. www.household-division.org.uk, ☎ **020/7839-5323.** Early June.

Hampton Court Palace Festival. High-end niche names (Burt Bacharach, Van Morrison, Russell Watson, Tom Jones) perform early in the month in a temporary theater on palace grounds. Tickets are around £50. www.hamptoncourtpalacefestival.com. ☎ **084/4412-2954.**

The Royal Academy Summer Exhibition. Artists have been in a frenzy to win entry to this blind competition for nearly 250 years.

Paintings, sculpture, drawings, architecture—if you can dream it, you can enter it, and if you're one of the most talented, your piece is anointed as the best that year. The show is what the Royal Academy is known for, and although it's not envelope-pushing, it's a seminal event in British art culture and shouldn't be missed if you're in town. www.royalacademy.org.uk.

Trooping the Colour. Never mind that the queen was born in April. This is her birthday party (92 in 2018!), and as a present, she gets the same thing every year: soldiers with big hats. A sea of redcoats and cavalry swarm over Horse Guards Parade, 41 guns salute, and a flight of Royal Air Force jets slam through the sky overhead. The queen herself leads the charge, waving politely to her subjects before they lose themselves in a hearty display of marching band prowess. Try for grandstand seats (£10–£35) instead of standing in the free-for-all along the route, where you'll only get a fast glimpse of passing royalty. The ticket policy is changing for 2018, so check its website early (in the past, tickets went out in Jan or Feb) for instructions. www.householddivision.org.uk/trooping-the-colour, ☎ **020/7414-2479.** Mid-June.

Taste of London Festival. The city's top chefs and the region's finest farmers convene in Regent's Park for 5 days of belly-stuffing. London.tastefestivals.com, ☎ **087/1230-5581.** Mid-June.

Pride London. A signature event on the world's LGBT calendar, in a good year London Pride can pull some 825,000 revelers, many of them heterosexual, with a buoyant roster of concerts and performances by famous names plus a parade (the U.K.'s largest) in the center of the City. The gay pride week, co-sponsored by the Mayor's office, also makes an excellent excuse for some blowout dance parties. www.prideinlondon.org, ☎ **0844/344-5428.** Late June or early July.

Wimbledon Championships. Why watch on television yet again? Check p. 185 for how to be one of the 500,000 to witness it in person. www.wimbledon.org, ☎ **020/8944-1066.** Late June to early July.

Greenwich and Docklands International Festival. An ambitious program of free theatrical and musical pieces, many of them developed by artists expressly for the spaces they're performed in. www.festival.org, ✆ **020/8305-1818.** Late June and early July.

Meltdown. A compendium of hip prestige arts held at the Southbank Centre, curated in the past by such notables as Patti Smith, David Bowie, or Yoko Ono. www.southbank centre.co.uk/meltdown, ✆ **020/3879-9555.** Late June

JULY

BBC Promenade Concerts. The biggest classical music festival of the year, held primarily at the Royal Albert Hall, "the Proms" consists of orchestral concerts for every taste. Seats start at £7.50. www.bbc.co.uk/proms, ✆ **020/7589-8212.**

Lovebox. The weekend-long music marathon held in Victoria Park in northeast London mixes newcomers with giants of sound, including past guests LCD Soundsystem, Mark Ronson, Frank Ocean, and Goldfrapp. The crowd is young and fun, starting with nitrous-huffing kids on Friday and morphing into a de facto gay pride day by Sunday. loveboxfestival.com.

New Look Wireless Festival. Held alfresco in Finsbury Park for 3 days, it books the best names in the biz. In 2017, those included Chance the Rapper, Nas, and The Weeknd. www.wirelessfestival.co.uk.

The Lambeth Country Show. A free, old-fashioned farm show overtakes Brixton's Brockwell Park (for a single weekend, anyway) with farm animals, jam-making contests, a fun fair, tractor demonstrations, and Punch and Judy puppet shows. Very English stuff. Free. lambethcountryshow.co.uk, ✆ **020/7926-7085.**

AUGUST

London Triathlon. Some 13,000 participants cycle through the City from Westminster, sprint around the ExCeL center in Docklands, and swim in Royal Victoria Dock in this annual event. Sir Richard Branson attends. www.the londontriathlon.co.uk, ✆ **020/8233-5900.** Early August.

Notting Hill Carnival. In August 1958, roving bands of white racists combed the slums of Notting Hill in search of Caribbean-owned businesses to destroy. Resulting community outrage and newly rediscovered cultural pride led to the formation of this festival, now Europe's largest street parade, attracting some 2 million people. It's a smorgasbord of cultures spanning the Caribbean, Eastern Europe, South America, and the Indian subcontinent. Sunday is kids' day, with scrubbed-down events and activities, but on Monday, the adults take over, costumes get skimpy, floats weave through small streets, and rowdy hordes celebrate into the wee hours. www.thelondonnottinghillcarnival. com. August Bank Holiday weekend.

Great British Beer Festival. Just like it sounds: More than 900 British ales and ciders are available to try at London Olympia—after all those tastings, you'll be relieved to learn the Tube is within easy reach. It runs 5 days. www.gbbf.org.uk. ✆ **01727/867-201.**

SEPTEMBER

The Great River Race. Always over too soon, the Race is the aquatic version of the London Marathon, with rowers vying to beat out 300 other vessels—Chinese dragon boats, Canadian canoes, Viking longboats, and even Hawaiian outriggers—on a morning jaunt upriver from the Docklands to Richmond. www.greatriverrace.co.uk, ✆ **020/8398-8141.** Saturday in mid-September.

Totally Thames. In conjunction with the Great River Race (above), nearly half a million souls attend London's largest free open-air arts festival, with more than 150 events. Southwark Bridge is closed for a giant feast, and there's a flotilla of working river boats, circus performers, and antique fireboats, tugs, and sailboats. Sunday sees the Night Carnival, a lavish procession of thousands of lantern-bearing musicians and dancers crawling along the water. Everything is topped off with barge-launched fireworks. totallythames. org, ✆ **020/7928-8998.** Mid-September.

Open House London. More than 800 buildings, all of them deemed important but normally closed to the public, yawn wide for free tours on a single, hotly anticipated weekend. Past participants have included the skyscraper headquarters of Lloyd's and Swiss Re (officially "30 St Mary Axe" but usually called "The Gherkin") and even No. 10 Downing St. The list of open buildings comes out in August. Some require timed tickets, but for most, the line forms at dawn. Open House also organizes year-round walking tours. www.openhouselondon.org.uk, ℭ 020/3006-7008. Mid-September

London Fashion Weekend. It's got nothing on its kin in New York or Milan, but here, pop-up shops from more than 100 designers are put on sale at deeply discounted prices in the hopes they'll build style buzz. www.london fashionweekend.co.uk. Mid-September.

Dance Umbrella. One of the world's best contemporary dance festivals, with plenty of standing-room seats for as little as £5. www. danceumbrella.co.uk. ℭ 020/7257-9380. Peaks in late September.

OCTOBER

Frieze Art Fair. More than 175 galleries vie for big money from collectors in a colossal 4-day tent show in Regent's Park. It has become influential in the contemporary art world. www.friezeartfair.com. ℭ 0871/230-3452.

Diwali. One advantage of visiting a multicultural city like London is that it affords you the chance to sample major international holidays in an English-speaking environment. One such treat is Diwali, the Indian "festival of light," when Trafalgar Square is transformed with lights, floating lanterns, massive models of the elephant god Ganesh, music, dance, and DJs. It's free. Mid- to late October.

BFI London Film Festival. An important stop on the cinema circuit, this event, sponsored by the British Film Institute, is geared toward media exposure, but there are plenty of tickets for the public, too. www.bfi.org.uk/lff, ℭ 020/7928-3232.

NOVEMBER

Guy Fawkes Night. In 1605, silly old Guy Fawkes tried to assassinate James I and the entire Parliament by blowing them to smithereens in the Gunpowder Plot. Joke's on him: To this day, the Brits celebrate his failure by blowing up *him*. His effigy is thrown on bonfires across the country, fireworks displays rage in the autumn night sky, and more than a few tykes light their first sparklers in honor of the would-be assassin's gruesome execution. Although displays are scattered around town, including at Battersea Park and Alexandra Palace, get out of the city for the weekend nearest November 5, also called Bonfire Night—the countryside is perfumed with the woody aroma of burning leaves on this holiday. Mount Primrose Hill or Hampstead Heath for a view of the fireworks around the city. November 5.

Lord Mayor's Show. What sounds like the world's dullest public access program is actually a delightfully pompous procession, about 800 years old, involving some 140 charity floats and 6,000 participants to ostensibly show off the newly elected Lord Mayor to the queen or her representatives. The centerpiece is the preposterously carved and gilt Lord Mayor's Coach, built in 1757—a carriage so extravagant it makes Cinderella's ride look like a Toyota Corolla. That's a lot of hubbub for a city official whose role is essentially ceremonial; the Mayor of London (currently Boris Johnson) wields the true power. All that highfalutin strutting is followed by a good old-fashioned fireworks show over the Thames between the Blackfriars and Waterloo bridges. www.lordmayorsshow.org. Second Saturday in November

London Jazz Festival. Some 165 mid-November events attract around 60,000 music fans. Many performances are free, and tickets are distributed by the venues. www. efglondonjazzfestival.org.uk, ℭ 020/7324-1880.

Remembrance Sunday. Another chance to glimpse Her Royal Highness. She and the prime minister, as well as many royals, attend a ceremony at the Cenotaph, in the middle of Whitehall, to honor the war dead and wounded, of which Britain has borne more than its share. Those red flowers you'll see everywhere—red petals, black centers—are poppies, the symbol of remembrance in Britain. Sunday nearest November 11.

DECEMBER

Carols by Candlelight. Royal Albert Hall's annual evening of sing-along Christmas carols, readings from Dickens, and music by Handel, Bach, Mozart, and Corelli played by the Mozart Festival Orchestra—in period costume. www.royalalberthall.com, ✆ **020/7589-8212.** Late December.

New Year's Eve Fireworks. As Big Ben strikes midnight, London rings in the New Year with 12 minutes of fireworks over the Thames and the Eye. It's so crowded that in 2015, the city began limiting attendance to 110,000 and requiring tickets (£10). A few tickets can be booked via www.london.gov.uk/nye in mid-June, with the rest available in September.

[FastFACTS] LONDON

Accessible Travel London can't seem to strike the balance between preserving old buildings and making sure they're accessible to all. With the laudable exception of the Docklands Light Railway, only a few Tube stations have lifts, and those with plenty of escalators still require passengers to climb flights of stairs. Research your options at **Visit London** (www.visit london.com/access), **Transport for London** (www.tfl.gov.uk/accessibility; ✆ **0843/222-1234**), and **DisabledGo** (www.disabled go.com). The website **UpDownLondon.com** keeps tabs on step-free access at Tube stations, including temporary maintenance obstacles.

Many London hotels, museums, restaurants, and sightseeing attractions have dedicated wheelchair access, all taxis and buses do, and persons with disabilities often get admission discounts. Generally speaking, the more expensive a hotel is, the more likely it is to be wheelchair accessible, but not always. The website

for **Nationwide Disabled Access Register** (www.directenquiries.com) lists the accessibility features of a wide range of facilities, from attractions to car renters.

Artsline (www.artsline.org.uk) has information about accessible entertainment venues, including which ones have infrared hearing devices for rental. Blind or partially sighted travelers will find useful advice from the **Royal National Institute of Blind People** (www.rnib.org.uk; ✆ **0303/123-9999**). **Tourism for All** (www.tourism forall.org.uk; ✆ **084/5124-9971**) has accessibility information for older travelers as well as travelers with disabilities.

The British agency **Can Be Done** (www.canbedone.co.uk; ✆ **020/8907-2400**) runs tours adapted to travelers with disabilities. **Wheelchair Travel** (www.wheelchair-travel.co.uk; ✆ **01483/23-76-68**) rents out self-drive and chauffeured chair-accessible vehicles (including ones with hand controls), provides day tours, and arranges city

sightseeing in special vehicles.

Area Codes The country telephone code for Great Britain is **44**. The area code for London is **020**. The full telephone number is usually 8 digits long. Businesses and homes in central London usually have numbers beginning with a **7**; those from farther out begin with an **8**. For more info, see "Telephones," p. 335.

ATMs/Banks See "Money," p. 331. One quirk to note: Retrieve your card immediately from ATM slots; many machines suck them in within 10 to 15 seconds, for security. Should that happen, you'll have to petition the bank to have it returned to you.

Business Hours Offices are generally open weekdays between 9 or 10am and 5 or 6pm. Some remain open a few hours longer on Thursdays and Fridays. Saturday hours for stores are the same; Sunday store hours are generally noon to 5 or 6pm. Banks are usually open from 9:30am to 4 or 5pm, with some larger branches open later on

Thursdays or for a few hours on Saturday mornings.

Cellphones See "Mobile Phones," p. 331.

Credit Cards Credit cards are accepted nearly everywhere, but if you can, bring **Visa** or **Mastercard,** because **American Express** is accepted less widely. (If you try to use it at a place that doesn't accept it, you may be mistakenly told your card has a problem; don't panic.) Many credit card issuers levy an annoying international transaction fee on top of your purchase—many **American Express** cards have dropped that fee, as have **Capital One Venture** (www.capitalone. com; ℓ **800/695-5500**) and several options from **Chase** (www.chase.com).

Small vendors may charge a transaction fee (3% is the norm) as a way of defraying the cost of dealing with credit card companies. Try not to use credit cards to withdraw cash—you'll pay a currency exchange fee, and worse, you'll be charged interest from the moment your money leaves the slot.

Europeans use **"chip and PIN" cards** requiring a code number. Some vending machines won't accept swipe-only cards and may incorrectly inform you that you were declined. Most U.S. cards now come with such a chip, but if yours doesn't, ask your lender to send you one for free. If you do have a swipe-only card, inform clerks you're using a "Signature card," as they

will usually have to scramble around for a pen (Europeans don't sign anymore). Restaurants will usually process your payment at your table wirelessly—the British consider it standard security practice not to let your card out of your sight and to check ID along with signature.

Customs Rules about what you can carry into Britain are standard but ever-shifting, so get the latest restrictions from **HM Revenue & Customs** (www.hmrc. gov.uk; ℓ **011-44/2920-501-261**). Your own government is responsible for telling you what you can bring back home.

Doctors Ask your hotel first. Then try the G.P. (General Practitioner) finder at **www.nhs.uk**. North American members of the **International Association for Medical Assistance to Travelers** (IAMAT; www. iamat.org; ℓ **716/754-4883** in the U.S. or 416/652-0137 in Canada) can consult that organization for lists of local approved doctors. **Note:** U.S. and Canadian visitors who become ill while they're in London are eligible only for free emergency care. For other treatment, including follow-up care, you'll pay £60 to £150 just to see a physician.

Drinking Laws Legal drinking age is 18. Children 15 and younger are allowed in pubs if accompanied by a parent or guardian. Drinking on London's **public transport network** is forbidden;

on-the-spot fines are issued to transgressors.

Electricity The current in Britain is 240 volts AC. Plugs have three squared pins. Foreign appliances operating on lower voltage (those from the U.S., Canada, and Australia use 110–120 volts AC) will require an adapter and possibly a voltage converter, although the range of capability will usually be printed on the plug. Many modern phone chargers and laptops can handle the stronger current with only an adapter. A few hotels provide North American-style outlets for a non-heating appliance such as a shaver, but don't count on one.

Embassies & Consulates In 2017, the **U.S. Embassy** moved from Grosvenor Square to an elaborate 4.9-acre complex in West London's Wandsworth district (Ponton Rd., SW8; http://london.usembassy. gov; ℓ **020/7499-9000;** Vauxhall tube). Standard hours are Monday to Friday 8:30am to 5:30pm. Most non-emergency inquiries require an appointment. You may not bring tablets or laptops. For passport information, call ℓ **877/ 487-2778** in the U.S.

The **High Commission of Canada,** 1 Trafalgar Sq., London W1 (www.canada international.gc.ca/united_ kingdom-royaume_uni/ index.aspx; ℓ **020/7004-6000;** Charing Cross tube), handles passport and consular services for Canadians. Hours are Monday,

Wednesday, and Friday 8 to 10:30am.

The **Australian High Commission** is at Australia House, Strand, London WC2 (www.uk.embassy.gov.au; ℭ **020/7379-4334;** Temple tube). Hours are Monday to Friday 9am to noon.

The **New Zealand High Commission** is at New Zealand House, 80 Haymarket, London SW1 (www.nz embassy.com/uk; ℭ **020/ 7930-8422;** Charing Cross or Piccadilly Circus tube). Hours are Monday to Friday 9am to 5pm.

The **Irish Embassy** is at 17 Grosvenor Place, London SW1 (www.embassyof ireland.co.uk; ℭ **020/7235-2171;** Tube: Hyde Park Corner). Hours are Monday to Friday 9:30am–12:30pm and 2:30pm–4:30pm.

Emergencies The one-stop number for Britain is ℭ **999**—that's for fire, police, and ambulances. It's free from any phone, even mobiles. Less urgent? Call 111.

Family Travel Attractions cater to the family market. The kingly treatment starts, at many places, with the so-named **Family Ticket,** which grants a reduced price for parents and kids entering together. For any length of stay, you can rent baby equipment from **Chelsea Baby Hire** (www.chelseababyhire.com; ℭ **07802/846-742**). If you need babysitting, **Sitting Pretty Babysitters** (www. sittingprettybabysitters.com; ℭ **07971/083-207**) will

come to your hotel for a minimum of 3 or 4 hours, depending on the time of week; rates are around £9.50 an hour with a £6.50 booking fee and a £ 16.50 membership fee.

If you are a **divorced parent** traveling with your children, bring proof to the airport that you are entitled to take your kids out of the country.

Some resources for family-specific travel tips include the **Family Travel Network** (www.familytravel network.com) and **Travel with Your Kids** (www.travel withyourkids.com), which has a section just about London's finds. **The Family Travel Files** (www.thefamily travelfiles.com) lists tour operators and packagers geared to families, but its suggestions aren't always the most economical or efficient. *Time Out* (www. timeout.com/london) includes a section on kids' activities.

When it comes to **baby supplies,** pacifiers are called "dummies," diapers are "nappies," a crib is a "cot," and Band-Aids are "plasters."

Health Traveling to London doesn't pose specific health risks. Common drugs are generally available over the counter and in large supermarkets, although visitors should know the generic rather than brand names of any medicines they rely on. *Note:* The general-purpose painkiller known in North America as

acetaminophen is called **paracetamol** in the U.K.

Pack **prescription medications** in carry-on luggage and in their original containers, with pharmacy labels—otherwise they may not pass airport security. Also bring copies of your prescriptions, just in case. If you require **syringes,** always carry a signed medical prescription. Don't forget an extra pair of contact lenses or prescription glasses.

If you need the advice of a doctor or a nurse, the national health care system operates a free, 24-hour hotline: **National Health Service Direct** (www.nhs.uk; ℭ **111**). Citizens of many European countries are entitled to free health care while in Britain (see www. dh.gov.uk/travellers), but not everyone is. Clinics were once known to treat tourists and then look the other way rather than deal with the paperwork required to bill them; private billing companies now police for every pound—to see a doctor you could pay between £50 and £150. Non-EU citizens should carry health or travel insurance.

Health Insurance U.K. nationals receive free medical treatment countrywide; visitors from overseas qualify only for free **emergency** care. **U.S. visitors** should note that most domestic health plans (including Medicare and Medicaid) do not provide coverage, and the ones that do often require you to pay for services upfront and file for reimbursement after you return home. You might want to buy international medical coverage from companies such as **United-Healthcare SafeTrip** (www. UHCsafetrip.com; ✆ **800/732-5309**) or **Travel Assistance International** (www.travelassistance.com; ✆ **800/643-5525**). **Canadians** should check with their provincial health plan offices or call **Health Canada** (www.hc-sc.gc.ca; ✆ **613/957-2991**) to find out the extent of their coverage and what documentation and receipts to bring home if they are treated overseas. For **E.U. nationals** (and nationals of E.E.A. countries and Switzerland), reciprocal health agreements ensure they receive free medical care while in the U.K., but you must carry a valid **European Health Identity Card** (EHIC).

Hospitals In the U.K., the ER is usually called A&E, or Accident and Emergency. If your need is urgent, dial ✆ **999** (it's free no matter where your phone is registered) rather than risk going to a medical center that doesn't offer A&E. You can search **www.nhs.uk** for the nearest A&E, or go to the 24-hour, walk-in A&E departments at **University College London Hospital,** 235 Euston Road, London NW1 (www.uclh.nhs.uk; ✆ **020/3456-7014** or 020/3447-0083; Warren St. tube) or **St Thomas's Hospital,** Westminster Bridge Road, entrance on Lambeth Palace Road, London, SE1

(www.guysandstthomas.nhs. uk; ✆ **020/7188-7188;** Westminster or Waterloo tube). For less urgent needs, visit **Central London Community Healthcare** (1 Frith St., W1; www.clch. nhs.uk; ✆ **020/7534-6500;** Tottenham Court Rd. tube), which is open Monday–Friday 8am–8pm, Saturday–Sunday 10am–8pm.

Innoculations Unless you're arriving from an area known to be suffering from an epidemic, inoculations or vaccinations are not required for entry into the U.K.

Insurance You may want special coverage for **apartment stays,** especially if you've plunked down a deposit, and for any **valuables** you may bring with you; airlines are only required to pay up to $2,500 for lost luggage domestically, less for foreign travel. Compare policies at **InsureMyTrip.com** (✆ **800/487-4722**), or contact one of the following reputable companies: **Allianz** (www.allianztravelinsurance.com; ✆ **866/884-3556**); **CSA Travel Protection** (www.csatravelprotection.com; ✆ **877/243-4135** or 240/330-1529); **Travel Guard International** (www.travelguard.com; ✆ **800/826-4919**); or **Travelex** (www.travelex-insurance.com; ✆ **800/228-9792**). Note that most insurers require you to purchase plans *before* you leave home.

Internet Wi-Fi flows freely at pubs, cafes,

museums, and nearly all hotels. Usually, you will have to fill in an email address to activate it, but often it's a data collection ploy and you can write dummy information. (See box on p. 321.) Virgin Media (www.virgin media.com/wifi) provides Wi-Fi in many Tube stations but not between them. Visitors can buy passes for £2 (1 day), £5 (1 week), or £15 (1 month). See "Mobile Phones" p. 331.

Laundry Launderettes are not easy to find in central London anymore, and expensive hotels will only do laundry and dry cleaning if you're willing to shell out. Look into the app **Laundrapp,** which will pick up and drop off to your hotel for free. Prices start at £2 per article or £2.50 for 1kg (2.2 lb.).

Left Luggage Useful if you're taking those cheap European flights with steep luggage fees, **Left Baggage** (www.left-baggage. com; ✆ **0800/077-4530**) has locations at Heathrow, Gatwick, and the big railway stations: It costs £12.50 per item per 24 hours for up to a week, then £5 per item per day thereafter.

Legal Aid If you find yourself in trouble abroad, contact your consulate or embassy (see "Embassies & Consulates," p. 328). It can advise you of your rights and provide a list of local attorneys (for which you'll have to pay if services are used), but they cannot interfere on your behalf in the English legal process. For questions about U.S. citizens who've been arrested abroad, telephone the **Citizens Emergency Center** of the Bureau of Consular Affairs in Washington, D.C. (✆ **202/501-4444** or 888/407-4747).

LGBT Travelers Gay and lesbian people have equality and marriage rights in England. Public displays of affection are barely noticed in the center of the city, although in the outer suburbs couples should show more restraint. Gay bashings are rare enough to be newsworthy, but it's true that an element of society can, once full of ale, become belligerent. Particularly in parks at night, be aware of your surroundings and give wide berth to gaggles of drunken lads. This advice holds irrespective of your sexuality.

For nightlife planning, the best sources for information are **Boyz** (www.boyz.co.uk), which publishes a day-by-day schedule on its website, and the free **QX International** (www.qx magazine.com). Both are distributed for free at many gay bars. Also see nightlife listings on p. 246.

Mail An airmail letter or postcard to anywhere outside Europe costs £1.17 for up to 10g (⅓ oz.) and generally takes 5 to 7 working days to arrive. Within the E.U., letters or postcards under 20g (⅔ oz.) also cost £1.17.

Mobile Phones Anytime you call a mobile phone in Britain, the fee will be higher than calling a land line, although there is no fee to *receive* a call or text.

Apart from renting a phone (not recommended to the casual visitor), many tourists simply enable their international **roaming** feature. Depending on your contract, your provider may bleed you—you'll pay as much as $2.50 per minute, even if someone from home calls you, and data is a killer. Check to see if your carrier offers a better option.

The other solution, if you have an unlocked phone that uses the GSM system, is to pop into any mobile phone shop or newsstand and buy a cheap **pay-as-you-talk** phone number from a mobile phone store. You pay about £5 for a SIM card, which you stick in your phone, and then you buy vouchers to load your new U.K. phone number with as much money as you think you'll use up (no refunds). That will give you a British number, which you can e-mail to everyone back home, that charges local rates (10p–40p per minute) and a deal on data that might allow 1GB in a month for about £5—much, much cheaper than roaming. Just call your provider before you leave home to "unlock" your phone (out-of-contract and last-generation phones are more likely to allow this), so that the British SIM card will function in it. That service is usually free. U.K. mobile providers with pay-as-you-talk deals, all comparable, include **Vodafone**

(www.vodafone.com), **O₂** (www.o2.co.uk), **Lebara** (www.lebara.co.uk), **EE/T-Mobile** (www.ee.co.uk), and **Virgin Mobile** (www.virgin mobile.com). Annoyingly, purchased SIMs come with automatic child content locks, which may block certain social sites. To remove the censorship, go to a mobile phone store run by your SIM provider to prove you're an adult. Bring your hotel's details—you must supply a U.K. address.

Even if your home mobile company won't permit you to unlock your phone, you can use its Wi-Fi features for Skype, FaceTime, WhatsApp, and the like.

Money British pounds are divided into 100 pennies (p), the plural of which is called "pence." Coins come in 1p, 2p, 5p, 10p, 20p, 50p, £1, and £2 (the 2-pound coin is commonly called a "quid"). Notes come in £5, £10, £20, and £50. The government is amidst a redesign of its money. The new British pound (£1), a small, chunky, gold-colored coin with silver faces, looks round but is actually subtly 12-sided. The previous version, truly round and golden without shiny faces, was phased out in October 2017. Paper £5 notes were replaced with a polymer version in May 2017, and in mid-2018 the paper £10 is also going plastic. If someone tries to pass you a paper £5 or £10, request a new one or spend it immediately. If you find yourself holding outdated money and a local bank refuses to exchange it, go to the Bank of England on Threadneedle Street (Bank tube) to exchange it. Now and then, you'll receive notes printed by the Bank of Scotland; they're valid, but an increase in forgeries means some shops refuse them. Banks will exchange them.

In past years, the exchange rate has hovered in the vicinity of £1 = US$1.50, but it trended to about US$1.30 after the U.K. decided to leave the European Union in June 2016; consult a currency exchange website such as **www.oanda.com/currency/converter** or the Oanda or XE apps.

All prices (including at most B&Bs but not at all hotels) are listed including tax, so what you see is what you pay. No guesstimating required.

Every visitor should have several sources for money, but cash is still king. The simple solution is to pull cash from an ATM upon arrival; rates are the cheapest there. Before leaving home, warn your bank and your credit card issuers that you intend to travel internationally so that they don't place a stop on your account. You may also need to adjust your PIN, since English banks require 4-digit codes. (If you know your PIN as a word, memorize the numerical equivalent.) Most banks hit you with fees of a few pounds each time you withdraw cash,

and your own bank may toss in a small fee of its own; gauge for yourself how much you feel comfortable withdrawing at a time to offset that fee. Also ask your bank if it has reciprocal agreements for free withdrawals anywhere. One institution that charges international usage fees below the industry standard is **Everbank** (www.everbank.com; ☏ **888/882-3837**); another is **Charles Schwab** (www.schwab.com; ☏ **866/403-9000**), which reimburses ATM fees.

Paying with **Apple Pay** on an iPhone is fast, but it only works up to £30.

Traveler's checks are dead—most places decline them—but creditors have come up with **traveler's check cards,** also called **prepaid cards,** which are essentially debit cards loaded with however much money you choose to put on them. They work in ATMs, and should you lose one, you can get your cash back in a matter of hours. You can reload the card mid-trip by calling a number or visiting a website, although there may be fees of a few dollars for ATM transactions. Try **NetSpend** (www.netspend.com; ☏ **866/387-7363**).

Changing cash is also on the outs. Old-fashioned cambios/bureau de change are few and far between, although you'll still find a few at the airport and around Leicester Square. If you must change money, better rates are offered by banks (open 9:30am–4pm).

Newspapers & Magazines London offers more publications than one would think a city of its size could support. The broadsheets, ordered from left to right, politically speaking, are the *Guardian,* the *Independent,* the *Daily Telegraph,* and the *Times.* On the Tube, *Metro* is free in the morning and *Evening Standard* is free in the afternoon. The salmon-colored *Financial Times* covers business. The tabloids are fluffier and more salacious: They include the *Sun,* the *Mirror, Daily Star,* the *Daily Mail,* and *Daily Express. Time Out* publishes a free listing of events and entertainments.

Other popular magazines include *Heat* (celebrity gossip), the *Big Issue* (written and sold by homeless and formerly homeless people), *Radio Times* (TV listings and celebrity interviews), and *Hello!* and *OK!* (fawning celebrity spreads usually planted by publicity agents).

Packing For your wallet's sake, pack sparingly! It's not as easy as it used to be to wink your way through the weigh-in. **British Airways,** for example, grants coach passengers a puny 23kg (51 lb.); if you exceed that, you will be smacked with a flat fee of £25 per flight (and it charges you more if you wait to pay the fee until you get to the airport). Bags over 32kg (71 lb.) will be rejected outright. Some airlines, such as **Virgin Atlantic,** can be ruthless about making sure even your *carry-on* baggage weighs

Newspapers & Magazines

PLANNING YOUR TRIP TO LONDON

no more than 10kg (22 lb.). If you're taking multiple airlines, stick to the tightest restrictions of the lot. Many airlines (even the no-frills) discount for booking baggage at least 24 hours early, and charge more at the airport.

Pare toiletries to essentials. You're not going to the Congo—you will find staples like toothpaste, contact lens solution, and deodorant everywhere. Women should bring a minimum of make-up; the British don't tend to use very much themselves. Brits are also more likely to wear trousers than blue jeans. If you plan to go clubbing, pack some fashionable duds—Londoners love to look natty.

You'll be most comfortable if you dress in clothing that layers well. Even in winter, London's air can be clammy, and dressing too warmly can become uncomfortable. No matter what the average temperature is (see weather box on p. 322), the air can grow cool after the sun sets; plan for that. A compact umbrella is wise year-round, as is an outer coat that repels water, since you never know when you're going to find yourself in one of those misty rains that make the British Isles so lush and green.

Don't bring illegal drugs (duh) or medical marijuana (duh), and also leave the pepper spray and mace at home; they're banned in the U.K.

Passports To enter the United Kingdom, all U.S. citizens, Canadians, Australians, New Zealanders, and South Africans must have a passport valid through their length of stay. No visa is required. A passport will allow you to stay in the country for up to 6 months. The immigration officer may also want to see proof of your intention to return to your point of origin (usually a round-trip ticket) and of visible means of support while you're in Britain (credit cards work). If you're planning to fly from the U.S. or Canada to the U.K. and then on to a country that requires a visa (India, for example), secure that visa before you arrive in Britain.

Pharmacies Every police station keeps a list of pharmacies (chemists) that are open 24 hours. Also try **Zafash,** a rare chemist that is open 24 hours, 233–235 Old Brompton Rd., SW5 (✆ **020/7373-2798;** Earl's Court tube). For nonemergency health advice, call the NHS at ✆ **111.**

Police Dial ✆ **999** or 112 if the matter is serious. London has two official police forces: the City of London police (www.cityoflondon. police.uk), whose remit covers the "Square Mile" and its 8,600 residents; and the Metropolitan Police ("the Met"), which covers the rest of the capital. Opening hours for all the Met's local police stations are listed at www.met.police.uk/local. In a non-emergency, you can contact your local police

station by dialing ✆ **101.** Losses, thefts, and other criminal matters should be reported at the nearest police station immediately. You will be given a crime number, which your travel insurer will request if you make a claim against any losses.

Safety Crossing the street is the most perilous thing you'll do. Always look down to see which way traffic is flowing—the street will be painted "Look right" or "Look left" so you'll know. Also, a steady-lit green man on the crosswalk signal means it's safe, but when the green man flashes, do not begin crossing—it means cars are about to gun it again.

Few places in London are unsafe. Neighborhoods that might be called sketchy are usually distant from the Tube lines, and they only feel tense after dark, when shops close. Simply be sensitive to who's around you and you'll do fine.

The biggest nuisance tourists might encounter—besides tipsy locals—is moped muggings. Each day, dozens of people are so absorbed in their smartphones that they don't notice the two-wheeled pickpockets zoom up, snatch their phone, and speed off. Simply be smart about how you use your phone and, of course, where you put your cash and what you leave sitting in the open.

London is always on the lookout for terrorist activity,

as it has been since the days of IRA violence. Don't leave a bag unattended even for seconds or you may lose it.

Guns are banned in London—even on most police officers—so you don't often see the kind of violence taken for granted in the United States. Londoners cite knife crime as a problem, but the victims are almost always young men who themselves carry knives. Some male tourists have gotten fleeced at "hostess bars" in Soho. If you do suffer a lapse of judgment and accept the barker's invitation to go into one, understand that you might have cash exacted by lunkheaded yobs with tattooed fingers.

Should you find yourself on the business end of the legal system, you can get advice and referrals to lawyers from **Legal Services Commission** (www.legalservices.gov.uk; ☏ **0345/345-4345**). Crime victims can receive volunteer legal guidance and emotional fortification from **Victim Support** (www.victimsupport.org.uk; ☏ **0808/168-9111**). In the unlikely event of a sexual assault, phone the **Rape Crisis Federation** (www.rapecrisis.org.uk; ☏ **0808/802-9999;** rcewinfo@rapecrisis.org.uk).

Senior Travel Don't hide your age! Seniors in England—usually classified as those aged 60 and over—are privy to all kinds of price breaks, from lower admission prices at museums to a third off rail tickets (to apply for the **Senior Railcard,** go to www.senior-railcard.co.uk). You may hear seniors referred to as OAPs, which stands for Old Age Pensioners, although that acronym is falling out of use—perhaps because it's rare to find a solvent pension fund anymore. Don't be offended if you're referred to as a "geezer"—in England, it's a compliment, meaning a fun-loving (if sometimes rowdy) bloke.

If you're over 50, you can join **AARP** (601 E St. NW, Washington, DC, 20049; www.aarp.org; ☏ **202/434-3525**) to wrangle discounts on hotels, airfare, and car rentals. Elderhostel's well-respected **Road Scholar** (www.roadscholar.org; ☏ **800/454-5768**) runs many classes and programs in London designed to delve into literature, history, the arts, and music. Packages last from a week to a month and include airfare, lodging, and meals.

Smoking Smoking is prohibited by law in any enclosed workplace, including museums, pubs, public transportation, and restaurants. If in doubt, ask permission.

Staying Fit **PureGym** (www.puregym.com) offers contract-free passes for 1 day, 3 days, or a week for as little as £10; it has facilities open 24 hours in Piccadilly (Rex House, 4–12 Regent St., SW1; ☏ **845/835-6936;** Piccadilly Circus tube) and Holborn (Lacon House, 84 Theobalds Rd., WC1; ☏ 0845/8356902; Holborn tube). Additional locations are in Marylebone, Victoria, and near Oxford Circus.

Student Travel Have ID on hand, and always mention you're a student—it'll save you cash. Attractions gladly offer discounts of around 25% for full-time students. However, your high school or university ID may not cut it where clerks haven't heard of your school: Before leaving home, obtain a recognized ID such as the **International Student Identity Card** (ISIC; www.isic.org). Those 25 and under who are not in school can obtain an **International Youth Travel Card,** also through ISIC, which performs many of the same tricks as a student discount card.

Before buying airline tickets, those 25 and under should consult a travel agency that specializes in the youth market and is versed in its available discounts: **STA Travel** (www.statravel.com; ☏ **800/781-4040**) is big.

Taxes Prices of all goods in the U.K. are quoted inclusive of taxes. Since 2011 the national value-added tax (**VAT**) has stood at 20%. This is included in all hotel and restaurant bills, and in the price of most items you purchase.

If you are permanently resident outside the E.U., VAT on goods can be refunded if you shop at stores that participate in the **Retail Export**

10

PLANNING YOUR TRIP TO LONDON | Senior Travel

Scheme—look for the window sticker or ask the staff. See p. 223 for details. Information about the scheme is also posted online at www.hmrc.gov.uk/vat/sectors/consumers/overseas-visitors.htm.

Telephones When dialing a number in this book from abroad, precede it with your country's international prefix (in the U.S. and Canada, it's 011), add the U.K.'s country code (44) and drop the first zero in the number.

To make an **international call** from Britain, dial the international access code (**00**), then the country code, then the area code, and finally the local number. When calling from a mobile phone, dial the full number including area code.

Directory assistance is at www.bt.com or ☎ **118-500.** Local calls start with 020.

The main **toll-free** prefixes are 0800, 0808, and 0500. Numbers starting with 07 are usually for mobile phones and will be charged at a higher rate. Numbers starting with 09 are premium-rate calls that will usually be very expensive (around £1.50 per minute) and may not even work from abroad.

Many attractions, hotel companies, and services have changed their standard phone numbers to profit-generating ones that charge for every minute you call them. You often can't reach 0845, 0870, and 0871 numbers (charged at 10p a minute or less) from abroad, and when you can, you're charged more. Use the Web instead to get information.

The majority of London's **payphones** are gone. You can barely find them, let alone rely upon them.

Phonecards, though rarely used today, can be an economical method for both international and national calls. They are reusable until the total value has expired. Cards can be purchased from newsstands and post offices, and offer rates of a few pence per minute to most countries.

Hotels routinely add outrageous surcharges onto calls made from your room. Rather than dial directly using a hotel phone, purchase a phonecard.

Time London is generally 5 hours ahead of New York City and Toronto, 8 hours ahead of Los Angeles, 11 hours behind Auckland, and 9 hours behind Sydney. It is 1 hour behind western continental Europe. Greenwich Mean Time is London time.

Tipping Waiters should receive 10% to 15% of the bill unless service is already included—*always* check the menu or bill to see if service was already added. At **pubs,** tipping isn't customary unless you receive waiter service (not food drop-off). Fine **hotels** may levy a service charge, but at the finest ones, grease the staff with a pound here and there. Staff at B&Bs and family-run hotels don't expect tips. **Bartenders** and **chambermaids** need not be tipped. There's no need to tip **taxicab drivers** but most people round up to the next £1, although a 10% to 15% tip is becoming increasingly standard.

Toilets London doesn't have enough of them. Washrooms can be found at any free museum in this guide, any department store, any pub or busy restaurant (though it's polite to buy something), and at Piccadilly Circus and Bank Tube stations. Train stations may also have toilets; they're free at Charing Cross, Victoria, and London Bridge but may charge 50p elsewhere. On weekends, open-air *pissoirs* for men are placed throughout the West End.

VAT See "Taxes," above.

Visas No E.U. nationals require a visa to visit the U.K. Visas are also not required for travelers from Australia, Canada, New Zealand, or the U.S. To be sure that hasn't changed, search "visa" at **www.gov.uk** long before your travel dates. The usual permitted stay is 90 days or fewer for tourists, although some nationalities are granted stays of up to 6 months. If you plan to work or study, though, or if you're traveling on a passport from another country, you'll need to obtain the correct paperwork.

Visitor Information Three official information units supported by British taxes are set up to help tourists, but only online: **Visit Britain** (www.visitbritain.com); **Visit**

England (www.visitengland.com); and **Visit London** (www.visitlondon.com). Visit London possesses the biggest database and publishes a free app with offline maps called **London Official City Guide** and an app collecting upcoming happenings, **London Official Events Guide.** The only official information bureau with a public office is across the road from St Paul's Cathedral north of Millennium Bridge: The **City of London Information Centre** (St Paul's Churchyard; www.visitthecity.co.uk; ✆ **020/7332-1456**) sells attraction tickets and Oyster cards, runs tours, and supplies brochures and counsel for day trips throughout the country. It publishes walking tours, a free City Visitor Trail audio walking tour app, and children's discovery trail maps. Opening hours are Monday to Saturday 9:30am to 5:30pm, Sunday 10am to 4pm.

Excellent independent sources for things to learn and things to do include **Londonist.com, LondonCalling.com, TimeOut.com/London, Townfish.com,** and the Twitter accounts Everything London (**@LDN**), **@LeCool_London,** and **@SkintLondon.**

Women Travelers First and foremost, lone women should avoid riding in **unlicensed London taxicabs,** especially at night. Flag down a black cab or call a minicab instead. The **Splitcab** app (www.splitcab.co.uk) allows women to find female-driven minicabs (and to share the cost with someone else going in the same direction). **Addison Lee** (www.addisonlee.com; ✆ **020/7407-9000**) has a huge, efficient fleet, and will text you the registration plate of your cab for added security. It has a free app for hailing rides.

A true club and not an agency, **Women Welcome Women Worldwide** (www.womenwelcomewomen.uk; ✆ **01494/46-54-41**) connects travelers worldwide and costs £37 a year to join, £27 a year to renew.

Index

See also Accommodations and Restaurant indexes, below.

General Index

Map List

MAP LIST

Photo Credits

p. i: © Stuart Monk; p. ii: © Luciano Mortula; p. iii: © nui7711/Shutterstock.com; p. iv: © anyaivanova; p. v, top: © MarkLG; p. v, bottom left: © visitlondonimages/britainonview/Pawel Libera; p. v, bottom right: © Joseph M. Arseneau/Shutterstock.com; p. vi, top left: © London and Partners/Visit Britain; p. vi, top right: © pio3/Shutterstock.com; p. vi, bottom left: © visitlondonimages/britainonview/Pawel Libera; p. vi, bottom right: © Paul Hudson; p. vii, top: Courtesy of Dennis Sever House/Roelof Bakker; p. vii, middle: © Jean-Pierre Dalbéra; p. vii, bottom: © Pawel Libera/London and Partners; p. viii, top left: © Elizabeth Blanchet; p. viii, top right: © Elizabeth Blanchet; p. viii, bottom: © visitlondonimages/britainonview/Pawel Libera; p. ix, top: © JuliusKielaitis/Shutterstock.com; p. ix, bottom: © Heather Cowper; p. x, top left: © visitlondonimages/britainonview/Pawel Libera; p. x, top right: Courtesy of Ronnie Scotts/David Sinclair; p. x, bottom left: © IR Stone/Shutterstock.com; p. x, bottom right: © visitlondonimages/britainonview; p. xi, top: Courtesy of Claridge's Hotel; p. xi, bottom: © IR Stone/Shutterstock.com; p. xii, top left: © Meghan Lamb; p. xii, top right: © Meibion/Alamy Stock Photo ; p. xii, bottom left: © Christian Mueller/Shutterstock.com; p. xii, bottom right: © Davide D'Amico; p. xiii, top: © pcruciatti/Shutterstock.com; p. xiii, bottom left: © Bikeworldtravel/ Shutterstock; p. xiii, bottom right: © Martin Pettitt; p. xiv, top: © aslysun; p. xiv, bottom left: © Premier Photo; p. xiv, bottom right: © Ritu Manoj Jethani; p. xv, top: © dahorsburgh; p. xv, bottom: © sloukam; p. xvi, top: © ian woolcock; p. xvi, bottom left: © Katie Sewall; p. xvi, bottom right: © Pawel Libera/London and Partners; p. 2: © elesi/Shutterstock.com; p. 3: © Pawel Libera/London and Partners; p. 4: © Michael Heffernan/London and Partners; p. 5, top: © James Petts; p. 5, bottom: © NigelSpiers/Shutterstock.com; p. 6: © ojohnson@maybourne.com; p. 7: © gnoparus; p. 8: © Vince Smith; p. 9: © chrisdorney/Shutterstock.com; p. 14: © Justin Black; p. 15: © Leonid Andronov; p. 16: © Luciano Mortula; p. 17: © PG_Payless; p. 18: © chrisdorney/Shutterstock.com; p. 19: © IR Stone/Shutterstock.com; p. 20: © Mike Fleming; p. 22: © CosminIftode/Shutterstock.com; p. 23: © littleny/Shutterstock.com; p. 38: © Meghan Lamb; p. 42: Courtesy of One Aldwych ; p. 43: © Have folder of images; p. 47: © The Goring, Belgravia, London; p. 53: Courtesy of Brown's Hotel; p. 54: Courtesy of The Stafford Hotel/Simon Brown; p. 55: © Gimas/Shutterstock.com; p. 56: Courtesy of 22 York Street; p. 74: © Bex Walton; p. 75: Courtesy of The Eagle; p. 77: © Garry Knight; p. 78: © Karl Florczak; p. 79: © Garry Knight; p. 81: © Ewan Munro; p. 83: © Alper Çuğun; p. 86: Courtesy of J. Sheekey; p. 90: © Ewan Munro; p. 93: Courtesy of Brown's Hotel; p. 94: © London on View; p. 96: © Tom Bastin; p. 105: © Stacy; p. 112: © Bikeworldtravel/Shutterstock.com; p. 120: © pisaphotography/Shutterstock.com; p. 129: © alessandro0770/Shutterstock.com; p. 131: © olavs; p. 132: © stu smith; p. 134: © Herry Lawford; p. 141: © scarriot; p. 144: © Loz Pycock; p. 146: © Bikeworldtravel/Shutterstock.com; p. 147: © cristapper; p. 148: © pio3/Shutterstock.com; p. 159: © MarkLG; p. 164: © Maria Morri; p. 173: © Karen Bryan; p. 175: © Dark Dwarf; p. 176: © ileana_bt/Shutterstock.com; p. 179: © Alexandra Reinwald; p. 190: © stefan m; p. 192: © Kamira/Shutterstock.com; p. 200: © Michael W. Pleitgen; p. 202: © Garry Knight; p. 203: © chrisdorney/Shutterstock.com; p. 207: © Justin Goring; p. 208: © Shou-Hui Wang; p. 211: © Wolfgang Heitzer-Krichel; p. 213: © Herry Lawford; p. 214: © gigijin; p. 216: © Lars Plougmann; p. 222: © Daniel Gale/Shutterstock.com; p. 228: © Kiev.Victor/Shutterstock.com; p. 229: © Andrew Baddeley; p. 230: Courtesy of Sadler's Wells/Tristram Kenton; p. 231: © Padmayogini/Shutterstock.com; p. 235: © Norio NAKAYAMA; p. 237: © Songquan Deng; p. 240: © Sophie McAulay/Shutterstock.com; p. 245: © Philip Sheldrake; p. 250: © Lewis Clarke; p. 253: © Kiev.Victor/Shutterstock.com; p. 255: © chrisdorney; p. 257: © Stuart Monk/Shutterstock.com; p. 264: © Ratikova; p. 269: © Marc Evans; p. 271: © Peter; p. 276: © Christian Mueller/Shutterstock.com; p. 278: © andersphoto/Shutterstock.com; p. 280: © David Terrar; p. 283: © Philip Sheldrake; p. 287: © Kiev.Victor/Shutterstock.com; p. 288: © Pete Spiro; p. 293: © iLongLoveKing/Shutterstock.com; p. 294: © e X p o s e/Shutterstock.com; p. 297: © Graham Taylor; p. 298: © e X p o s e/Shutterstock.com; p. 300: © David Evison; p. 301: © Dutourdumonde Photography/Shutterstock.com; p. 303: © littlesam/Shutterstock.com; p. 304: © chrisdorney/Shutterstock.com

Frommer's EasyGuide to London 2018, 5th edition

Published by

FROMMER MEDIA LLC

ISBN 978-1-62887-358-0 (paper), 978-1-62887-359-7 (e-book)

Editorial Director: Pauline Frommer
Editor: Holly Hughes
Production Editor: Heather Wilcox
Cartographer: Roberta Stockwell
Photo Editor: Meghan Lamb
Cover Design: Howard Grossman

For information on our other products or services, see www.frommers.com.

Frommer Media LLC also publishes its books in a variety of electronic formats. Some content that
appears in print may not be available in electronic formats.

Manufactured in the United States of America

5 4 3 2 1

ABOUT THE AUTHOR

Jason Cochran was twice awarded Guide Book of the Year by the Lowell Thomas Awards (Society of American Travel Writers) and once by the North American Travel Journalists Association. His voice has reached millions of travelers, starting in the mid-1990s, when he wrote one of the world's first travel blogs, to his familiarity as a commentator on CBS and for AOL, to his work today as editor-in-chief of Frommers.com and co-host of the *Frommer Travel Show*. He lives in New York City and Los Angeles.

ABOUT THE FROMMER TRAVEL GUIDES

For most of the past 50 years, Frommer's has been the leading series of travel guides in North America, accounting for as many as 24% of all guidebooks sold. I think I know why.

Though we hope our books are entertaining, we nevertheless deal with travel in a serious fashion. Our guidebooks have never looked on such journeys as a mere recreation, but as a far more important human function, a time of learning and introspection, an essential part of a civilized life. We stress the culture, lifestyle, history, and beliefs of the destinations we cover, and urge our readers to seek out people and new ideas as the chief rewards of travel.

We have never shied from controversy. We have, from the beginning, encouraged our authors to be intensely judgmental, critical—both pro and con—in their comments, and wholly independent. Our only clients are our readers, and we have triggered the ire of countless prominent sorts, from a tourist newspaper we called "practically worthless" (it unsuccessfully sued us) to the many rip-offs we've condemned.

And because we believe that travel should be available to everyone regardless of their incomes, we have always been cost-conscious at every level of expenditure. Though we have broadened our recommendations beyond the budget category, we insist that every lodging we include be sensibly priced. We use every form of media to assist our readers, and are particularly proud of our feisty daily website, the award-winning Frommers.com.

I have high hopes for the future of Frommer's. May these guidebooks, in all the years ahead, continue to reflect the joy of travel and the freedom that travel represents. May they always pursue a cost-conscious path, so that people of all incomes can enjoy the rewards of travel. And may they create, for both the traveler and the persons among whom we travel, a community of friends, where all human beings live in harmony and peace.

Arthur Frommer

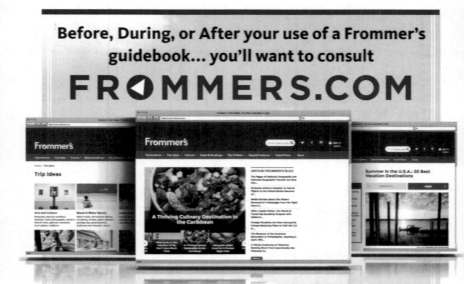